FAT
&FURIOUS

The Primal way to live *Healthier* for *Longer*

SUPPORTED BY THE EVIDENCE OF

23 LEADING MEDICAL PROFESSIONALS

STEVE BENNETT SHARES THE INFURIATING
TRUTH BEHIND WHAT MAKES US FAT
AND THE STEPS NEEDED TO
LIVE LONGER IN BRITAIN

STEVE BENNETT

Published December 2019

Book Design: Dan Morris
Cover Design: Theo Johnson
Insert Design: Kati Elliott

ISBN: 978-1-9999071-5-0

www.healthdaddy.com
www.primalliving.com

*What are the secrets to losing weight and living healthier,
happier and for longer?*

*We first accept that we have little evolved since our primal ancestors
and then optimise our nutrition, environment and lifestyle.*

We have to live primally.

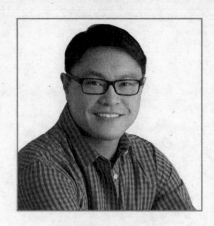

FOREWORD

Caloric reduction is a harsh and bitter disappointment. Yet all the 'experts' still agree that caloric reduction is the key to lasting weight loss. When you don't lose weight, they say, 'It's your fault. You were gluttons. You were sloths. You didn't try hard enough. You didn't want it badly enough.' There's a dirty little secret that nobody is willing to admit: The low-fat, low-calorie diet has already been proven to fail. This is the cruel hoax. Eating less does not result in lasting weight loss. It just does not work. It is cruel because so many of us have believed it. It is cruel because all of our 'trusted health sources' tell us it is true. It is cruel because when it fails, we blame ourselves. Let me state it as plainly as I can: 'Eat Less' does not work. That's a fact. Accept it. It's the very reason why Steve Bennett was fat for so many years and why he is now furious!

Dr Jason Fung
Author of *The Obesity Code, The Complete Guide To Fasting* and *The Diabetes Code*
www.dietdoctor.com

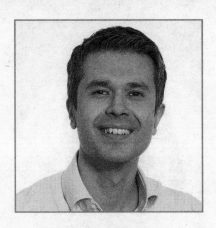

PREFACE

As a qualified doctor for over 18 years and a practicing cardiologist, I have come to realise that much of modern medical practice has become no better than putting a sticking plaster on a severed artery. As doctors, we are trained to treat the symptoms of disease, rather than addressing root causes. This, in combination with commercial influence on dietary guidelines and health advice, has resulted in a complete healthcare system failure and an epidemic of misinformed doctors and harmed patients.

Consequently, healthcare is in crisis; over 60% per cent of the UK adult population are overweight or obese. The roots of obesity, type 2 diabetes and CVD are firmly embedded in the food environment. Poor diet contributes to more disease and death globally than physical inactivity, smoking and alcohol combined. The role of poor dietary advice, however, is often ignored; specifically, the advice to consume foods that are "low fat" and "low in cholesterol." The low-fat dietary guidelines were based on flawed science when they were introduced 40 years ago, and the result has been catastrophic, increasing the consumption of low-fat junk food, refined carbohydrates and polyunsaturated vegetable oils. The conspicuous rise in obesity immediately following their introduction suggests they are the root cause of the problem.

Steve Bennett's personal journey in how he overcame his own health problems from changing his lifestyle is both powerful and compelling. Driven by a sense of injustice and drawing on his own research interviewing a wide variety of the most forward-thinking and respected experts in their chosen fields, Steve has produced the most detailed and comprehensive book on diet, lifestyle and their impact on health that I've read to date. This is all the more impressive that it comes from a non-scientist and also an extremely intelligent and articulate man who is understandably furious about how we've all been lied to by Big Food and Bad Pharma; two of the most powerful industries who, by spreading misinformation for profit, are directly responsible for our current healthcare crisis. This book is empowering, helping us to be able to choose and enjoy foods that we can be confident will confer wellness not illness.

Dr Aseem Malhotra
Consultant Cardiologist and international bestselling author of *The Pioppi Diet*

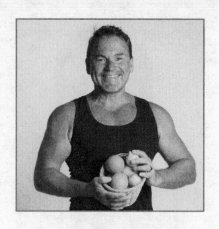

INTRODUCTION

When my seventh child Louie was born (yes I have seven, I know that's a lot), I was obese, unhealthy and approaching my fiftieth birthday. Like all parents, I want the best for my children and just as important for me, I want to be around to see them grow up, and to be in their lives for as long as possible.

Five years ago, I was so frustrated and terrified by being very fat and what that could mean to my health (and ultimately when I would die), I decided to step back from my businesses and spend my days researching health. The more I studied, the more furious I became. Furious that for all of those years of bouncing between being fat and obese, I had been fed a big fat lie about what was causing my weight and ultimately how to get rid of it. It wasn't that I hadn't tried, I had always exercised regularly and had continuously eaten what I was told should help me shift my weight, but for 25 years I had always lost the bulge battle. None of the diets I went on worked. I tried really hard, I became a slave to them and yet no matter what I tried, I was imprisoned in my fat body.

Since I discovered the truth, my stubborn belly has gone, and so have all of the health issues associated with it. The infuriating thing is, pretty much everything I thought I knew about food before was wrong. My thinking, much like nearly everyone else in Britain, had been shaped by big food and pharmaceutical companies that, as it turns out, have no interest in my health at all. They regrettably only care about making a profit and then protecting it with their lies. To them, it's simply about corporate wealth and not consumer health.

What I uncovered was that my previous food choices had been shaped by misinformation and brainwashing from corporate advertising. And, with the onslaught of fast and packaged food with their highly addictive ingredients, it wasn't just me they had made fat, it was the nation too. So much so, that the average adult in Great Britain today is two and a half stone heavier than adults were in the year I was born! Or look at it another way. In the past 50 years, we have put on more weight than in the past 2.5 million years!

Today, we have an absolutely insane governmental guideline telling us what we should eat. The cold hard fact, however, is that it's making Britain sick. According to researchers, the life expectancy of my children's generation is expected to be ten years shorter than my generation, and that makes me furious! With seven wonderful children, I will not just accept this, and neither should you.

In search of the truth about both what makes us fat and what steps we need to take to help us live longer, I have met and interviewed many of the world's most forward-thinking medical professionals, including doctors, authors, scientists, investigative journalists, and nutritionists. I have analysed hundreds of health books, even more white papers and what I have uncovered is going to be revealed throughout this book. But just in case you are only flicking through the introduction, while in a bookstore or waiting for a flight, with no intention of buying it, here is the infuriatingly simple answer in a nutshell...

The wave of obesity sweeping our country and the tsunami of chronic disease has primarily been caused by us not eating real wholesome foods. As a nation, we are starving our bodies of good nutrition, and poisoning ourselves with mass-produced, artificially modified, sugar-loaded nonsense. Also, we are using shampoos, antiperspirants and creams made with substances known to cause harm. Furthermore, we are stressed, don't sleep enough, and are sedentary.

Our human body was not designed to live like this.

How do we live healthier, happier and for longer? We must first accept that we have little evolved since our primal ancestors and then optimise our lifestyle, environment and nutrition to the fundamental needs of the human body. I call this the LEON principle of primal living. They are the principles for living healthier for longer and they are yours to own. They are both beautiful in their simplicity and reassuringly easy to remember.

The LEON principle of living primally:

1. Lifestyle
We need to optimise our happiness, sleep, exercise and more. That begins with 'how' we spend our days and 'what' we do to take care of this amazing body of ours.

2. Environment
How do we optimise our environment? Well, it begins with avoiding toxins wherever we can, such as chemicals in beauty products, potions, lotions, and pesticides in food. It also means radically changing the relationship that we have with technology and, in particular, our mobile phones (sorry).

3. Optimise
Throughout this book, you'll hear me use the word 'optimise' because it is an important aspect of a primal lifestyle. *Fat & Furious* is packed to the brim with

advice from some of the most respected health professionals in the world, and if you're anything like me, the moment you understand the secret to living healthier and for longer, you will want to optimise each and every nugget of information.

4. Nutrition

I believe in a low carbohydrate diet. One that focuses on eating organic and natural foods. I believe that natural fats are healthy and that eating meats from animals who have lived in their natural habitat is not only good for our health, but good for our planet's health too. I believe only by consuming real food, together with quality supplements, can we optimise our nutrition and provide our body with what it needs to thrive.

Please use the LEON principles to look after yourself and those whom you love. It's not complicated, the changes are reassuringly simple and once you understand the difference they make, you'll never look back. Throughout *Fat & Furious*, we have the remarkable privilege of the advice and wisdom of 23 pioneers in the field of health all in one place. All you need to do is to take their guidance and optimise it in every possible aspect of your lifestyle, environment and nutrition.

By providing you with the truth about what we eat and by revealing what I believe is a secret agenda of governments, food and pharmaceutical giants, I am going to dislodge the effects of corporate indoctrination and conditioning. I will provide you with the knowledge and hopefully the motivation to control the destination of your health, happiness and longevity.

As George Orwell once said, "In a time of universal deceit, telling the truth is a revolutionary act". This book sets out to pass on the proven truth behind weight loss and living a long healthy life.

And finally, here is the really good news. The conclusion I have come to from all of my research - and it's so exciting - is that if we live more primally, we have so much more control over our health, happiness and both our longevity and that of our planet than you could ever imagine.

Steve Bennett
Dad, Author and Nutritional Activist

CONTENTS

MEET THE CONTRIBUTORS

I have had the honour of meeting and interviewing the true health pioneers of the global medical stage. Some are risking their careers in pursuit of unveiling the truth and in no small way, I owe this book, my life (and that of my family) to them. They are not only leaders in their respective fields, but they have also given up their time without sponsorship or payment, removing any conflict of interest, which is sadly often rife in medical research.

The by-product is a body of work which gives you, and I, unparalleled access to these forward-thinking medical revolutionary professionals in one place.

It took me four years to piece together what their combined work truly means to our health and wellbeing, but today, in a little over 300 pages, I'll help you connect the dots on how their life-changing work and research could change the course of your own personal lifespan, starting today.

These remarkable individuals have simply passed on their knowledge with one singular motive – to help you and those you love to live healthier for longer. Some you may recognise from their own books, others may be new to you, but each are world-class leaders in their respective fields, and it's been a privilege to have spent time with them all. Some have become good friends, all have been remarkably generous with their time, and I am, without exception, in bewildered awe of each and every one of them.

The text is taken pretty much verbatim from their incredibly insightful interviews and podcasts and therefore is generally written as spoken. Anything in brackets I have added for better comprehension. To listen to the full interviews that we recorded, please search for the podcasts or the videos under the same name as they are in this book or visit our website *www.primalliving.com*.

To give you an insight into each remarkable contributor, I have provided a quick profile on each of them:

Dr David Unwin

David is a GP in Southport, where he has been practising for over 30 years. During that time, he has become fascinated by how people can become really healthy without using medication. In 2016 David was bestowed the NHS Innovator of the Year award. He is Ambassador for the all-party Parliamentary Group on Diabetes, the Senior Medical Advisor to *www. diabetes.co.uk*, who have helped over 50,000 people put their diabetes in remission and is a founding member of The Public Health Collaboration. David says that one of the things he enjoys most is helping patients make lifestyle changes in order to make it possible to deprescribe their medication.

Dr Patrick Holford

Patrick is a leading spokesman on nutrition in the media, specialising in the field of mental health. He is the author of 40 books, translated into over 30 languages and selling millions of copies worldwide, including *The Optimum Nutrition Bible*, *The Low-GL Diet Bible*, *Optimum Nutrition for the Mind* and *The 10 Secrets of 100% Healthy People*. Patrick is the Founder of the Food for the Brain Foundation and a director of the Brain Bio Centre, a treatment centre that specialises in helping those with mental health issues, ranging from depression to schizophrenia. In 1984 he founded the Institute for Optimum Nutrition (ION), an independent educational charity, with his mentor, twice Nobel Prize winner Dr Linus Pauling, as a patron.

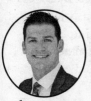

Dr James DiNicolantonio

James is a cardiovascular research scientist and a doctor of pharmacy. He is the author of the international bestseller *The Salt Fix* (a brilliant book carrying the subtitle Why the Experts Got it All Wrong and How Eating More Might Save Your Life) and co-authored *Super Fuel* and most recently *The Longevity Solution*. He is a well-respected and internationally known scientist and an expert on health and nutrition that once testified in front of the Canadian Senate regarding the harms of added sugars. He is an Associate Editor of British Medical Journal's (BMJ) *Open Heart*, a journal published in partnership with the British Cardiovascular Society.

Dr Aseem Malhotra

Aseem is both a practising Cardiologist and a Professor of Evidence-Based Medicine. He is a founding member of Action on Sugar and has led work highlighting the harm caused by excess sugar consumption in the United Kingdom, particularly its role in type 2 diabetes and obesity. Aseem has written for several publications including the BMJ, The Guardian and Observer, BBC online, Huffington Post, The Daily Mirror, Daily Mail, The Daily Telegraph and the Washington Post. In 2018 he was ranked by Onalytica as the number 1 doctor in the world influencing obesity thinking. His first book, co-authored with Donal O'Neill, *The Pioppi Diet*, published 2017, is already an international bestseller.

Nina Teicholz

Nina is an investigative journalist who, for over a decade, has specialised in food and nutrition. Her international best-seller *The Big Fat Surprise, Why Butter, Meat and Cheese Belong in a Health Diet*, was book of the year for The Times, Wall Street Journal and BBC Food Programme. The British Medical Journal appraised the book saying, "Deeply disturbing in showing how overenthusiastic scientists, poor science, massive conflicts of interest, and politically driven policymakers can make deeply damaging mistakes". Nina has also written for the Economist, Washington Post, New York Times, and many others. She served as associate director for the Centre for Globalisation and Sustainable Development at Columbia University. Teicholz studied biology at Yale and Stanford and earned a graduate degree from Oxford. She lives in New York City with her husband and their sons.

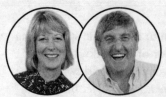

Katie and Giancarlo Caldesi

The Caldesi's are owners of Caffé Caldesi in London and La Cucina Caldesi Cookery School. They first came to public attention when they featured in the BBC Two series Return to Tuscany in 2006. They are both regular visitors to our screens appearing as guests on a vast array of food programmes such as BBC One's MasterChef, Saturday Kitchen, Sunday Brunch and more. The Italian Government has awarded Giancarlo the honour of Cavaliere for his work and along with Katie has written many critically acclaimed cookbooks.

In 2011, aged 59, Giancarlo's vision became blurry. Soon after, he couldn't even play football with his young sons. Sadly, he was diagnosed with type 2 diabetes. By 2014 his weight had bloomed to 17 stone, and his HbA1c levels were dangerously high. Even worse, later that year it was established that he had a severe gluten intolerance. It felt like his world of food, and everything he loved was forbidden, and although determined to fight, he was very low. No pasta, no pizza, no bread.

Imagine an Italian master-chef, who for over 60 years was used to eating his beloved pasta at least once and often twice a day, being told to stop. What he didn't realise is that his diagnosis would probably save his life. Now, five years on, his diabetes is in remission. It's been a difficult journey, but Giancarlo feels that if he can do it, then anyone can.

Dr Jen Unwin

Dr Jen Unwin (BSc, MSc, DPsy, FBPsS) is a consultant clinical health psychologist and has been working in the NHS for over 30 years helping people with chronic illness to live well with their conditions. She has researched the importance of hope in health and wellbeing. Jen has been actively involved with the British Psychological Society, of which she is a fellow and also the UK Association for Solution Focused Practice, of which she is a past chair. Jen also sits on the advisory board of the Public Health Collaboration.

Patrick Holden CBE

After studying biodynamic agriculture at Emerson College, Patrick established a mixed community farm in Wales in 1973, which today is the longest-running organic farm in the country. Patrick was the founding chairman of British Organic Farmers in 1982, before joining the Soil Association, where he worked for nearly 20 years as a director and during which time the organisation led the development of organic standards. Patrick is the founding director of the Sustainable Food Trust, working internationally to accelerate the transition towards more sustainable food systems. His advocacy for a major global transition to more sustainable food systems now entails international travel and regular broadcasts and talks at public events. He is patron of the UK Biodynamic Association and was awarded the CBE for services to organic farming in 2005.

Deborah Colson MSc

Deborah has been specialising in nutritional support for mental health and wellbeing since 2002. She undertook her initial training at the Institute for Optimum Nutrition in London and went on to complete an MSc in Nutritional Therapy at the University of Westminster. Deborah has co-authored several books, including *Optimum Nutrition for Your Child* and *The Alzheimer's Prevention Plan*. She has worked with a wide range of organisations and institutions, including special needs schools and colleges, delivering health improvement programmes.

Gary Taubes

Gary is an investigative science and health journalist and co-founder of the non-profit Nutrition Science Initiative (www.*NuSI.org*). He is the author of *The Case Against Sugar* (2016), *Why We Get Fat and What to Do About It* (2011) and *Good Calories, Bad Calories* (2007), published as *The Diet Delusion* in the UK. Gary is the recipient of a Robert Wood Johnson Foundation Investigator Award in Health Policy Research and has won numerous other awards for his journalism. These include the International Health Reporting Award from the Pan American Health Organization and the National Association of Science Writers Science in Society Journalism Award, which he won in 1996, 1999 and 2001. He is the first print journalist to win this award three times.

Dr Robert Lustig

Dr Robert is Professor Emeritus of Paediatrics, Division of Endocrinology at the University of California, San Francisco. He specialises in the field of neuroendocrinology, treating hormonal disorders in children, and he is interested in how the brain controls hormones and how hormones control the brain. He was head of the UCSF paediatric obesity program for 17 years. Dr Lustig has fostered a global discussion of metabolic health and nutrition, exposing some of the leading myths that underlie the current pandemic of diet-related disease. He believes the food business, by pushing processed food loaded with sugar, has hacked our bodies and minds to pursue pleasure instead of happiness; fostering today's epidemics of addiction and depression. Robert is a global best-selling author and his presentation on YouTube, *Sugar, the Bitter Truth*, has had 8.9 million views.

Professor Tim Noakes

Tim Noakes is a South African scientist and an emeritus professor in the Division of Exercise Science and Sports Medicine at the University of Cape Town. He is a proclaimed author, amongst his best-sellers are *The Real Meal Revolution*, *The Lore of Running*, and *The Lore of Nutrition*. In 2012 he received the Lifetime Achievement Award from South Africa's National Research Foundation for his contribution to sports science research. His most recent book, *Real Food on Trial*, tells the true story of his four-year-long court hearing in South Africa, where the establishment tried to silence his dietary opinions. Tim was victorious. He is ranked on Twitter as the 4th most influential scientist across the globe!

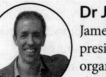

Dr James Goolnik

James qualified in 1992 from King's College London. He is a past-president of the British Academy of Cosmetic Dentistry, the largest organisation dedicated to advancing the art and science of cosmetic dentistry in the United Kingdom. James has twice been voted the most influential person in dentistry in the UK by trade magazine Dentistry. His book *Brush* is a number one bestseller on Amazon, from which James donates all of his profits to the charity Dentaid. The first project was in Malawi, where James installed a two-surgery dental practice and led a dental team to deliver a skills transfer workshop. His latest charitable project is tackling sugar being used as a reward for children.

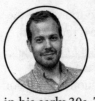

Dr Dan Maggs

As a general practitioner (GP), you'd think Dr Dan Maggs would know how to get his weight problems under control. Yet despite several attempts – adhering to a 'balanced diet' as specified in the UK's national dietary guidelines – he found himself clinically obese in his early 30s. Thankfully, a chance encounter while on holiday in 2016 led to him discovering the power of a primal diet, built around a low carbohydrate intake. In the following six months, he lost an incredible five stone (31kg) and rapidly normalised his weight! Losing so much weight by going against government advice and ignoring mainstream dietary guidelines led him to question much of what he learned during medical training. Quickly, he'd discovered these guidelines aren't based around robust medical evidence at all and that his experiences prove we should be adopting a primal approach to the way we eat and live. He spreads his powerful message both to his patients and via his website *www.carbdodging.com*.

Dr Joanne McCormack

Joanne McCormack has been a GP for 24 years. She has always been interested in weight and nutrition, having wondered why on her journey following dietary guidelines she was getting heavier, and why the same was happening to many of her patients. Joanne founded the website *www.fatismyfriend.co.uk* and is one of a group of 12 founder doctors of the Public Health Collaboration charity. She holds frequent low carb, behavioural change meetings in multiple locations to aid patients in losing weight, improving their diabetes control and improving their general health.

Dr Shan Hussain

Practising as a GP for 18 years, Dr Shan Hussain has become a renowned author, health coach, wellness advisor and ambassador to the World Health Innovation Summit. He is the founder of The Health Studio, believing in a holistic approach to health, centred around our collective physical, mental and social wellbeing. As such, he has a particular interest in health promotion and disease prevention. During his career, Dr Hussain has developed several coaching programmes and mentorship schemes designed to help reverse the symptoms of many stress-related health problems, working with individuals and organisations to help naturally improve health in a sustainable way. His bestselling book, *The Big Prescription*, serves as a guide for readers to learn about evidence-based holistic health practices that create the foundation of his work. Shan's podcast Enduring Health, is one of the most listened to health podcast series on the internet.

Dr Emer MacSweeney

Dr Emer a leading London neuroradiologist with experience in both the NHS and the independent sector. Currently, she is the CEO and Medical Director of Re:Cognition Health. Her previous posts include director of neuroradiology at Atkinson Morley's Hospital, St George's Healthcare Trust and managing director at MedTel UK. Dr MacSweeney has a special interest in neuroradiology of cognitive impairment disorders, with considerable experience in imaging of neurovascular diseases and traumatic brain injury.

Dr Jason Fung

Jason is a Canadian nephrologist, a medical doctor who specialises in kidney care and treating diseases of the kidney. He's a world-leading expert on intermittent fasting and low carbs, especially for treating people with type 2 diabetes. He has written three best-selling health books, *The Obesity Code*, *The Complete Guide to Fasting* and *The Diabetes Code*, and he co-founded the Intensive Dietary Management programme. His *www.dietdoctor.com* website features a wealth of information on health.

Dr Malcolm Kendrick

Dr Malcolm is a practising GP living in Macclesfield. Malcolm is a three-time best-selling author. Two of his books, *The Cholesterol Con* and *A Statin Nation*, are a must-read for anyone thinking about taking statins. Malcolm's third book, *Doctoring Data* is so insightful that when you next see a questionable newspaper headline about health, you should download an electronic version, and it will help you better understand how it was dubiously crafted. Malcolm's area of expertise is in studying the heart and what actually causes heart disease.

Ivor Cummins

Since 2012 Ivor has been intensively researching the root causes of modern chronic disease. His particular focus has been on cardiovascular disease, diabetes and obesity. He shares his research insights at public speaking engagements around the world, revealing the key nutritional and lifestyle interventions which will deliver excellent health and personal productivity. He has recently presented at the British Association of Cardiovascular Prevention and Rehabilitation and also at the Irish National Institute of Preventative Cardiology annual conferences. Ivor's 2018 book *Eat Rich, Live Long* details the conclusions of his research and his website *www.thefatemperor.com* has a wealth of information.

Dr Peter Brukner

Peter is a medical doctor and specialist sports and exercise medicine physician. In March 2010 he was appointed Head of Sports Medicine and Sports Science at Liverpool FC, and also that year he accompanied the Australian National Football Team to the World Cup in South Africa. In 2013, Peter became the team doctor of the Australian Cricket Team. More recently, Peter has become interested in lifestyle issues and their relationship to health. In particular, he is interested in the role of diet, especially a low carb diet, in both health and athletic performance. Peter has established the not-for-profit campaign *SugarByHalf* with the aim of reducing the intake of added sugar in Australia. He is also a noted author, his best-selling book *Clinical Sports Medicine* is a must-read for all athletes and professional sportspeople.

Hannah Richards

Hannah is the author of *The Best Possible You*, a best-selling book about how nutrition and lifestyle choices can help you heal and renew your body. As a nutritionist and lifestyle coach, Hannah encourages us to listen to our body and reconnect with the signals it sends that we may have learned to ignore. She is also an expert in gastrointestinal health and has written a course on how to manage gut clients in private practices. She is the founder of The Gut Clinic in Mayfair.

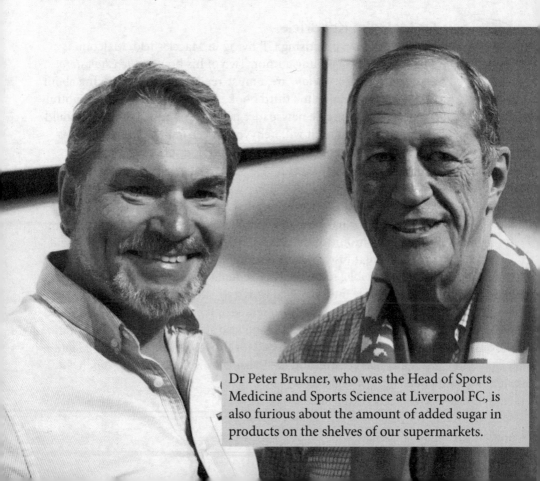

Dr Peter Brukner, who was the Head of Sports Medicine and Sports Science at Liverpool FC, is also furious about the amount of added sugar in products on the shelves of our supermarkets.

CHAPTER 1

EVOLUTION

*"Although nature needs thousands or millions of years to
create a new species, man needs only a few dozen years to destroy one."*
VICTOR SCHEFFER

In this chapter, I am going to set out the background to why I believe that we need to look back through history to discover how to live healthier and happier for longer.

Our environment, our lifestyle and the Great British diet has changed more over the past 100 years than over the past 1 million and there are now more sick Brits than ever. These changes have led to an epidemic of disease; cardiovascular disease, cancer, high blood pressure, type 2 diabetes, dementia, fatty liver disease. These aren't just scary headlines, these killers have become a 'local problem'.

I say this more out of embarrassment than anything else. For years, I was the same as most people. I followed the advice that should have been trustworthy. If it said 'healthy' on the packaging, I bought it. If the doctor told me that I needed to cut out certain foods to lower my cholesterol, I'd listen and do as I was told, because well… why wouldn't you?

Through the advice of some true health pioneers, I have learned that almost all of what we have been conditioned and brought up to believe about food and health is simply wrong. By the end of this book, you will wholly understand the truth about our health, wellbeing and longevity. You will likely be furious, but at least you will know the truth.

Furious, simply because I'm willing to bet you will recognise almost all of the following myths. Like me, you may have even passed some of them on to your children and I'll save you the suspense, the truth is as embarrassing as it is terrifying. Here are some of the biggest health misconceptions of modern times:

Fat & Furious Facts Plus Convenient Corporate Myths

"Don't skip breakfast – it's the most important meal of the day." Wrong! It's the most dangerous meal of the day and does not set us up properly as we have been taught.

"Our governments want us to live long lives". Really! If we all lived healthily for an extra 20 years, it's pensions that could cripple the economy, not the NHS.

"Our health is predominantly hereditary." Wrong! It's our diet, our lifestyle and our environment that ultimately shapes our health and longevity.

"We should eat a balanced diet." Wrong! If you uncover something that's bad for your health, you should avoid it. The only place we should occasionally balance is on the bathroom scales!

"Never eat red meat or fat as it causes heart conditions." Wrong! Organic grass-fed meat is one of the healthiest foods we can consume. In fact, it is what we are designed to eat.

"Never sunbathe as it causes skin cancer." Yes it can, but there is a far greater chance of developing other internal cancers, osteoporosis or heart conditions by avoiding sun.

"Eat three meals a day and eat little but often." Wrong! Eating this way triggers disease as our body never goes into repair mode. Intermittent fasting is how we were designed.

"Consume 0% or low-fat everything." Seriously wrong! We now understand that quality fats are not our enemy. Food labelled as low fat, or zero fat, are stuffed full of sugars to replace these missing fats, and it's these sugars that are deadly.

"Don't skip meals because your metabolism will slow down." Wrong! Unless we go a whole three or four days without food, skipping meals actually speeds up our metabolism.

"Brown bread, brown rice and whole-grain cereals are all healthy." Wrong! For many, they are actually unhealthy foods dressed up in a nutritional outfit. They still turn into potentially life-threatening sugar in our body and could cause many to develop type 2 diabetes, cancer, heart disease, Alzheimer's and more.

"Artificial sweeteners help you lose weight." Wrong! They might not in themselves be very calorific, but they may damage our healthy gut bacteria and switch off the satiety hormone, which informs us when we are full.

"Type 2 diabetes, cancer, heart disease, strokes, dementia, obesity and Alzheimer's are at an epidemic level globally." Wrong! They are local epidemics in countries eating

unnatural and carbohydrate-heavy diets. There are still remote, self-sufficient communities where they are unheard of.

"Counting calories helps us to lose weight." Wrong! The body processes calories from carbohydrates, fat and protein differently, therefore using calories as a measure is, in the main, futile. Plus, who wants to spend their entire life doing maths?

"Slogging our hearts out by jogging for endless hours is healthy." Wrong! It's potentially detrimental to our heart, and instead, we should just move more and exercise in short intervals. Plus, you can't out-exercise a bad diet!

"Having high cholesterol is a major cause of heart attacks." Wrong! Many leading heart specialists believe having high cholesterol is not at all even linked to heart disease. And recent studies show in the over 60s a lower LDL (the so-called bad cholesterol) reduces lifespan! The complete opposite of what your doctor might tell you.

"Educate yourself on what food labels mean." Wrong! Real food does not need a label.

"There is a pill for every ill." True! But over-prescription is responsible for one of the largest increases in hospitals admission across Great Britain.

"Prawns, eggs and other food high in cholesterol will raise your cholesterol levels and should be avoided." Wrong! Just because a certain food type is high in dietary cholesterol has little correlation to what happens when you have consumed it. And as you will learn shortly, high LDL cholesterol isn't actually usually the problem.

"Don't eat meat. It causes global warming". Very wrong. Meat from cattle that are allowed to graze in fields are not part of the problem, but part of the solution.

I am sure at this point, in fact, I hope you are sceptical about some of these alternative viewpoints. After all, as Charles Darwin once said, "Great is the power of steady misrepresentation", so it's very natural for you at this point to feel that some of these challenges to conventional wisdom must be wrong. By the end of the book, with the help of my 23 magnificent contributors, I anticipate that you will feel both furious and motivated for real change.

To understand how to live healthier for longer by avoiding the onslaught of modern diseases, we are going to discuss how our caveman ancestors survived and thrived, and how we have very little evolved since man first set foot on the planet. We will then cover some basic biology to help you develop a better understanding of what happens to various foods when they enter our body.

How is it that while contagious diseases that caused so much devastation 100 years ago have been virtually eradicated, we now face a completely new array of deadly conditions? This book will reveal all.

Major Killers	
100 Years Ago	**Today**
Pneumonia	Heart Disease
Tuberculosis	Cancer
Diarrhoea	Stroke
Polio	Diabetes
Measles	Alzheimer's
Syphilis	Respiratory Disease
Scarlet Fever	Liver Disease
Typhoid	Influenza
Whooping Cough	Pneumonia

How sick are we in Great Britain today? In just 50 years, cancer has gone from being fairly rare to now something that has had a devastating effect on most families. Diabetes has gone from virtually unknown to an epidemic. And boy have we put on weight. Look at these current British sickness statistics:

- The average adult in the UK is now 2.5 stone (nearly 16kgs) heavier than they were just 50 years ago, and it won't be long before one in two is obese. Is it a coincidence that over the past 50 years, there has been a three-fold increase in sugar consumption in our country, most of it hidden in food?
- Half of people living in Britain today, at some point in their life, will be diagnosed with cancer.
- Dementia has grown at an epidemic rate to become the biggest killer of women.
- Over the last 20 years, the number of people with diabetes has more than doubled.
- Almost four in five adults in England have a 'heart age' older than their actual age.
- A third of elderly patients may be being prescribed unnecessary medication, putting them at needless risk of side-effects and costing the NHS millions.
- We are currently the only European country with a declining life expectancy.

Please re-read those statistics. Do they make you feel frightened? Don't be. Believe it or not, they are all, in the main, linked to the same thing. This book is going to help you side-step becoming a sick statistic. With a great National Health Service, our chances of living healthily and for a very long time are actually better now than ever before.

However, to avoid the current tsunami of chronic illness that has a vice-like grip on our nation, it is crucial that you begin to live your life more in line with the needs of the human body. In practice, the more primal you become, the happier, healthier and longer you should live. All being well, you might even become a centenarian or even a supercentenarian.

To understand the principles of living a primal lifestyle, we need first to develop a basic understanding of our evolution. Here is a very stripped back timeline of Earth and the progression of our species. Later we will explain at which point in time our current DNA evolved, which is the period I believe we should all base our food and lifestyle choices upon. This is the spirit, the heart, the core, the foundation of living primally.

The Primal Timeline

- Our Earth is 4.5 billion years old
- 3.6 billion years ago, the first microscopic organisms (bacteria) formed
- 6 million years ago, bipedal apes developed the ability to walk on two legs
- 3 million years ago, some human-like apes began using two legs as their main method of movement
- 2.5 million years ago, humans started to use hand tools, and for many paleoanthropologists this event marks the true beginning of the human race
- 200,000 years ago, Homo Sapiens (Latin for 'wise man') emerged in Africa
- 100,000 years ago, Homo Sapiens learned to create fire to heat food
- 12,000 years ago, we experienced an agricultural revolution
- 6,000 years ago, saw the beginning of agricultural carbohydrates
- 2,500 years ago, man discovered that you could extract sap from sugar canes
- 300 years ago, sugar still accounted for less than 1% of calorie intake
- 75 years ago, the first pesticides were introduced
- 70 years ago, plastic was first used commercially
- 50 years ago, the average adult in Great Britain was 2.5 stone lighter
- 40 years ago, our government introduced guidelines on eating more healthily for the first time
- 2 years ago, the first report of declining life expectancy in Great Britain

While the human race can be traced back to 2.5 million years ago, for the vast majority of that time we were not at the top of the food chain. For most of our existence, we have been the hunted rather than the hunter. Certainly, for the first 1.5 million years, we lived off foraging, collecting plants, and eating small animals. About the only time we would enjoy feasting on a larger beast would be when an even larger carnivore had moved on from its prey, leaving behind scraps for us humans.

Both before and after we developed the ability to heat our food, meat from small animals such as rabbits and wild sheep, bugs, snails and insects were the backbone of our natural diet. Around 100,000 years ago, we moved to the top of the food chain when we began to create fire and cook our food and with it came the ability to eat more fibrous and tough foods.

When meat could not be found or caught, then berries, figs, mushrooms, nuts, roots and leaves were consumed. At this point in our history there were no settlements, and all human life was nomadic. From season to season our ancestors would travel looking for new sources of food. What they ate in the summer would vary dramatically from what they ate in the cold winters. This brings us nicely to our first principle that is crucial for both our wellbeing and longevity. Our primal ancestors' diets were very diverse and provided a wide array of crucial nutrients.

12,000 years ago there were just a few million humans on Earth. That's like the population of Birmingham spread across the entire planet. With so much space and freedom, why would any human want to settle down? But for some reason, 12,000 years ago they did. As our distant ancestors migrated from East Africa, they came across what we today know as Turkey and Iran. They seemed to like it there and decided to settle. They started to raise sheep and goats and began to plant seeds. This was the beginning of the Agricultural Revolution and the turning point in our evolution. This became our first step away from eating what we were designed by nature to eat.

6,000 years ago saw the first development of agricultural carbohydrates. Their arrival in Southern Europe has been associated with an average decrease of six inches in height and a shortening of lifespan by ten years. Yes, you read that correctly! Isn't it infuriating that we have had evidence for 6,000 years that carbohydrates shorten lifespan? Interestingly, during the same period the nomadic cultures of America that ate buffalo and the meat-eating Maasai of Tanzania and Kenya, who all avoided agriculture carbohydrates, remained tall and lean.

The Speed Of Evolution

As a species, we evolve very slowly. Have you ever wondered why it is that when we get out of the bath, our fingers and toes are all wrinkly? It's because thousands of years ago we used to catch fish with our bare hands and feet. Our toes and fingers went wrinkly so that our feet could grip onto the rocks, and fish did not slip through our fingers. Do we need to do this today? Of course not! It is, however, going to take our DNA a very long time to catch up. Because as a species we humans evolve so slowly, we should consume foods and undertake a fitness regime as closely in tune with the requirements of our DNA as possible. Optimising our nutrition is not about counting calories or doing what the big food corporations with their misguided and sometimes dishonest research tell us we should do. It's simply doing what nature has designed us to do.

Because evolution, in the main, takes thousands of years, my starting point for most of my advice on health is in searching for ancestral precedence. Asking 'how long does it take for us to evolve?' is similar to asking 'how long is a piece of string?' The scientist François Jacob, who won the Nobel Prize in Physiology or Medicine in 1965, said, "Evolution is a tinkerer, not an engineer". So, as evolution is not an exact science, we should focus on 'food that is natural to eat'. For that, we should look at the period before our ancestors started planting foods and, without any question, before we started to mess with them genetically.

Think of evolution in another way. The further we live away from the equator, the paler our skin has become in order to maximise the diminishing amount of sunshine. So, if evolution were a quick process, within a few generations people of African descent would start to develop paler skin. Yet scientists suggest that it can take more than 1,000 years to witness even the tiniest degree of change. Still, I would assume that lightening skin tones in order to absorb more sunlight, and therefore create more vitamin D, would not be as big a challenge for evolution as trying to deal with new types of incoming foods.

Today, so many people are on medication mainly because they are consuming foods that the body was not designed to deal with, and we haven't yet evolved to adapt to them. An analogy would be that it's like putting the wrong type of fuel in a car and then stuffing it full of additives to try to make it perform!

Professor Tim Noakes
Tim, as evolution is such a slow process, should we be looking at the diet of our distant ancestors, to rediscover what diet we are effectively designed to eat?

I have had a fascination with anthropology from a very young age. And because South Africa has such a long history in discovering the origins of humans, it's something that has always been close to my heart. But my family is originally from Liverpool, and it's important to remember that not so long ago the north of England was covered in ice! What were people eating then? They were eating sheep and meat and other stuff, they weren't eating fruit, vegetables, cereals and grains. So, as I originate from Liverpool, I have tailored my own diet progressively to more just meat, fish, dairy, nuts and eggs, and that is essentially what I eat. And the closer I have come to mirroring my ancestors' diet, the healthier I have become. I actually think it's important to look at the recent history of food in your own country. This is an important diet for England.

But I meet a lot of people from grain baring countries. I know some Iranian people, which is probably where the wheat started, and they are very happy to eat lots of wheat, and it seems that they are possibly more adapted, because they were the first populations to eat wheat. They have been exposed to it for 18,000 years. The key point is that in those days if they weren't able to eat wheat, they would have died. But if the wheat had come along only two or three thousand years ago, then they would have had much less time for the selection process to happen. I always tell people to look back at what their great, great grandparents were eating, or even further back than that.

Life Expectancy is Reducing in Britain
Surely, looking back into history to discover how to live healthier for longer is flawed logic. Aren't we now living the longest lives ever in human existence? Well, Paul Clayton and Judith Rowbotham wrote in the *International Journal of Environmental Research and Public Health*, an excellent yet shocking article explaining why life expectancy today, especially for men, is shorter than it was 130 years ago.

The article was titled How the Mid-Victorians Worked, Ate and Died. In it they discussed the golden era of British health, a period between 1850 and 1880 where farmers were over-producing real foods, such that all classes were able to afford good nutrition. As a result, life expectancy in 1875 was equal or even better in Great Britain than it is today. In fact, for adult men living 130 years ago, the average life expectancy was three years longer than it is today. How furious does that make you feel? The authors concluded the article with the following. "It shows that medical advances allied to the pharmaceutical industry's output, have done little more than change the manner of our dying. The Victorians died rapidly of infection and/or trauma, whereas we die slowly of degenerative disease. It reveals that with the exception of family planning, the vast edifice of twentieth century healthcare has not enabled us to live longer but has in the main merely supplied methods of suppressing the symptoms of degenerative disease which have emerged due to our failure to maintain mid-Victorian nutritional standards".

Professor Tim Noakes

The British were at their healthiest in the mid-Victorian Era, between 1840 and 1880. That is when they were the tallest and the healthiest. And their life expectancy was also very good. But then Britain started to implement the industrial diet and health started to deteriorate. By the time of the Boer War, which happened right at the end of the 19th century, the British couldn't find enough tall soldiers, and they had to change the rulings of who they could take. And that is how quickly deterioration in health can happen. That took just one generation and sadly it has accelerated even faster more recently.

In a nutshell, the overwhelming majority advice in this book is based on the varied diets and lifestyles of the human race, from before the agricultural revolution, which took place 12,000 years ago. A time when everyone lived more primally.

CHAPTER 2

PRIMAL PRIMER

"It is not the strongest or the most intelligent who will survive but those who can best manage change."
LEON C MEGGINSON

This chapter is going to set out the primal scene. It's part biology, part nutrition and provides background information that will prove useful as you continue on your journey.

A New You

Every five or six years, you and I almost become an entirely new person. Our skin is constantly dying and being replaced, in fact our entire outer covering is replaced every single month. Our complete skeleton is regenerated every ten years or so. Our lungs are replaced every six weeks, our liver in less than six months, and our tongue's 9,000 taste buds are rejuvenated every ten days. Sadly, the one body part most of us would love to be self-regenerating at high speed – our brain – is, in the main, as old as we are. In fact, most things in our head are permanently ours. The eyes don't replace themselves and once our adult teeth come through, that's our lot. The rest of our body, cell-by-cell, day-by-day, is in a state of continual repair, rebuild or replace... or it should be.

All of this replacing, regenerating and rejuvenating is fuelled by one thing and one thing only: what we consume. Hence the saying, 'we are what we eat'. If we eat junk food, our new body parts will be created by junk and will not be quite as good as the cells they are replacing. That's what causes ageing. Rubbish input equals rubbish output, or as computer geeks say 'garbage in, garbage out'. However, eat the right foods, drink enough water and consume sufficient vitamins and minerals, and we are going to make some pretty good body parts and at the same time, delay the ageing process.

Dr Shan Hussain
I believe that you are not only what you eat but also what you absorb and assimilate from your environment.

How Long Could We Live?
To answer this question, let me take you on a journey around the world. Soviet gerontologists say that Russia's oldest man, Shirali Mislimov, who lived in the mountain village of Barzavu, lived to 168!

Dr David Davis, a gerontologist from University College in London, spent 1971 to 1973 in the Vilcabamba valley in the Andes. He discovered death certificates for four people that had lived to 150, and at the time he was there, one person was 126! Dr Davis also wrote that there was no cancer, heart disease, diabetes, high blood pressure or any other westernised diseases. Yet in villages just 50 miles away, where they had been infiltrated by westernisation, chronic illness was at normal westernised levels.

In 1971, Dr Leaf, a lecturer at Harvard University, visited the remote town of Abkhazia in Georgian Russia, he interviewed a lady by the name of Khaf Lasuria who was more than 130 years old. She had only retired two years earlier and when she was 100 years old, was still the fastest tea leaf picker in the village. Dr Leaf checked the records, and it was true. In the 1940s, she held the farm record! An article was written about her in the January 1973 edition of National Geographic, quoting her words, "Every day is a gift when you are over 100". The doctor was amazed that the women drank alcohol regularly, but most importantly, she was always walking and working.

Another Russian gerontologist studied 15,000 people over 80 years old in Georgia and found that more than 70% regularly walked in the mountains and over 60% still worked. A nine-year study of 123 people, all of whom were over 100 years old, in Abkhazia, revealed that not one of them had cancer, and the vast majority were described as in a state of neurological and psychological stability.

The History of British Obesity
What we are told we should eat by our government is dangerous and is wrong. The foundation of the UK's current Eat Well Guidelines can be traced back to nonsense guidelines assembled in the USA where I deem the story to have begun in 1948; the year when Proctor & Gamble funded the fledgling American Heart Association (AHA) with a whopping $1.7 million. At the time the company peddled, amongst other things, their man-made lethal fats. Just one corporate-funded event acted as a catalyst for our own government's nutritional guidelines. These guidelines turned their back on the very foods that had been the natural, stable diet of humans since the beginning of time.

This absurdity accelerated to the point of complete insanity with the mismanaged research conducted by an American physiologist, Ancel Keys. The AHA must have been jumping for joy at his findings that we needed to avoid saturated fats and cholesterol. It must have delighted their corporate sponsors. By 1961, Keys achieved stardom when the America Heart Association announced that saturated fat increased the likelihood of heart disease. The sugar associations clapped their hands with glee and lobbied the Department of Health to stick with Ancel Keys view, burying and slurring all research that proved otherwise. This included discrediting the courageous British physiologist and nutritionist John Yudkin, who had written a book called *Pure White and Deadly*, subtitled 'How Sugar is Killing Us and What We Can Do to Stop It'. Yudkin was ridiculed by Ancel Keys and silenced by the sugar trade.

Back to the USA. In the early 1970s, Richard Nixon drove down the cost of food and, with the help of his agricultural secretary Earl Butz, they massively funded farmers to produce cheap wheat, soy and maize. But they ended up with a vast stockpile and the solution was to export it en-masse to Great Britain. In 1977, to further support farmers and continue to keep food prices low, the US dietary guidelines totally demonised fat. But the removal of fat made the new grain and wheat food taste bland, and so began the infusion of sugar into almost everything!

By 1980, the American Dietary Guidelines were upgraded to a food pyramid, of which the base of all daily consumption was recommended to be bread, pasta and potatoes. But these are the very foods that prominent English undertaker William Banting advised people who needed to lose weight to avoid. He wrote this in the very first book ever to be written on diet in 1863. As it did in the USA, the obesity epidemic in Britain and our tsunami of modern chronic illnesses was born!

Nina Teicholz

In America we have spent hundreds of millions of dollars on vast nutritional studies; huge big rigorous studies, the exact trials that you are supposed to do, and every time they finish them, they find that cutting out fat from the diet does not work. They reveal that cutting out saturated fat and cholesterol didn't spare people from heart disease. In fact, the more that men lowered their cholesterol in the biggest ever heart disease study aimed at confirming Ansel Keys cholesterols/heart disease hypophysis; it revealed the total opposite, and that men were more likely to have a heart attack with lower cholesterol.

It's like everything came out wrong, and the people in our health institutes, just couldn't handle it. They couldn't believe the outcome. They thought they must have done something wrong in the trial. So, they published neither the studies nor the results. We found documents in basements from the National Institute of Health, that hadn't been published saying that saturated fats have no effect on heart disease whatsoever. We did all of these rigorous studies, and they were all ignored. You see, for the researchers and the policymakers, by this point, it had already become the policy of the American Heart Association, and then the policy of the government, and they were unable to reverse out of their policies. They didn't want to be seen as weak; there is so much cognitive dissonance in your mind, you can't believe that you might have been wrong, you don't want to be seen as flip-flopping on the public. That's not good for your reputation, and the food industry was invested in your policies at this point, so there were all sorts of reasons why they felt they couldn't reverse out of their policies.

So saturated fats, just like a jury trial, have been tested and tested and found over and over again not to be guilty, the evidence was never ever there, so now it's time to let them out of jail! Since the release of my book and also the works of Gary Taubes who also wrote about these buried and unpublished studies, there have now been more than 17 independent teams of scientists from all over the world that have looked at those clinical trials again. They looked at the most rigorous types of data and conducted what is called a systematic review of them, and found zero effects of saturated fats on heart disease.

Gary Taubes
With so much evidence proving that the current government guidelines are flawed, how long do you think it will take before governments tell the truth?
It's a very good question. It's the $64 billion question. There are a lot of forces acting against us. There are 50 to 60 years of bad science. There is a famous saying in science, from Max Planck, that 'science progresses funeral by funeral'. The older generation dies off, and the younger generation grows up with the new belief. One of the problems here is that the older generation were just bad scientists. They didn't know how to do really rigorous critical science, to think critically and sceptically about their beliefs. And they conveyed that belief system, that bad science, the term is pathological science (an area of research where people are tricked into false results, by subjective effects or wishful thinking) to the younger generation. So we are always fighting their science. And there is no way in the system for the scientists to say 'stop, we made a mistake'. It's virtually impossible for them. The funding system will pass them by. It's the quickest way for them to be marginalised as 'quacks' in this field. And in fact, I know some really good scientists that believe like I do, but because they want to be able to influence the system - as slow as it takes, don't say anything. And you are up against the food industry with all of their powerful lobbies.

Fat, Protein & Carbohydrates
Everything that lives – whether it be a tree or a human, a dog or a strawberry – is made of the same basic ingredients: fat (fatty acids), carbohydrates (dressed-up sugars) and proteins (amino acids). Fat, carbohydrates and protein are the three macronutrients (derived from the Greek word 'macro', meaning large) that, either by themselves or combined, make up all of the food we eat. The human body needs both fat and protein to survive and flourish but - contrary to popular belief and even government guidelines - not a single ounce of carbohydrate is necessary to sustain human life. Not today, tomorrow or ever!

Everything we eat - no matter what it looks like, its texture or its taste - is broken down in our gut into one of the three components mentioned above. Later in this book we will learn about micronutrients - which are other foodstuffs such as minerals, phytonutrients, and vitamins - but first we need to get a clear and simple understanding of fat, protein and carbohydrates.

Understanding Macronutrients

While there are three macronutrients, natural whole foods generally only contain a combination of two. If the food (or drink) is derived from something that once had a face, it is made up of protein and fat, the exception being a small amount of carbohydrate in eggs and milk. If the food came out of the ground, it generally consists of protein and carbohydrates. Note how everything has protein! This is because protein is the building block of life.

A few exceptions to the two macronutrient rule are nuts, seeds, milk and avocados, which feature all three macronutrients. There are also a few foods made of just one macronutrient: table sugar (although it's less a food, more a poison) is made up of just carbohydrate, and oils such as coconut and olive are made from just fat.

What Do Macronutrients Do?

In all humans and animals, all three macronutrients can carry out energy-related roles:

- Carbohydrates – are converted to sugar for energy
- Fats – are converted to fatty acids, in the main to repair cells or to use as energy
- Proteins – are converted to amino acids, to repair and rebuild cells or to use as energy

Let me start this section on macronutrients with something that came as a shock to me, and something that I still have the hardest time in convincing some of my more stubborn friends. Of the three macronutrients, it's not fat that makes us fat, it is carbohydrates. We could buy the flabbiest cut of meat on sale in our butcher's and serve it with a baked potato, and it would be the potato that makes us fat, not the flabby meat. You see, it's quite simple, our body has no intention of storing fat as fat! Our body has a preference to use fat as fuel.

Sadly, while there are many wonderful natural healthy fats, there are some deadly man-made ones too, but we will get to these later. We will also learn later that for the body to store fat as fat, it needs the presence of lots of sugar to glue (glycerol) it together, but for now it is important to understand these two very important and life-changing facts:

1. As long as we cut down our carbohydrate intake, eating fat does not make us fat.
2. Carbohydrates and other sugars are the only macronutrients that are easily converted into body fat.

Dr Dan Maggs

Natural fats are not the enemy. We have demonised and vilified the good guy for more than 50 years, and all the while the sickly sweet kid has been getting away with murder!

Dr Patrick Holford

Professor Paul Kenny (a professor specialising in neurobehavioral disorders, who in 2018 conducted the following research) fed a group of rats nothing but fat for a month, and they gained a little bit of weight, but nothing much. They would eat the fat, feel satisfied and then stop. He then fed them nothing but sugar and they gained some weight, maybe not as much as we might have expected. They would eat the sugar, feel satisfied and then stop. In the third experiment, he fed them a diet of 50% fat and 50% sugar, which is basically what junk food is, and they went ballistic. They just binged; they couldn't stop eating. Junk food just fools the brain. You see, in nature, you never find high fat with high carbs. You get fat and protein, you get carbs and protein, but you don't get high fat and high carbs. That is junk food, and it affects the brain in a certain way, and you can't stop eating. And I noticed one other thing. He was actually feeding them cheesecake. And what we know about milk, is that it is sort of addictive and it is meant to be; you know, when a baby is breastfeeding, they need to become a sort of addict. And that's why the milk chocolate bar, with dairy, high fat and high carbs, you just can't stop eating. We can run on fat, we could run on carbs, but put the two together, and we create a food that people won't stop eating.

Fat – Fatty Acids

While proteins and carbohydrates are fairly straightforward to understand, fats are a little more complex. Rather than provide chapter and verse straight away, we will cover just the basics right now and then build up the picture throughout the remainder of *Fat & Furious*.

Let me again state that if we are overweight, fat in food is not our enemy but our friend. Or, more precisely, good fats should become our new best friends. Fats don't make us fat, and never have done. It's carbohydrates and to a far lesser degree protein that causes us to pile on weight, but not fat. I remember how I would always cut the fat off my beef, lamb, chicken and duck in the belief it was the fat that made us fat, when in reality, leaving it on meat means we drop it from our waistline.

Quality fats correct our hormones and keep them in balance so that we feel more energetic. They actually help us burn more energy (not store it) and make us feel fuller so that we stop overeating. And, more importantly, quality fats reduce the likelihood of us falling victim to six out of ten of the most common causes of death in Great Britain!

Sources of good fats include anything rich in omega 3 such as salmon, nuts, avocado, coconuts, olive, lamb and organic butter. Deadly fats to avoid include all trans-fats (normally food labels call them 'partially hydrogenated oils'), fats in processed and packaged foods and vegetable oils, which believe it or not, are rarely derived from vegetables.

Fat Facts

Here is a brief scientific explanation of the different types of fat:

Saturated fats: which in the main are solid at room temperature, have their bonds filled with hydrogen (i.e. they are literally saturated). Despite all that you have read and heard, saturated fats cannot be bad for us because breast milk – without which many of us wouldn't be here right now – is rich in saturated fats. So too is my beloved coconut oil!

Unsaturated fats: include the hugely beneficial omega 3 and olive oil. They're not unhealthy either. These can be further broken down into monounsaturated and polyunsaturated:

Monounsaturated fats/oils: (usually liquid at room temperature) have one double bond of hydrogen missing. As long as they are natural, these aren't unhealthy either. They can't be, as all health-conscious individuals will be aware of the many benefits of both avocados and nuts.

Polyunsaturated oils: (usually liquid at room temperature) have two missing bonds (I know 'poly' normally means many, but when it comes to fat, it means just two). The hugely beneficial omega 3 is indeed a polyunsaturated oil.

In principle, all fats are incredibly healthy, as long as they are real fats and not manufactured fake fats, which can be very toxic and dangerous. The health concern should not be whether a fat is saturated or not, but whether it is real or manufactured. Seriously, you don't need to concern yourself with which type of fat you are consuming, as long as you ensure it is real!

Trans-fats: be extremely cautious of trans-fats. While natural trans-fats are produced in the guts of some animals, such as beef, lamb and some dairy products, the vast majority of trans-fats are artificial fats, hydrogenated to make them last longer. If the ingredient list says hydrogenated or partially hydrogenated, then it's not a healthy fat and should be avoided! Artificial trans-fats or hydrogenated oils are toxic, ugly and deadly.

Dr Aseem Malhotra

As a result of Ancel Keys misguided research, he became the most influential person in changing dietary guidelines in 1977 in the USA and 1983 in the UK, and those dietary guidelines said that we should consume less than 30% of our calories from fat and less than 10% from saturated fat. The food industry jumped on the back of this and started to promote and market low-fat foods which had added sugar. If you take the fat out, it doesn't taste as good, so you add sugar. And now when we reflect on the evidence, and I look at all of that myself, saturated fat does not cause heart disease, it's a complete myth. It's complete nonsense, it's not about saturated fat, and we are talking here about foods such as butter, cheese, red meat and I have analysed this and published on this research. I have taken the evidence in its totality, I haven't cherry-picked things, and what does it tell us? It tells us that there really is no link at all. No link with death rates, type 2 diabetes, with strokes, with heart disease, with heart attacks, even if you are a heart attack patient and you reduce saturated fats, it doesn't have any benefit for you.

Dr Malcolm Kendrick

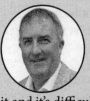

The world is obsessed with telling us that saturated fats are bad for us because that's just a message that has gone on and on and on! There is no evidence for it. It is just something people say. The most powerful parasite is an idea. Stick an idea in someone's head, get them to believe it and it's difficult to shift it. It's not there because the evidence is there, it's not there because of science, it's just there because people have just said it so many times for the last 60 years and its stuck. That's it.

Dr James DiNicolantonio

What are the bad and ugly fats?
The ugly fats are the trans-fats, where they oxidise the seed oils to make a more solid fat, high in omega 6, like your soybean oil and corn, a.k.a. vegetable oil (you will learn later in the book, that unlike omega 3, too much omega 6 is harmful). They are a huge part of the American diet and the UK diet too. When you guys cook fish and chips, they are very commonly deep-fried in these omega 6 oils. And the reason why they are bad for you is, one, they are very susceptible to oxidative stress because they have so many double bonds which are very susceptible to free radical attack. The second thing is that they are low in antioxidants, which compounds the problem. When you extract oil from these tiny seeds, you have to use a high amount of heat, hexane and toxins, which even start oxidising the oils before our bodies start oxidising it. The best fats are your extra virgin olive oil, as well as your marine omega 3, from either algae or from fish. MCTs, medium-chain triglycerides, are also very healthy fats, the body burns these fats even better than long-chain saturated fats, and you find these in coconut oils.

Protein – Amino Acids

This is the basic building block of all life forms. Its name is derived from the Greek word 'proteios', meaning 'primary' or 'first'. Protein is the driving force of change within our body. It comes to our aid when we need repairing – it rebuilds many of our organs, body tissue and muscles. It is responsible for growth in the young and is the creator of our hormones.

Protein is made up of amino acids. There are 22 different types of amino acids and they are all created from the elements carbon, hydrogen, nitrogen or sulphur. Our body can actually produce most of the different proteins that it needs, but there are nine that it can't make and these are very important to our health. For this reason they are named the 'essential proteins' and it is imperative that they form part of our diet.

In 2007 the World Health Organisation published a report scoring the quality of proteins from various food sources. As animals contain similar combinations of proteins to humans, it's not surprising that food derived from animals topped the list, with eggs, poultry, meat and fish the clear winners.

Once the body receives amino acids from foods rich in protein or from supplements, using the 22 different incoming varieties it is able to make more than 50,000 different varieties of protein inside our body. Once these new proteins are synthesised they form, among other things, our organs, bones, blood, and replace or repair muscle tissue. They are responsible for the creation of essential hormones such as insulin, melatonin and human growth hormone.

Carbohydrates - Sugar

Once we start living primally, in addition to carefully dodging the poisonous oils, our new dietary enemy becomes sugar and processed carbohydrates. Carbohydrates are almost exclusively derived from plants (plus a few dairy products) and are not found in meat, fish or poultry.

Throughout this book you will see carbohydrates written as CARBS. The reason for this is that I want you to see carbohydrates for what they are, with a very apt acronym: 'Carbohydrates Are Really Bad Sugars'. What do I mean by this? Basically, carbohydrates are just sugar in disguise.

Potatoes, pasta, bread, cereals and rice all convert to sugar in the body, and when it enters our bloodstream, sugar is poisonous! They might be dressed up in fancy packaging, and often carry labels with misleading health benefits, but we need to realise our body was never designed to consume them.

Whether they are simple or complex, all CARBS are still eventually turned into sugar by our body. The complex ones just take a little longer. Every time we eat CARBS, complex or not, we are eating sugar. Too much CARBS/sugar makes us fat, and will eventually lead to a whole host of problems, illnesses and diseases.

 Professor Tim Noakes

Carbohydrates are not an essential component of the human diet. There is no known medical condition that is caused by a deficiency of dietary carbohydrate. As a result, the influential US National Academy of Medicine concludes: 'The lower limit of dietary carbohydrate compatible with life apparently is zero, provided that adequate amounts of protein and fat are consumed.' Hence, no human and especially not anyone with an impaired capacity to metabolise carbohydrate needs to eat carbohydrate. This is to be expected, because, until the Neolithic period, which began with the agricultural revolution about 12,000 years ago, carbohydrates provided a minority of the food energy ingested by humans.

Dr Aseem Malhotra

As a result of incorrectly cutting down on saturated fats, we have increased our consumption of carbohydrates, particularly low-quality carbs. I am not talking about fruit and vegetables, I am talking about bread, pasta, rice and potato. As with much of what we are told in the government's Eat Well Guidelines, what you are getting is foods that are relatively poor in nutrition, combined with being very starchy and high in glucose. And the problems we are dealing with are related to consuming too much glucose. Type 2 diabetes is a problem of carbohydrate intolerance related to too much glucose over time, which affects your body's ability to metabolise it. 50% of high blood pressure is related to insulin resistance, I would describe it as having excess body fat related to diets that are high in starch and sugar. And that is at the roots of most of the problems.

The Carbocoaster

With the exception of fibre, all CARBS are converted to sugar, and any excess sugar in the blood is bundled up by insulin and stored as body fat. This can happen so quickly that shortly after a CARB-loaded meal, that we feel hungry again. We call this the Carbocoaster.

The Carbocoaster works like this. We eat a sandwich and the body converts the bread to sugar. Our brain summons insulin to quickly grab any excess sugar, which to our body is pure poison, and stores it as body fat. Because the bread is now no longer in circulation, we feel hungry again, so consume another. The Carbocoaster effect is enhanced because both the blood sugar levels keep getting topped up and then depleted quickly, and after the initial surge of insulin this too plummets as it finishes hiding the sugar. This rollercoaster only happens with CARBS and other sugars. There is no fatocoaster or proteinocoaster, just the dangerous, highly addictive, adrenalin-rushing, body-crushing, high-speed Carbocoaster.

CARBS and other sugars work on the brain the same as cigarettes. We get a craving and we eat a pack of crisps, mints or a doughnut or two. It satisfies us for a short while, but not for long. Before we know it, we want more. One biscuit becomes two biscuits becomes three biscuits and so on. CARBS are addictive and just like cigarettes they have the power to cause chronic illness and kill us!

You are going to come across the phrase 'Metabolic Syndrome' several times in this book. It is a phrase used a lot in medical circles today, relating to the fact that most chronic illnesses we face in Great Britain including cancer, heart disease, Alzheimer's, type 2 diabetes, strokes, obesity and more, can all, in part, be related to the release of too much insulin. This modern onslaught of insulin is caused by one thing and one thing only, the consumption of far too many CARBS.

When we want to lose weight, different authors, different experts and different doctors all offer varying advice on how many CARBS we should consume each day. Some will say 70g, some 100g and some very specific amounts such as 73g. But the reality is the body doesn't actually need any CARBS at all! Put simply, the fewer CARBS we eat, the quicker we both lose weight and regain our metabolic health.

When we get down to our ideal weight, if we want a couple of apples or bananas then we can go for it. We won't want bread because once we start living without it, we become as averse to it as we would if we were forced to eat a dead rat! If we start eating too many CARBS in fruits (which is, after all, nature's candy) and vegetables and our weight starts to pile back on, we simply just cut them down again. It really is as straightforward as that.

Dr Dan Maggs

The most nutritional part of a doughnut is the hole. Processed/refined carbs and sugar are void of nature's nutrients, minerals and vitamins. They do nothing for the body other than to provide it with energy. And excess energy is stored as body fat, normally around the waistline.

Types Of CARBS

Let's look at CARBS in a little more detail. Depending on the size of the molecule, they may be known as either simple or complex. As well as breaking down into simple or complex, CARBS are also categorised as refined or unrefined.

Simple CARBS

These are the CARBS with the smallest molecules, so they are quickly absorbed and give a rapid boost in energy, a rapid increase in blood sugar levels and cause a spike in the production of insulin. As they are converted to energy so quickly, if we don't burn off this energy promptly it is quickly stored as fat in our body's favourite fat store. Simple CARBS include virtually all types of sugar. They are also found in natural products such as milk and fruit. But most of all, we are going to find them hidden in all sorts of processed foods, sweets and fizzy drinks.

Complex CARBS

These CARBS are composed of long strings of simple carbohydrates and are therefore bigger. As they are bigger they have to be deconstructed into simple CARBS before they can be absorbed. As a result they provide energy more slowly. Because complex CARBS are digested more slowly, with a slower release of energy, there is more opportunity for our body to use the fuel and they are therefore less likely to be stored as body fat. However, the energy from complex CARBS is still released faster than both protein and fat. Potatoes, peas, whole grain, wheat, rice, pasta and beans are all complex CARBS.

Now before you rush out and eat loads of potatoes, rice, pasta or grains because I have informed you that they are called complex CARBS, I want you to remember that they still convert to sugar (it just takes a little longer).

Refined CARBS

These are CARBS that have been highly processed in a factory. Any goodness that the CARBS might have been hiding, such as fibre, minerals and vitamins, are normally removed, or at best dramatically reduced, in the refining process. On the packaging of refined CARBS, we will often read that they have vitamins and minerals added, but these are only putting back some of the goodness that resided before being processed.

Unrefined CARBS

As you will have correctly guessed, these are CARBS that have not been processed. As well as vegetables and brown rice, foods labelled as wholegrain or multigrain are generally unrefined. Here is the good news: unrefined CARBS from vegetables and fruits (as long as they are organic) come complete with all of the vitamins and minerals that Mother Nature intended for us to consume. That said, if CARBS are over cooked, then their nutritional values start to diminish and in some cases disappear completely.

Complex & Unrefined CARBS

So if someone eats complex CARBS that are unrefined, then surely they won't put on weight – right? It's a nice idea, but unless we are keeping portion sizes extremely small, then most likely we will. You see, if we consume any more CARBS than we can burn at that time, while the body will store a small amount in the liver and muscles, it will send the rest to our fat stores.

If you are still not convinced that it's CARBS that make us fat with their constant and continual conversion into sugar, and their quick release into the bloodstream causing a spike in insulin, then why is there such a thing called the Glycaemic Index? Food labels index all CARBS based on how quickly they perform this task. There is no glycaemic index for either protein or fat. Why? Because protein rarely converts into poisonous sugar and fat never does.

Dr James DiNicolantonio

What happened in the early 1900s was we started to get an infusion in the diet of seed oils, trans-fats and sugar. Then, because of the invention of the steel roller mill, we started refining our carbohydrates, which basically gave us all these very refined powders, instead of eating real whole carbohydrate foods. From that moment on and forward, there has been a steady incline in heart disease, diabetes, fatty liver disease and even our children are now being diagnosed with fatty liver disease. We have invented all these medications and surgical devices that may help some people to live longer, but we are living with all of these chronic diseases. So our quality of life has gone down, and now ever our life expectancy is starting to dwindle.

Glycaemic Index

First of all, the name 'glycaemic' is derived from the medical term 'glycaemia' meaning 'the presence of glucose in the blood'. All CARBS receive a glycaemic index (GI) score from 1 to 100. The lower the number the better - or should I say, 'less horrible'. A score of 1 is the lowest and slowest and 100 is the highest and fastest to convert CARBS to glucose (a type of sugar). Therefore, pure glucose obviously scores 100. However, it is not as black and white as the GI score might suggest, as it assumes we are only eating the food being scored in isolation and not combining it with other foods, which when bound together after digested may change the speed of conversion into sugar.

The other limiting factor of GI is that it doesn't look at portion sizes. There are some items with a fairly low GI score, where the portions sizes are by definition big and therefore still not recommended if we are either trying to lose weight or stay healthy. A more reflective index is the glycaemic load (GL). While GI is useful to know how quickly glucose will enter the bloodstream, the GL informs us how dangerous that load will be.

The GL index is calculated simply by multiplying the typical grams of carbohydrates in a serving by the GI index for that type of CARB and then dividing it by 100. For an easy and comprehensive list, I have added a combined GI & GL chart to the colour insert section.

A Spoonful of Sugar

Dr David Unwin talks about how he often comes across patients who can't understand why their diabetes hasn't gone into remission, even though they have cut out all sugars. He then has to explain that while they may have removed the obvious sugars, like sweets and sodas, they often aren't aware that starchy carbohydrates, such as bread, pasta, rice and potatoes, digest down into surprisingly high amounts of glucose.

David realised some time back that many people struggled to visualise the GI and GL charts and began to research what effect certain popular foods had on the bloodstream. To get the message to really sink in, he had the idea of comparing the effect of popular food choices to eating spoons full of sugar.

I have added a 'Spoonful of Sugar' graph in the colour insert section. David's Spoonful of Sugar infographics have become so widely appreciated in medical circles, that the National Institute for Health and Care Excellence (NICE), a government body which provides national guidance and advice to improve health and social care, have now formally adopted them.

As you will repeatedly see throughout this book, when excess sugar enters the bloodstream, our body views it as poison and releases insulin to usher it to our fat stores. And too much insulin has an association with cancer, type 2 diabetes, heart disease, Alzheimer's and many more chronic illnesses that we today face in Britain.

Before they went to school each day, I always fed my young children what I thought was healthy cereals and apple juice and I am furious that nobody told me that these turned into sugar! Please use the chart in the colour section of the book, to avoid making the same mistakes as I did.

Fructose

Later we will learn about the different types of sugar. We have just discussed glucose and its effect on blood sugar levels, now it's time to look at fructose. When we eat table sugar (sucrose), it is made up of 50% glucose and 50% fructose. When these simple sugars arrive at the liver for processing, one of three things happen. First, they can be released into the blood to be used for energy. Next, they can be either stored in the liver or sent to the muscles and stored as glycogen (a secondary source of energy which we will come to later). Thirdly, the liver will convert excess glucose and all fructose (yes, all fructose) into saturated fat. The vast majority of the fat, if not all of the fat that ends up in the arteries and in LDL, is synthesised in the liver from sugars (fructose and glucose) in a process known as 'de novo lipogenesis'. All of the fat synthesised is saturated fat and most of it palmitic acid. What makes this interesting is that the type of saturated fat synthesised is palmitic acid, which is the fat most likely to cause cardiovascular disease (CVD). This is really critical to understand, because many dietitians tell people to cut down on any food that includes palmitate acid. However, the palmitic acid in the arteries that can cause CVD, biologically has to have originated from CARBS.

What is interesting is that of the two simple sugars, the one that is usually turned into saturated fat is fructose. In fact, it seems that no fructose is released from the liver into the bloodstream. Think about this logically; we have blood glucose measurements and a glycaemic index, but never fructose measurements. It's also why people with diabetes only ever measure glucose in the blood.

This fat fact is vital to understand if you are to recognise that all of those headlines you hear about the dangers of eating saturated fat are wrong. The dangerous saturated fat is the one that, through lipogenesis, we synthesise ourselves, as a way to deal with deadly sugar. It is important to understand that it is almost impossible for fat that we eat to create very low-density lipoproteins (VLDL), which then becomes LDL. It is the synthesis of CARBS, in particular fructose, that is the sole contributor and building block of LDL. This is basic human physiology.

An investigation recently found that in 1960 the American Sugar Industry paid Harvard researchers to produce a clinical paper stating that it was the intake of fat, not sugar, that causes CVD. Once you understand basic human physiology and novo lipogenesis, you realise this is entirely untrue. In fact, it is believed that over time, it is fructose that is a contributing factor to both CVD and to non-alcoholic fatty liver disease (NAFLD). Where does fructose come from? Table sugar, soft drinks, fruit and high fructose corn syrup.

Dr Robert Lustig

Fructose is very sweet. It's the reason why we like sugar, and it is the reason we crave sugar. It is addictive. Fructose is the addictive component of sugar. It goes to the reward centre of the brain and activates it. We have a limited capacity to metabolise fructose. But our livers have to metabolise it because fructose does not enter any other cell. So when you take a fructose load like Coca-Cola, it's basically all going to your liver. And the liver gets overwhelmed because basically, it has a fixed capacity to deal with it, and if you overwhelm your liver, it doesn't know what to do with the rest. So, the liver will turn that extra fructose into fat, and that is called 'de novo lipogenesis', new fat making. And that fat then has one of two fates. It can either be exported out of the liver, which in this case you have now got substrates for obesity and heart disease, or it will precipitate within the liver, and then you get fatty liver disease. And now you have liver dysfunction, insulin resistance and metabolic syndrome. You can think of fructose as the ageing compound; it causes wrinkles.

In defence of fructose in fruit, it comes with fibre. The fibre stops all of the fructose from being absorbed. The sugar is what makes it taste sweet, but it is the fibre that makes it healthy. The fibre is setting up a gel on the inside of your intestines. You need both soluble and insoluble fibres, and fruit has both. What's happening is that you are setting up a latticework on the inside of your intestines, cellulose is setting up like a fishnet. And the soluble fibre like the pectins and the inulin are plugging in the holes in that latticework to provide this gel, which is then reducing the rate of absorption and therefore protecting your liver. And if you don't absorb it early, it goes further down the intestine, and your microbiome bacteria will chew it up. So even though you consumed it, you didn't get it because your bacteria did.

So the two rules of diet which people do not understand:
- Protect the liver
- Feed the gut

Foods that do both are healthy. Those that do neither are unhealthy. Those that do one or the other are in the middle. Examples of food that do both include anything with fibre. Fruit is good, but not fruit juice. Real food works, processed food, doesn't.

Leptin vs Ghrelin

Armed with a basic understanding of the macronutrients - fat, protein and CARBS (a.k.a. sugar) - it's time to discuss hormones. First of all, what is a hormone? For now, let's think of it in its simplest form: it is a chemical that is released by one part of the body to deliver a memo to a different part. How does the hormone know where to deliver the message? Most biology books suggest that the hormone is like a key, and it only opens one lock. In other words, the intended recipient has a shape/lock that only the intended hormone/key fits into.

If you are guilty of overeating and are overweight or obese, it might not be your fault at all. The guilty party might be a little-known hormone called leptin. After we have eaten a meal, our body is supposed to release this little fella and send him off to our brain to tell us that we're full – to basically tell us to stop eating. Leptin is actually dispatched from our fat stores with a clear message to say we're stuffed, stop sending us more supplies, we're overcrowded.

If something goes wrong with our leptin and it doesn't want to get out of bed and go to work, then we will crave food all day and pile on weight. Not only that, when leptin is having a lie-in, his colleagues in the metabolic department slow down too. It's a double blow for our body. We feel hungry, we consume more food, and our slowed metabolism isn't going to use much of it for fuel.

As Dr Michael VanDerschelden explains in *The Scientific Approach to Intermittent Fasting*, "When we eat a meal under normal conditions, leptin rises, blocks hunger and causes the thyroid to release thyroid hormones to increase metabolism".

When we eat too many CARBS, there is a heightened possibility of developing type 2 diabetes. This is where fat cells can become insulin resistant due to a constant bombardment over a prolonged period of time. Sadly, for those who are overweight or obese, it's the same story with leptin. Over time as you get heavier and heavier, your body cries out for help and dispatches more and more leptin to the brain in an attempt to rein in appetite and stop us from eating. With so much leptin knocking on the door, the brain refuses to listen. It then doesn't realise that it has been fed and thinks it's starving. Not only do you carry on eating, but also the brain warns the thyroid that you are in a period of starvation and tells it to slow down your metabolism. Doubly unhelpful whammy! So now with your slow metabolism, feeling tired and constantly hungry, you sit on the sofa and scoff more foods high in sugar, because they're what's going to make you feel fuller faster. It's a race to the bottom in more ways than one!

If you are overweight, there is every chance that your body has become resistant to leptin. So how do you get the brain to start acknowledging it again? Simply by following these four important primal beliefs: eat healthy fats and not CARBS; intermittently fast; get more active; and consume plenty of fibre - as it is believed to help repair leptin resistance.

Throughout this book, you are going to discover how vital it is to develop the right type of bacteria in your gut. One way to nurture leptin is to develop colonies of bacteria that support it and remove those that can damage its production. Put another way, some varieties of bacteria can sabotage leptin production, causing us to overeat.

Ghrelin is the opposite of leptin. This hormone is the one that informs us that we are hungry. Ghrelin is essentially our hunger hormone. Before we eat, he runs around screaming to be fed. But after we have eaten, he is sent to the bedroom to awaken leptin and tell him to go to work.

Most people go and eat as soon as they hear ghrelin and his stomach rumblings demanding to be fed, but if we can resist these demands, wonderful things start to happen inside our body. First of all, we kick-start our automated repair process, we begin to fight inflammation (which is one of the biggest factors of modern disease) and we stimulate human growth hormones (HGH). What's best is Mr Ghrelin gets a little angry when we don't listen to him, so recruits more and more of his ghrelin family to assist him in trying to get us to eat and the more ghrelin there is in our body the more good it does. Combine this with exercise and we will increase our HGH even more.

As you will read later, there are great gains for most people in skipping breakfast. One of the scientific reasons for this is that there is a lot of ghrelin in our bodies after a good night's sleep and if we can resist its calls for food and exercise in this fasted state, then our health is really going to reap the benefits.

Professor Tim Noakes

Carbs do not satisfy hunger – they stimulate it. Most of the food in question is processed and developed with one purpose in mind: to make you want more. They are tested and refined to the point where they are as addictive as they are destructive. Scientists even have a name for this: they call it the 'bliss point'. Addictive foods produce continual hunger, and so are the key drivers of the obesity/diabetes epidemic.

I was talking to a lady who had lost 60kg, and she told me that when she was fat, she woke up in the morning hungry and the only thing that drove her all day was hunger and that it was always there, it was incessant. Sadly, if you ask fat people that, that's what they will tell you. They say the key driver is hunger. And the tragedy is that you can reverse it so quickly by cutting the carbs and controlling the sugar addiction.

Dr Dan Maggs

A low carb diet in part works by removing hunger. Once you reduce your carb intake, you no longer feel hungry, even when you are fasting.

Microbiome

For easier comprehension I will keep the explanation brief at this point, but will build on this 'crucial to our health' subject throughout the book.

'Microbiome' is the name given to the collective array of more than 10,000 different species of microscopic living organisms residing in and on our body. Known as microbes, these organisms are too small to see with the naked eye, but rest assured we humans are all home to a colossal quantity of them - in fact, so many of them that they vastly outnumber or own body cells. These microbes include bacteria (good and bad), fungi, protists, archaea, viruses and even microscopic animals.

There is a good reason why I have followed leptin vs ghrelin with a small section on our microbiome. Today, there is much research that suggests that the type of microbes that are most prevalent in our gut actually play a large role in controlling our feelings of fullness or hunger. In other words, it's not just our brain telling us that we are hungry or full, but also the colony of microbes that, via our diet, we have allowed to gain a disproportional critical mass in our digestive system.

While there are said to be more than 10,000 different species of microbes in our body, adding up to some 100 trillion in total and meaning that statistically we are 90%

microbe and only 10% human, just two groups dominate our guts. I didn't just pluck these numbers out of thin air - there is a fascinating and wonderfully written book by biologist and zoologist Dr Alanna Collen called *10% Human*, which is certainly worth getting hold of. *10% Human* brilliantly details the intertwined lives of microbes and humans and provides an insight into what is happening inside our guts and what a huge contributing factor to body weight and obesity our microbes play.

Let's get back to the two varieties of microbes that play a dominating role in our gut, Firmicutes and Bacteroidetes. These two strands of microbes alone can control whether we stay lean or get fat.

First, let's talk about Firmicutes. Even though their name might sound as if they make us firm and cute, they are actually responsible for the total opposite! These bacteria are experts at extracting as much energy (calories) as possible out of the food that we eat. Of course, the more calories that are absorbed, the more weight we will put on. If we can keep our not-so-cute Firmicutes under control, and let our Bacteroidetes flourish, we are less likely to put on weight. Bacteroidetes carry out the opposite task to Firmicutes. After extracting vital nutrients and vitamins from food in our intestines, they let many calories slip through the net and exit the body by catching a ride on the fibre in our poo.

An article in the Huffington Post in December 2014 stated, "Avoid sugars and processed carbs. Firmicutes are so well-suited to grow on sugar that they're known to grow rampantly in factories that process sugar cane into table sugar".

If you're still not convinced that the difference from being fat or slim could be as simple as taking care of our gut microbiome and ensuring our Bacteroidetes triumph over our Firmicutes, then let me tell you about a biological study involving human twins and a group of healthy slim mice. One of the twins had become obese, and scientists injected bacteria from her gut into the gastrointestinal tract (the gut) of half of the mice. The other twin had remained svelte and the scientists injected her bacteria into the second group of mice. Guess what happened. Those mice given the bacteria from the obese twin became obese and those that received the bacteria from the slim twin remained lean.

What is this research telling us? If we are overweight or obese, it might not be our fault at all, instead we could have developed a faulty microbiome. It might not have anything to do with a lack of willpower, or genetics, but the fact our bad bacteria are constantly rinsing every last calories out of the food we consume and at the same time messing with the signals we send to our brain, making us always feel hungry. It's yet another good reason to cut out CARBS and other sugars, and to start eating healthy fibrous foods.

There is a lot more to come about our microbiome later on in the book, but for now let's move on.

Fibre

It's important to have lots of fibre in our diet as it works in partnership with bacteroidetes to literally flush many calories down the toilet.

On my last visit to Tanzania, I started to wonder if it was just a lower intake of food that made everyone look so lean and healthy, or whether something else was stopping their obesity rates rising like they are in Great Britain. I asked if anyone had a secret to tell me, but sadly nobody understood that there was any other way to be. When I showed a classroom of children photos of fat British people (just type 'fat British people' into Google and click 'images' to experience what the kids saw), they burst out laughing and ran around the classroom, sticking their bellies out as far as they could! That night, back in my hotel, I found a report by the National Academy of Sciences of the United States of America titled, 'Impact of diet in shaping gut microbiota revealed by a comparative study in children from Europe and rural Africa'. It began by stating the methodology: "We compared the faecal microbiota of European children (EU) and that of children from a rural African village in Burkina Faso (BF), where the diet, high in fibre content, is similar to that of early human settlements at the time of the birth of agriculture".

The results were staggering, and the whole report is online and worthy of a read. Here is just a small snippet from their conclusion: "Both in the Western world and in developing countries diets rich in fat, protein and sugar, together with reduced intake of unabsorbable fibres, are associated with a rapid increase in the incidence of non-infectious intestinal diseases". Don't assume this is suggesting that we shouldn't eat fat, protein or sugar, because if it was there would be nothing left to eat. What it is suggesting, is that eating a combination of all three causes problems, especially in the absence of fibre. We will discuss fibre in more detail later.

Dr Shan Hussain

How important is fibre to our health? According to *The American Journal of Clinical Nutrition*, consuming 35g of fibre was associated with a lower risk of cardiovascular disease by as much as 54% and death from all causes by 37%.

From Our Lips to Our Bottom: Gut Business

'A taste on the lips, forever on the hips' goes the saying and, of course, if we are talking about CARBS and other sugars then that is extremely apt. But what we need to develop is a heightened awareness of what happens once food has left our mouth. It's amazing that the vast majority of humans (including me for 48 years) eat stuff every day and only ever think about how it tastes. Most people only ever think about the very first step of the process, because it's the only step that they misguidedly believe they actually experience. The reality of course is very different.

Let's first look at how we digest food. The act of digestion is the breaking down of food by a combination of chemical and physical means. If we can understand the basics, then we will begin to understand how important it is that we eat the right things. When we talk about digestion, it all starts in our nostrils. We rev up our digestive machine the moment we smell the aromas from food. Whether it is sweets, Sunday dinner or a ripe fruit, our mouths begin to produce saliva, our bellies rumble and our intestinal glands set in motion the secretion of various chemicals. Our eyes can also kickstart our digestive system by sending positive messages to the brain.

Then, as we chew our food, our teeth and tongue work in partnership with saliva to break it down for delivery into our body. The mush then travels down from our throat into a 25cm long tube called the oesophagus (also called the gastro-intestinal tract or GI tract) and drops into our stomach. It might surprise you that food doesn't just sit still in our stomach, but is churned like a washing machine, with its contents constantly hitting the sidewalls until they break down into much smaller particles. The physical motion is aided by enzymes (molecules that speed up chemical reactions) and acids that are strong enough to dissolve some metals. The length of the stomach spin cycle varies depending on what we have eaten. Simple CARBS virtually pass straight through, but more fibrous foods and meats can take five or six hours before they are ready to leave the stomach on their way to the small intestine.

Our small intestine is a massive 7m (23 feet) in length, and it is way more complex than we might at first imagine. On the inside its surface is not smooth, but looks like a valley full of billions of little cactus plants. These enable the small intestine to create a huge surface area that is bigger than a tennis court! Each square millimetre of our small intestine is filled with 30 or so of these cactus-like structures known as villi. But what purpose does our small intestine fulfil? It breaks down all of the food we eat into the three macronutrients: fat into fatty acids, carbohydrates into sugar and protein into amino acids. The villi then absorb these molecules, placing the sugar and amino acids into our bloodstream, and dispatching them to the liver to perform a safety check before being passed into the main circulatory system.

The small intestine has to process fat differently. Fat is insoluble and therefore can't be dispatched into the bloodstream. Instead the small intestine sends fats (along with insoluble vitamins A, D, E and K) on a different highway known as the lymphatic system. This works alongside the blood vessels that carry protein and CARBS (sugars). It's like a dual carriageway running alongside the motorways of the body.

Although the two run alongside each another, there is one major difference. While the liver performs a safety check on the sugar and amino acids in our blood before allowing it into the stream, the lymphatic system does not pass its produce through any organ for a safety check. This is one of the reasons why it is important to understand the difference between healthy and unhealthy fats. The fats go straight to the heart to be pumped out into our system. The heart can't perform any detoxification process like the liver does – it can't tell the difference between healthy coconut oil or the deadly highly processed so-called vegetable oils found in packaged food - it just simply injects it into our bloodstream.

If you try to picture the small intestine, you might think that, with its complex cactus-like lining and its job of making all different types of food - from curries to cakes - disappear, it is a pretty smelly and dirty environment. However, at the end of each process, it actually goes through its own cleaning and cleansing routine. The problem is that, if we constantly eat food, it never gets time to finish the job properly. This is one of the many benefits of intermittent fasting – it lets our small intestine finish its cleaning routine properly.

Let's recap on the function of the small intestine (also known as the small bowel). It acts like a giant cheese grater and breaks down food into the three main macronutrients and dispatches the energy to fuel our body. Picture it as our internal food processor – it's quick and efficient, and with some types of food gets straight to work after we have eaten. But not everything we consume can be digested by the small intestine, and what it can't cope with is passed into the large intestine.

The large intestine is our wellbeing centre. Its job is to process all the micronutrients and vitamins that our body requires to operate correctly. It is slower and more precise and sifts through all the leftovers passed on by the small intestine. In terms of length, our large intestine is approximately 1.5 metres long (far shorter than the small intestine) but receives its 'large' prefix because of its diameter, which is a gigantic 6 to 7cm (2.3 to 2.8in). Yes, we have a pipe inside us that's as long as a pogo stick and as wide as a drainpipe. When we stop and think about how massive these two organs are, our first impression might be to question the reason for their vast size. After all, their role doesn't sound as vital as the lungs that keep us breathing or the heart that pumps blood around our body – both of which are tiny by comparison. But their vast size should act as proof of how vital what we eat is to our overall wellbeing.

Let's get back to the role of our large intestine. Its job is to deal with all of the undigested stuff, and it does this in several ways. Firstly, it tries to reclaim all of the fluids that have been used in the digestive process and put them back into the body. The part of the large intestine responsible for returning water and salts is known as the colon. Another vital role for the large intestine is to process nutrients. It is also home to huge colonies of microbes known as our gut flora, which believe it or not weighs more than our brain. Yes, you read that right, the bacteria in our intestine weighs more than our brain! So maybe it stands to reason that our gut control far more of our health and wellbeing than we realise.

Once the entire digestive tract has finished its job, the large intestine signals to the brain that it's home time, and together they converse with both the final part of the large intestine, the rectum, and our circadian body clock on the exit strategy for the leftovers, i.e. faeces! The whole procedure of processing food varies in length based on several things, including what we have eaten, our age, stress levels and exercise. On average, assume it's a 16 to 24-hour cycle.

Metabolism

Let's now look at what happens when we eat from a metabolic point of view - metabolism is the process of converting food and drink into energy and unlocking nutrition. As we already know, we are designed to eat a certain diet, and the evolution of our species hasn't yet progressed to consume the manufactured and lab created stuff that we all too often put into our body. We were designed to eat free roaming-animals and naturally-growing plants. It's that simple. After all, fresh plants and wild animals were the only food available to our caveman forefathers.

As we eat food, our body digests each meal and breaks it all down into the macronutrients. For example, the smallest component of fat is known as fatty acids, the smallest component of proteins is amino acids (the good stuff that builds muscles), and for carbohydrates they simply become sugar. The body processes different nutrients in a particular order, based on how easy the task is. Alcohol is absorbed very quickly and around a quarter of what we drink can be transferred into the bloodstream and hit the brain in less than one minute! Next come carbohydrates, which easily break down into sugar, followed by the conversion of protein into amino acids. Fats are left until last, as it is quite a complex task for our body to convert them to fatty acids.

Insulin (The Fat Building Hormone)

Dr David Unwin

What does insulin do? It's a hormone that we produce that helps us deal with sugar. It is produced by the pancreas gland, and it deals with sugar. It pushes sugar from the bloodstream into cells, where you need sugar in your muscles for energy. But if you eat more sugar than you need for energy, insulin pushes excess sugar either into your belly fat or your liver. But what happens if that insulin does not work very well? Well, then the blood sugar levels, known as glucose, starts rising and you end up with a higher blood sugar level. And high blood sugar levels are dangerous, certainly over time it attaches to proteins in an irreversible way and starts damaging your circulation. It damages the small circulation in your eyes and your kidneys and over time damages your larger circulation in your arteries. And that's why we worry about hearts and strokes with diabetes. So, having a high glucose level over time isn't good news, because it almost ages your body.

Let's start with a basic understanding of insulin. When glucose levels are too high - such as what happens after eating sugary foods, carbohydrates or a huge amount of protein - the pancreas releases a hormone known as insulin which binds to the liver and muscle cells, signalling for them to remove glucose (a liquid form of sugar) from the bloodstream and store it as insoluble glycogen (a solid). The problem is that, depending on our build, the liver and muscle stores combined only hold around 300–500g of glycogen, which in terms of calories is just 1,200 to 2,000, after which all excess glucose becomes stored as body fat (also known as adipose tissue).

On the other hand, when our blood sugar levels are too low, the pancreas releases a hormone know as glucagon that breaks down insoluble glycogen (solid) into soluble glucose (liquid), allowing it to be released into the bloodstream for use as energy or when it breaks down glycogen in a muscle that itself needs energy, it uses it as its own fuel.

Glucagon; what I call the slender hormone, works in the opposite direction to insulin. The two of them need to work in partnership to ensure the right amount of glucose is in the blood.

The role insulin performs in the human body is similar to the role of nacre inside an oyster. Pearls are formed in oysters, when a foreign body such as a grain of sand enters the shell and begins to irritate the fleshy little creature inside. In an act of self-defence, the oyster excretes a layer of nacre over the intruder. Trouble is - with its new, shiny, larger coating -this little intruder becomes even more irritating. So the oyster, which obviously isn't overly bright, excretes another layer of nacre over the original layer. This event is repeated over and over again, until eventually the oyster is prised open and a gleaming pearl pops out.

The way a pearl is created is very similar to the role of insulin in the body. After we have eaten food with a sugary content, or after the body has converted CARBS into sugar, the body cries out for help in getting rid of the poisonous interloper. Yes, our body sees sugar as a poison. The pancreas steps up and secretes the hormone insulin all over the sugar, in an action not dissimilar to the oyster, secreting nacre over its unwanted intruder. But our body is brighter than the oyster and decides not to leave it in a place where it's going to constantly irritate us, but instructs insulin to march off, carrying excess sugar to our fat stores.

The trouble is, when we keep sending lots and lots of insulin to our fat stores, they get overcrowded and often become what is known as insulin sensitive or insulin resistant. It's a bit like being in a noisy office – we notice the distraction at first, but eventually we just block it out. For those who eat too frequently, and who consume lots of CARBS, the end result might be hyperglycaemia (chronically elevated sugar in the blood) or hyperinsulinemia (dangerously high amounts of insulin in the blood).

This is what often causes type 2 diabetes, when overconsumption of CARBS leads to the cells shutting up shop and not letting insulin do its job. Incidentally, type 1 diabetes is much rarer and is a very different condition. For those suffering with type 1, the body isn't able to generate sufficient or any insulin to transport the CARBS and other sugars from the blood and into the body, and therefore most sufferers have to inject themselves with insulin.

For those who have type 2 diabetes, while the medical profession once regarded it as a chronic, progressive and irreversible disease, thousands of people in Great Britain are now putting their type 2 diabetes into remission by living more primally. Please be aware that I am not claiming that living a primal way of life will reverse everyone's type 2 diabetes, as it varies from person to person. However, if a sufferer strictly follows a high (quality) fat, medium protein and extremely low CARB eating regime - adhering to the primal foods that we recommend later - and intermittently fasts (which we also cover later), there is a strong likelihood that they can reverse their type 2 diabetes.

Before we start to look down on insulin, we should remember that the hormone is only doing the job nature designed it to do! When we are eating healthily, rather than seeing it as a prison officer escorting a villain to the fat cells, we should view insulin as an usher in a church, accompanying energy to each and every seat. Insulin is one of the most critical hormones in the metabolism of food, and our cells are unable to process glucose without it. As long as we don't consume too many CARBS, just as it has for more than 2 million years, our insulin system functions perfectly. But when we regularly eat a diet too rich in CARBS – a diet that we were not designed to eat, just like a Harley Davidson is not designed to run on diesel – it causes serious damage to our engine. Let's keep it as simple as possible with an equation:

CARBS lead to sugar in the blood and the creation of insulin
Too much insulin = insulin resistance
Insulin resistance + overweight = type 2 diabetes

Looking at the above equation, it's logical to come to the conclusion that type 2 diabetes is in fact the intolerance of too many CARBS!

Dr David Unwin

Insulin is kind of a boss hormone. Insulin is designed to get rid of sugar because sugar in the blood is dangerous. So, in a sugary environment, insulin switches off your ability to burn fat. Our body is like a hybrid car. It can either burn sugar or fat, but not at the same time. Before I knew all this, I used to eat biscuits all day. I wouldn't be able to burn fat. My own insulin had switched off my ability to burn fat. And in a way that would explain very interestingly why, while I was eating biscuits all day, I was continually hungry and yet I had got a big tummy. Because I had got fuel there, but I could not reach it. Because I was in a sugary environment, that same sugar stopped me from burning my own belly fat. And now I have gone low carb, I am quite slim, simply because I can now burn my own body fat.

Let me explain further about hormones. As I mentioned earlier, they are chemicals that send messages from one part of the body to another. The intended recipient of the hormone has what are known as receptors on its surface. Often, the analogy of a key and lock is used to explain their function. The hormone being the key, which floats around the body until it finds a receptor (the lock), which it can open. When cells are constantly offered sugar from the bloodstream, they may become insulin resistant.

Picture it as the locks freezing up and rejecting the keys. The result is that the sugar can't enter the cell and therefore it stays in the bloodstream. Too much sugar in the bloodstream confuses our immune system - which had worked flawlessly for Homo Sapiens in our hunter/gatherer days - so the body instructs the pancreas to keep producing more and more insulin. But that obviously doesn't solve the issue, because once the cell's receptors aren't working, no matter how many keys we throw at the locks, they just won't open and let the glucose in. So now it's a twofold problem. There are now high levels of both glucose and insulin roaming around creating havoc in the bloodstream. For the caveman, at the end of summer stuffing his face full of ripe, sugary apples, this was not an issue. While he would still experience a huge spike in insulin, without refrigerators to keep the fruit fresh, it would all have been consumed over a week or two and then his food would revert back to his normal low carbohydrate staples. But in Great Britain, where we can have whatever food we want 365 days a year, it's not so much a short spike in insulin that causes the problem, but the on-going daily consumption of sugary foods over a prolonged period.

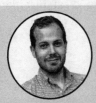

Dr Dan Maggs

After consuming a meal, our blood sugar level will rise, and insulin gets to work. While all foods have an effect on insulin, carbs and other sugars cause insulin to work overtime. While insulin is active, the last thing our body will want to do is to burn off any energy from our fat stores. Put simply, when sugar is in our bloodstream, no matter how hard we exercise, we aren't going to lose weight. Insulin and fat burning work almost exclusively on their own.

Energy Sources and Storage

Our body can run on three types of fuel. For immediate use, it burns glucose. When that's not readily available it calls upon glycogen and eventually, when it is out of both glucose and glycogen, it consumes fat.

- Bloodstream – Glucose (liquid sugar) is burnt for energy.
- Liver – Can store approximately 100g (400 calories) of glycogen (kind of a solid sugar).
- Muscles – Can store 300 to 500g of glycogen. That's approximately 1,200 to 2,000 calories, enough fuel for an hour or so workout.
- Body fat - Can store 10,000 to 25,000g of fat. That's a whopping reserve of energy, some 40,000 to 100,000 calories.

Recap Of Insulin, Glucagon and Glycogen

When we eat CARBS/sugar, the pancreas creates insulin to get rid of the excess sugar in the bloodstream and insulin converts glucose (the liquid form of sugar) to glycogen. If the two glycogen stores are full, excess CARBS/sugars are converted to body fat. On the flip side of the coin, if there is too little sugar in the bloodstream, the pancreas creates a different hormone called glucagon which does the opposite to insulin: it informs the liver to convert stored glycogen back to glucose and then stored fat back into usable energy.

They sound ridiculously similar, but it's crucial to remember the difference between glycogen and glucagon:

Glycogen (pronounced gly-co-jen) – is a type of solid sugar (a starch/ polysaccharide) and is the first storage form of sugar in the body. It is stored in the liver and muscles.

Glucagon (glue-ka-gone) – is a hormone sent to the liver with an instruction to reconvert solid glycogen to liquid glucose. Glucagon performs the opposite task to insulin.

Dr Jason Fung

Glycogen is like a wallet, in that money goes in and out constantly. But like a wallet, while it is easily accessible, it can only hold a limited amount of money. Like the wallet, glycogen is able to quickly convert back to glucose to provide energy. Whereas fat is like a bank account, it's harder to access but has unlimited storage space.

Cholesterol

What is cholesterol? Firstly, despite what you have previously believed, cholesterol isn't evil and in fact we can't live without it. Dr Malcolm Kendrick writes in *The Great Cholesterol Con*, "Why do you think that an egg yolk is full of cholesterol? Answer: Because it takes one hell of a lot of cholesterol to build a healthy chicken. It also takes one hell of a lot of cholesterol to build, and maintain, a healthy human being". Although there are many more, let me give just two reasons why we need cholesterol. Later you will read about how vital it is to get out in the sun, as it provides an invaluable source of vitamin D - which among other things helps to prevent certain cancers. The vitamin D delivered by sunshine is actually created (synthesised) by cholesterol. And we would not be here at all without cholesterol, as it is a building block for most sex hormones.

However, while cholesterol is essential for life, some doctors believe that it can become dangerous, by assembling inside our arteries. Known as atherosclerosis, this is a disease in which plaque builds up inside our arteries (blood vessels that carry oxygen-rich blood to our heart and other parts of our body). It starts off with a gunk-like substance that can eventually calcify, making the arteries stiff and narrow. Nobody knows how long this takes, but it is believed to be a couple of decades. However, the most dangerous period seems to be before the arteries calcify. This intermediate stage is known as unstable plaque. These plaques don't just build-up in arteries leading to the heart (the coronary arteries), but in many other areas of the body too.

When plaques build up in the carotid arteries in the neck they often break off into chunks and are carried in the arteries towards the brain. As they get into the smaller arteries they get stuck, and the result is often a stroke.

If we simplify it a little, there are four main cholesterol measurements we might get from our doctor:

- The good cholesterol (HDL – high-density lipoproteins)
- The so-called bad cholesterol (LDL – low-density lipoproteins)
- The ratio between our good and so-called bad cholesterol
- Total cholesterol

Technical Stuff

Lipoproteins are made of fat (a.k.a. lipo) and proteins. Our body produces three main types of lipoproteins: Very low-density lipoproteins (VLDL), low-density (LDL) and high-density (HDL). The amount of lipid (fat) in a lipoprotein is what affects its density. Fat is less dense and lighter in weight than protein and as a result LDLs contain more lipid relative to protein. Fundamentally, LDLs carry cholesterol into blood vessels, while HDLs transport them out of the body.

So the burning question is not what causes high cholesterol per se, but what causes the so called bad guy, LDL. It appears that it's not by avoiding certain foods that are themselves high in cholesterol. It turns out that the biggest preventative measures we can take are to lose weight, exercise and avoid excessive levels of stress. I confess that when I was diagnosed with high levels of LDL cholesterol, I was the heaviest I had ever been and after launching a new company just several months before my medical examination, I was so stressed out, and working such long hours that I had no time to exercise. From personal experience I fully agree with the current thinking on the causes of elevated LDL cholesterol.

Dr Aseem Malhotra

I co-authored some original research with Malcolm Kendrick and 16 international scientists, where we looked at the association of the so-called bad cholesterol LDL, with heart disease in people aged over the age of 60. So, one: we found no association and two: strangely, there was an inverse association with death. In other words, the higher your LDL, the less likely you were to die. I remember when we published the paper, I wrote about it in The Telegraph and I talked about a lady who came to see me. She was in her early 60s, and when she walked into the consultation room, she was as white as a ghost. I asked her what was wrong and she said she was really worried because her doctor had told her that her cholesterol was high. I turned to her and said, congratulations, you are going to live longer. I explained everything to her, and she left the consultation reassured and happy.

Throughout this book we repeatedly learn that CARBS pile on the weight, and constantly scoffing rather than giving our body a break from eating prevents the body from going into self-repair mode so, indirectly, LDL is fuelled by CARBS and by not fasting. All that said, it appears obsessing about cholesterol levels, whether it be total cholesterol or bad LDL, might actually be barking up the wrong tree. A tree that is making the pharmaceutical industry super rich. Statin business is big business. It's now a £23 billion industry, with more than 40 million people around the world currently being prescribed the drug.

An interview with cholesterol expert Barry Groves PhD, which can be found online, indicates that there is more evidence to support that an overall low cholesterol level is actually more harmful than overall high cholesterol. He cites recent research, which suggests that a low cholesterol increases the risk of numerous other diseases and, overall, leads to an earlier death. He explains that we are more likely to get infectious diseases, cancer or Alzheimer's if our cholesterol is too low.

Here is another huge medical U-turn. Until recently, virtually the entire medical professional arrived at the same hypothesis about how to avoid cholesterol. The hypothesis went something like this: "When we consume too much food containing cholesterol, the cholesterol levels in our blood will rise too." But the hypothesis is wrong. It is now believed that, just like eating fat does not make us fat, reducing our intake of cholesterol does not lower blood cholesterol. So avoiding eggs, prawns and meat, all of which are high in cholesterol, isn't necessary even if you have a high cholesterol level (which might turn out to be a good thing anyway).

If you are already on statins for high cholesterol, one of the best things you could ever do for your health is to quickly go out and buy *The Great Cholesterol Con*, and form your own opinion whether the £23 billion statin industry may have led you up the wrong path. Or consider research carried out in 2009 that revealed how Switzerland had the highest levels of cholesterol in the world, but the 4th lowest rate of death from CVD. Or consider the 'HUNT2 Study' in Norway. A study of 50,000 people over 15 years actually found the opposite to what your doctor might tell you, in the fact that older people with a higher LDL lived as long, if not longer!

Dr Malcolm Kendrick

LDL, the so-called bad cholesterol, cannot penetrate the endothelium, which is the internal single lining of all blood vessels, including veins, arteries, small arteries, arterials and capillaries. And if it can't get past the endothelium, then it can't get into the artery wall, and therefore it can't be the cause of heart disease. Now that's a very simple idea, but I must have read 20,000 papers trying to understand the function and relationship of the endothelium and LDL and could it get through or could it not get through. I think a huge pack of wolves have been howling at the wrong forest.

Dr Aseem Malhotra

Scientists universally accept that trans-fats – found in many fast foods, bakery products and margarine – increase the risk of cardiovascular disease through inflammatory processes. But saturated fat is another story. The mantra that saturated fat must be removed to reduce the risk of cardiovascular disease has dominated dietary advice and guidelines for almost four decades. Yet scientific evidence shows that this advice has, paradoxically, increased our cardiovascular risks. Furthermore, the government's obsession with levels of total cholesterol, which has led to the overmedication of millions of people with statins, has diverted our attention from the more egregious risk factors.

After you finish reading this book, if you have very high LDL, or want to reduce it just to keep your doctor happy, then before making a lifelong commitment to funding the pharmaceutical companies, why not try eating more of the following foods:

- Oily fish
- Broccoli
- Spinach
- Nuts (especially walnuts and almonds)
- Avocado
- Coconut and coconut oil
- Olives and olive oil
- Tea
- Garlic
- Dark chocolate

Cardiovascular

Ask anybody in the gym flogging their guts out on a running machine why they are doing it, and most will respond that it is to improve their cardiovascular system. In chapter 6, I will explain why, according to research, endless hours on the treadmill are just not necessary. But first, let's start with a basic understanding of what cardio or cardiovascular really is.

Our cardiovascular system refers to the way our heart and blood vessels transport approximately five litres (eight pints) of blood around our body - all day, every day. Cardiovascular originates from Greek 'kardia', meaning heart, and 'vasculum' from Latin for 'small vessel', which relates to the blood vessels. Driven by the heart (which is not much bigger than our fist), blood is used as a vehicle to transport nutrients, oxygen and hormones to every part of the body. Our arteries carry blood away from the heart and our veins bring it back. The heart has a left side (left ventricle) and a right side (right ventricle). The left ventricle pumps blood out of the heart. People that are sedentary tend to have a smaller left ventricle than those who exercise. Put simply, those who exercise regularly can turn their low-powered engine from a Mini into a Ferrari. Obviously, the more powerful the engine, the better it deals with stress, such as going up inclines.

Let's assume we are now taking regular exercise, and our heart has increased in size and power, the next thing we want is our transport system, (a.k.a. our arteries), to enlarge, so that pressure doesn't build up. If we can become less stressed, and therefore more relaxed, then our arteries won't be uptight and our blood pressure will therefore drop. Both sprinting and weightlifting are what we call interval training, which helps the heart to grow strong and arteries to become more elastic. In contrast, we now understand that - despite what was originally believed - the endurance sports we were encouraged to do, such as running (the very activity that was first called aerobic), do not help strengthen the heart after all and instead completely stress out our hormones and immune system. Sorry joggers, but it's true. There is a lot more to come on the dangers of endurance sports later.

Cell Powerhouse

Each cell in our body is made up of trillions of atoms. In each cell there are various tiny cellular structures that perform specific tasks and functions. These groups are known as organelles. Their name explains what they do very well – what organelles perform inside the cell is similar to the role organs perform in our body. One of the most important organelles within each cell is the mitochondria, which are found in all cells with the exception of red blood cells. Their job is to provide energy to the rest of the cell. If each body cell were a city, mitochondria would be the energy plant or electricity board. If a cell were a toy, the mitochondria would be the battery that brings it to life. Alongside the nucleus (another vital organelles that holds our DNA), maintaining healthy mitochondria is vital to our health and wellbeing.

While mitochondria organelles can use glucose as an energy source, they actually prefer to use fat. It is now believed that looking after these key components to each cell and feeding them what they like to eat – healthy fats – is of paramount importance to a healthy body. By example let's consider multiple sclerosis (MS), which is an autoimmune disease where the body's immune system breaks down and starts attacking the central nervous system. When Dr Terry Wahls became wheelchair bound, she decided to take matters into her own hands and began researching the effects of nutrition. In her brilliantly insightful book, *Minding My Mitochondria*, while introducing her readers to what they do she says, "If those little maintenance workers don't have all the proper nutrients, like amino acids, then they can't build according to the DNA blueprints". In other words, the mitochondria, the powerhouse of each cell, must receive the right nutrients.

Some cells have just a handful of internal mitochondria, while others like those in our brains can have hundreds. In fact, it is estimated that 10% of our entire body weight can be attributed to mitochondria. One of their most vital tasks is their role in informing the rest of the cell when it is time to die. If cells don't die at the appropriate time, and instead continue growing, they can become a cancerous tumour.

It's In The Genes - Or Is It?

If our parents suffered from a heart condition, Alzheimer's or cancer, does that mean that our fate is sealed? Is it just destiny that we will fall victim to the same bad luck? In this topic I want to demonstrate that, through the choices we make and the actions we take, it is us who are ultimately in control of our destiny - and not our genes. Let's start with a little caution, and then move on. There is an elevated risk that we might be more susceptible to the same conditions as our parents and grandparents. In Patrick Holford's brilliant *Optimum Nutrition Made Easy*, he says,

"In studies tracking the health of 44,000 sets of twins, 27% of the risk was due to inherent factors. That means that in 73%, the risk is due to external factors such as diet and lifestyle. Alzheimer's is another good example. Only one in 100 cases of this debilitating disease is caused by genes".

While our genes might be predisposed to a certain condition, it means we need to follow a healthier lifestyle to balance our odds. By eating well, fasting intermittently and exercising, in most cases any rogue genes we might have inherited should stay dormant for our entire life. Our genes don't dictate our future, but instead increase our susceptibility to various diseases. If I tell you that sugar can cause cancer, it might be the case for some and not for others. It also doesn't mean that sugar is the only cause of cancer. What it does mean is that consuming sugar, just like smoking cigarettes, increases our chances of getting cancer just as it does with most of the other almost exclusively Westernised diseases we will discuss later. If cancer, Alzheimer's, gout, diabetes, thyroid problems or heart disease runs in your family, then it's your susceptibility that rises. If we have a heightened susceptibility to a modern disease, then living primally, reducing our intake of CARBS and other sugars, and intermittently fasting and exercising are actions we should take to mitigate our susceptibility.

We discussed earlier in the chapter that it takes thousands and thousands of years for evolution to take effect and hence the need for us to eat the food that our primal ancestors used to eat. Anything else is most likely to cause an imbalance and lead to ill health or disease. Anyone who has accidentally put diesel in a petrol car (or vice versa) will know what happens. As soon as the wrong fuel is sucked into the engine, it splutters, struggles and eventually stops. Yes, genes play a background role, but what's leading the rapid growth in modern diseases are the actions and choices we humans are making. If it was all the fault of our genes, then common sense says cancer rates could not have exploded in the UK, from one in 20 people a century ago, to one in two people now contracting the disease during their lifetime.

Dr Mark Hyman provides a great analogy in the foreword of *Hashimoto's Protocol* by Dr Izabella Wentz: "'Genes are not your destiny' is something I truly believe in. I tell my patients that genetics load the gun, but environment pulls the trigger. The way you eat, how much you exercise, how you manage stress and your exposure to environmental toxins all contribute to the formation and progression of chronic diseases". Another way to think of it, is to use a poker analogy, "Our genes deal us our hand, but it's how we play our cards that defines our outcome".

If ill-health runs in your family, and you are of the mindset that it is futile looking after yourself because you're doomed anyway, then check out *www.epigenetics.com*. The word 'epi' is Greek for 'over' or 'on top' and genetics of course relates to that which we inherit, something transmitted from one generation to another. Those who study epigenetics are trying to discover how much of who we are is actually inherited or induced. After spending a lot of time researching epigenetics for myself, I believe we have far more control over our outcome than we realise. It is worth remembering that, many of the diseases we fear – Alzheimer's, heart disease, diabetes etc – are all fairly modern illnesses. Just a century ago they virtually didn't exist. Three of my four grandparents, plus my wonderful auntie Avis, all died from cancer. But several decades ago, when they passed away, they weren't fully aware of what caused the diseases. On paper it might look like the dreaded cancer is a very probable outcome for my family, but I believe that it isn't. I believe that genes have very little influence over modern diseases. Sure, they govern the colour of our eyes, hair and how tall we become, but are they really that responsible for passing on diseases that have come about because we have changed our lifestyle so much from that which nature designed for us? If we subscribe to Dr Hyman's analogy that, 'genetics load the gun, but environment pulls the trigger', that still leaves us in full control. Or as I teach my children, 'If it's to be, it's up to me'.

What about being overweight, surely that is in the genes? Apparently not. We can understand why people believe this, as we will often see entire families being overweight or obese. However, in 2010 it was proven that our genes do not predetermine our weight. In that year, in order to try to discover what genes were associated with being overweight, more than a quarter of a million people had their DNA analysed. Of the 21,000 genes in our body, only 32 appeared to play any role in weight gain. Such a small number led scientists to suggest that the difference in weight between those with the very lowest genetic likelihood and those with the absolute highest likelihood was just 7.7kg (17lbs). That means, even if we are extremely unlucky and the permutation of our genes is the very worst possible outcome, then at most we can only blame our parents for a little more than one stone of our weight. The realistic chances of all of our DNA lining up in this combination is lower than winning the jackpot on the National Lottery!

As Dr Jeffrey S. Bland writes in *The Disease Delusion*, "We are not hardwired to come down with the diseases that undermined the later years of our parents or grandparents". His outstanding book also states, "The bottom line is that genetic inheritance is not fate. Your lifetime health was not predetermined at your conception. On the contrary: you have the opportunity – and the power – to shape your own pattern of health and longevity".

One final thought on genetics. When I was born in 1966, only 1.5% of Brits were obese, yet less than two generations later 28% of the population are obese. Therefore, obesity is invented and not inherited.

The Vicious Obesity Cycle

The obesity equation is not as simple as many would have us believe, and it is not as I read the other day where it was described as, 'Greediness + Laziness = Fatness'. Of course, we have to take some responsibility for occasionally overindulging, and sitting on the sofa watching TV when we could be outside walking in the park, but this is only part of the story. There is a lot more to the obesity epidemic than meets the eye. If it were as simple as cutting back on our food and moving a little more, then I am confident that we wouldn't be in our current predicament, where two out of three British adults are overweight!

I firmly believe that most people who are overweight or obese have just become trapped in what I call the vicious obesity circle. It revolves like this: big food corporations, just like the cigarette companies, fill their produce with ingredients that are addictive. We see the misleading adverts, showing beautifully fit and healthy people consuming these goods, and go out and purchase them. The more we buy, the more the supermarkets feature them in what they call 'end caps' and at the checkout, which further leads to more purchases. We then consume all these unhealthy products and get fatter, but as we are still exposed to the adverts of slim models pretending to eat them, we assume it can't be their produce that is making us fat... so we carry on buying. The government at this point are earning loads of tax from the sales and therefore either turn a blind eye, or even worse sometimes endorse the wrong stuff!

How do we bring a halt to the vicious obesity circle? We need to get a better understanding of what makes us healthy and what does not, and then tell the big corporates where to stick their evil produce. We need to kick their CARBS and sugary produce into touch. Together we need to stop buying their hugely profitable packaged foods stuffed full of dangerous oils and infused with chemicals. Breaking the vicious obesity circle will mean that I won't get to write another book, but it will mean our kids will all live longer, happier and healthier lives.

Jen Whitington, the author of the brilliant book *Fixing Dad*, writes, "So do we still believe that the responsibility for this disease [type 2 diabetes] lies with the individual sufferers or do we share Professor McGregor's opinion that it lies as much if not more with the food industry? Or is it that the government has seriously let us down? After all, how many people knew that government nutritional guidelines had, for years, been funded by industry and had nothing to do with World Health Organisation (WHO) recommendations?"

As mentioned above, when I was born in 1966 only 11% of the British public were overweight and only 1.5% were obese. Today those numbers have risen to 64% being overweight and 28% obese. The average weight of an adult in the UK is approximately 2.5 stone heavier than it was 50 years ago. If we keep expanding our waistline at this rate, a few generations from now everyone in Britain will weigh more than 30 stone!

Now here is an interesting thought. With more than half of the British population being overweight, should we not recalibrate the scales and change what constitutes as overweight? Currently, if more than 25% of our body mass is fat, we are described as overweight, and if it is more than 30%, we are obese. Some people are suggesting that as we are now so fat as a nation, it is the time to change the qualifying criteria. But I believe we shouldn't! Make no bones about it: being overweight shortens lives. Being overweight can cause diabetes, cancer and much more. We must not just accept this epidemic. We must not simply accept the unacceptable.

We have increased our weight more in the past 50 years than the previous 1 million! If our primal ancestors had put on weight at the same rate as we have over the last two generations, each human would weigh more than the planet itself! Of course, that's nonsense, but it demonstrates that something has gone very wrong in recent decades and something must be done about it.

Should We Measure Weight, BMI, or Body Fat Percentage?

This is a really good question and the answer will be different for different people. Personally, I feel the best measure is our percentage of body fat, but let's go through the four main measurements that people use to determine if they are a healthy weight.

Weight

In isolation, this is a pretty useless measurement. If you are 6 feet tall and weigh the same as your mate who is 4 foot 8, then the likelihood is one of you is not a healthy weight for your height.

Body Mass Index (BMI)

Devised in the 1830s by Belgian mathematician, statistician and sociologist Lambert Quetelet, the Body Mass Index is just one measurement that can provide a rough indication of how healthy we are. However, it only considers our height compared to our weight, and therefore it might incorrectly tell us that we are overweight, when we have a big frame or lots of muscle mass. It is important to remember that muscle weighs more than fat. That's not strictly true, as a ton of feathers weighs the same as a tonne of lead. But what is true is that three extra stones of fat will undoubtedly make us look fat, but if they were three stones of muscle, we would look lean and ripped!

Let's use me as an example. I am 1.73m (5 foot 8) tall (or short depending on your view) and I currently weigh 81.3kg (12 stone 8lbs). To calculate BMI we divide our weight by our height squared.

$$BMI = 81.3 / (1.73 \times 1.73) \ 2.99 = 27.19$$

The BMI Index guidelines are as follows:

- <18.5 - Underweight
- 18.5 to 24.9 - Normal
- 25 to 29.9 - Overweight (fat)
- 30 to 34.9 - Moderately obese
- 35 to 39.9 - Severely obese
- 40 plus - Morbidly obese

Based on BMI only I am overweight and halfway to becoming obese! In addition, BMI does not differentiate between males and females, which is a little strange as women tend to carry less muscle than men and have more slender frames. Therefore, overall it is likely to underestimate females and overestimate males.

Waistline

Call it what you like: 'beer belly', 'spare tyre', 'jelly-belly', 'muffin top' or 'love handles', they are all nicknames for visceral fat. Measuring visceral fat via our waistline might be more beneficial than it first appears. While it is only one measurement, it's by far the most important. Without doubt, the fat we carry around our waist is considered to be the most dangerous of all. While we might be desperate to reduce our bingo wings, oversized buttocks or large hips for appearance reasons, it's the size of our belly, regardless of our height, that is an important indicator of our overall health.

The waist measurement should be taken just above the belly button and is often referred to as an anthropometric measurement. Anthropometry is derived from Greek 'anthropos' for 'human' and 'metron' meaning 'measure', suggesting that just this one measurement provides an overview of an individual's health.

The size of our waist reflects the amount of fat deposited around our heart, kidney, liver, digestive organs and pancreas. Fat around these vital organs can lead to a wide range of illnesses including heart diseases, type 2 diabetes, cancer and strokes. It is said that a waistline of more than 37 inches (94cm) for men, and 31.5 inches (80cm) for women, indicates that there is too much fat surrounding organs, and the NHS website would describe you as 'at risk'. The same website states you are at very high risk and you should contact your GP if your waist is:

- 102cm (40ins) or more for men
- 88cm (34ins) or more for women

To better understand the correlation between our waistline and health, over a period of nine years researchers across the Mayo Clinics in America studied more than 600,000 patients between the age of 20 and 83 years. Their findings suggested that the risk of mortality increased by 7% in men and 9% in women for every 5cm (2in) in waist circumference!

What's more startling is that men who had a waist of more than 109cm (43in) had a 50% increase of mortality compared to those with a waist of 89cm (35in) or lower. Even more alarming is that women with a waist of more than 94cm (37in) had an 80% increase in mortality than those with a waist of less than 68cm (27in).

Just as BMI is inaccurate as it doesn't take into account muscle mass or frame, the problem with just looking at waistline is it doesn't look at any other factor. While it's an accurate indicative measure for those of a fairly normal height, it might not be terribly precise for those that are very short or very tall.

Body Fat Percentage

One of the most useful indicative measurements of a healthy body is to find out what our percentage of fat is, compared to our total body mass. There are several ways to measure this. First, there are lots of websites where we can enter multiple body facts and stats, and they will perform a calculation for us. We could invest in a pair of digital scales that send a pulse through our body and estimate the amount of fat we have. Alternatively, we could go to our doctor and have them analyse our fat for us. Then there are a whole range of callipers and various other devices we can purchase that we place on various parts of the body, and they provide a measure of the body fat in that particular region.

The calculation is very simple. For example, if you weigh 81kg (180lbs) and have 8kg (18lbs) of fat, then your body fat percentage is 10%. However, getting an accurate measurement is surprisingly challenging. Obviously, if we put on more weight our percentage goes up, and if we lose fat our percentage goes down. But also, increasing or decreasing muscle or retaining or losing water content can dramatically alter the measurements. For example, if I measure my body fat as soon as I get out of bed I get a reading of around 16%, but this can drop dramatically to 13% just two hours later if I have been to the gym or played tennis.

The key thing if you are going to measure your percentage of body fat is to do it at exactly the same time each day. My recommendation is to get out of bed, go to the toilet and then take your measurement. On mornings when we get out of bed much earlier than normal or have a long lie-in, then we shouldn't weigh ourselves that day as the body fat percentage reading will be misleading.

Why Calories In/Calories Out Isn't The Answer

'Move more, eat less'. 'Just ensure that the calories going in are less than we burn, and then we will lose weight'. You must have heard this hundreds of times, but it really is a very dangerous over-generalisation. Firstly, the body utilises the calories it receives from CARBS, fat and protein in different ways. While it is true that, in a test tube known as a calorimeter, we can burn different types of food and measure the amount of heat they give off (remember that calories are measurements of heat/energy), it's only loosely relevant to how the body utilises calories. What is a calorie? It is the amount of heat it takes to raise the temperature of one gram of water by one degree Celsius.

By the gram, it's true that CARBS have fewer calories than fat. Per gram CARBS contain four calories, protein sits in the middle at five and the previously vilified enemy, fat, possess a much larger nine calories per gram. Looking at calories per gram, you can see how so many people have reached the wrong conclusion for so long, blaming fat for making us fat, and not CARBS. But the human body does different things with all three macronutrients. For example, it pretty much uses protein to grow our hair and replace blood, skin and nails, so these calories aren't exactly going to make us fat. Likewise, it uses fat not just as energy, but to create vital hormones and acids that we need to survive. But with CARBS, unless we are burning more than we consume each day, the body just doesn't use them for anything other than storing energy in the form of body fat, i.e. they make us fat. Remember, if we're not planning on getting marooned on a desert island, or going into hibernation for six months, we don't actually ever need to consume a single CARB to survive.

Most importantly, as you are going to read repeatedly through this book, insulin plays a vital role in our health, or lack thereof. What really makes us put on weight is insulin and this book is going to show you how to be the master of it. What we should be focusing our attention on is whether the body is more likely to store the calories that we consume or burn them.

Any conversation regarding 'eat less – move more' is futile without an understanding of both the role insulin plays in the body and the bacteria in our gut. Let me labour this point for a moment because it's very important if we are looking to lose weight. A certain species of bacteria strips more energy from food than others. If we allow them to dominate the space in our gut, then losing weight becomes extremely difficult. It is for this reason that subscribing to the basic law of thermodynamics – energy in = energy out – is just plain wrong!

Medical research now suggests that by getting a better balance of microbes in our stomach, even when consuming the same amount of daily energy, we can absorb 50 calories less each day. Over three years that equates to a stone in weight and over ten years to more than three stone. That's enough to turn someone who is obese into a streamlined specimen or, of course, vice versa!

Gary Taubes

You can't compare the caloric value of carbs, protein and fat. It's like saying if I hit you over the head with $100 of notes, or if I hit you over the head with $100 in coins or $100 in gold, it's going to have an entirely different effect, even though it's the same measurement. Even if I was to hit you over the head with $500 in notes, it's still not going to do as much damage as the $100 in coins, because these are fundamentally different forces at work. The nutrition community keep repeating this mantra that a calorie is a calorie is a calorie, but each of these micronutrients, fat, protein and carbohydrates, influence your body in a very different way. Your body secretes totally different hormones for each of these nutrients.

Don't Count Calories

There is a dirty immoral little lie that corporations and governments just won't admit, and that is neither counting calories, nor the low-fat diets work. Inevitably, in the long run, they both invariably lead to obesity.

It's not just calories in/calories out that's a waste of time. Counting calories consumed in isolation is pretty meaningless too. Let me tell you a short story. A few years back, I was skiing with my uncle Dave. We rounded a corner on the slope, and we saw down the mountain a class of small children enjoying a skiing lesson. I turned to Dangerous Dave (we call him Dangerous Dave because he is very accident prone) and as we descended I kept repeating, "Don't-hit-the-kids-don't hit-the-kids-don't-hit-the-kids-don't-hit…" and you can guess what he did. He took out every single one of them. By the time he came to a stop, there was not a single child left standing. After a number of apologies and 15 minutes helping them put their skis back on, luckily without injury, they were on their merry way.

Later that night I tossed and turned in bed wondering why Dave had ploughed into them and then it struck me. It is like what happens when we get told not to think of a pink elephant. I kept yelling "Don't hit the kids!" and all Dave could focus on was the kids. If I had said "Ski left, keep left," then he most likely would have done it and avoided them all together.

So here lies the problem with most diets: they focus on food, food, food. In reality, when we count calories we're thinking more and more about food. What a primal life is about is stopping us from overthinking about what we eat. When we fast we are not thinking about it. When we are eating natural food, we're not thinking about having to read food labels, we just enjoy our meals. It's easy once we get into living primally – we don't have to read heaps of diet and fitness magazines every month, we don't need to go to slimming clubs and instead of reading labels we just avoid them!

Plus, as we discussed in the previous topic, there is a gross misunderstanding with those who count calories in that no two calories are the same. On paper, the same number of calories from bread or meat should provide the same amount of fuel for the body. Wrong! Wrong for so many reasons. For example, protein is thermogenic, which means it produces heat as we digest it. When our body creates heat, we burn more calories. Therefore, for this reason alone (and there are many more) it is incorrect to assume that calories are an accurate measurement at all.

Athletes, trekkers, adventurers and sportspeople are not lean because they exercise; it is their leanness that allows them to exercise. Whereas fat or obese people are not overweight because they don't exercise, it is their size and therefore lack of energy that prevents them from doing so. This is why the old 'eat less - move more' just doesn't work. By the way, if you are counting calories, are you calculating kilocalories (kcals) or the international standard for energy kilojoules (kJ)? While kilojoules are more accurate, most people and food labels in the UK count kilocalories, which are the equivalent of 4.18 kilojoules. Confusing, hey?

My advice to religious calorie counters: if you insist on counting calories, then you should take a helicopter view and only think about them in the following two ways. The first calorie number is 2,000 calories. That is the approximate number of calories from CARBS and several other food types that our body can store in the liver and muscles in the form of glycogen. Any further intake of calories that aren't immediately used to fuel activity just increases the waistline and several other fat stores.

The second is 3,500 calories. That is because one pound of body fat is 3,500 calories. Therefore if we want to lose a pound of body fat, we must burn 3,500 more calories than the combination of what our human body and the trillions of micro-organisms in our gut extract from what we consume.

Dr Dan Maggs

When we start evaluating the nutritional value of food that we eat, we want as high a percentage as possible to be in the form of vitamins, minerals and phytonutrients (much more on these later), as well as plenty of fibre and oils such as omega 3.

Food Labels

Cigarettes kill us - it even says it clearly on the packets. Packaged foods, highly processed lab-created foods, CARBS and other sugars kill us too, but as of yet, the warnings are not that explicit on food labels. Cancer, Alzheimer's, gout, tooth decay, heart attacks, obesity and many more nasties can be attributed to the wrong diet.

When we struggle to pronounce all those added chemicals on food labels then we can, with a fair degree of certainty, assume that our body will be just as confused by the ingredients once we have consumed them. Long shelf-life packaged foods are often so full of complex preservatives and chemicals that they could survive a nuclear war.

We won't find a label on organic steak or celery. If we want to get our health on track, we should keep our food choices simple and avoid as much labelled food as possible. This includes sauces, ready meals, tinned beans and almost anything with a label. On the occasion when we feel the need to buy something to complete a meal and it has a label on it, or if it contains long words that we don't understand, we can bet our bottom dollar that it's not going to be good for our health. And, of course, here we are talking about what goes on the label. What's often just as frightening is the information they leave off.

I firmly believe that if food has a label, it has most likely been engineered for addiction and manufactured for overeating. It has been created solely for corporate wealth and not public health.

Professor Tim Noakes

Most of the foods in question are processed and developed with one purpose in mind: to make you want more. They are tested and refined to the point where they are so addictive as they are destructive. Scientists even have a name for this: they call it the 'bliss point'. Addictive foods produce continual hunger, and so are the key drivers of the obesity/diabetes epidemic.

Diseases vs Self-Inflicted Harm

I remember once when working with the Colourful Life Foundation in a tiny village outside of Moshi in Tanzania, we visited a young man named Eric in his tiny mud-built home. Eric had been receiving nutritional flour from our foundation after he was diagnosed with AIDS. Now before you ask why my charity provides very sick people with flour, which is completely un-primal, it is because most people we support that are suffering with AIDS are very underweight and malnourished. Our flour helps them rapidly put weight back on. If you like, this is further proof that the fastest way to gain weight is to eat lots of CARBS.

Anyway, as we talked, he explained that he also had tuberculosis, and the previous week he had contracted malaria. That evening I was having dinner with Jo Waddington, whose magnificent charity Ace Africa we partner with for projects in Tanzania, and we started discussing how terrible a hand Eric had been dealt. Jo was born in England but has now been in Africa for more than 17 years, and she started to explain her view on diseases. Jo explained that in Africa, almost without exception, every person her charity was treating had caught his or her illness. Most of the conditions they suffered from were virtually cured in the modern world through vaccinations or avoided through education. But while people suffering from syphilis, meningitis, malaria, tuberculosis and AIDS were seen on a regular basis, they virtually never came across a patient with high blood pressure, Alzheimer's, heart disease, cancer or diabetes.

As different as the way of life is from rural villages in Africa to that in a British city, so too are the illnesses people suffer. Together, Jo and I arrived at the conclusion that virtually all of the diseases in the modernised world must come down to a combination of lifestyle, pollution and diet. Since beginning my primal journey, I have found that the vast majority of the medical experts I have consulted also believe that it is the food we consume in Great Britain that is the biggest contributor to virtually all chronic diseases in this country. So much so, these modern diseases that we now face in our so-called modern society are now what we refer to as 'locational diseases'.

The medical fraternity in the westernised world have done a brilliant job of virtually wiping out cholera, dysentery, smallpox, diphtheria, whooping cough, polio, meningitis and many more deadly infections that we might have caught in the past. But as we have transcended from natural foods to processed foods, they have simply been replaced with new diseases such as cancer, Alzheimer's, heart disease, obesity, diabetes, ADHD, multiple sclerosis, Parkinson's and a host of other illnesses.

Dr Shan Hussain

In the developing world, people die prematurely from contagious infections and diseases. In Great Britain, we die prematurely, mainly because of our food and lifestyle choices. The top five causes of death, namely cancer, heart disease, stroke, lung and liver disease, all have preventable elements to them.

Teeth

Dr James Goolnik

Tooth decay is all down to diet. There is an enzyme called amylase. Everyone has it, and when we chew bread, it breaks it down into sugar (amylase secreted in saliva, help break down starches into simple sugars). Try this at home, put a piece of bread in your mouth and try and chew it for about a minute. You will notice how sweet it becomes. That is the enzymes turning it into sugar. If you have bread three times a day, you are literally dipping your teeth into sugar, three times a day!

Unfortunately, our Western diet now has become more and more processed. When you go to the supermarket, probably more than 80% of products have added sugar in some way, and as dentists, we see more and more tooth decay problems. Sadly, most people don't even realise that there is sugar added to these things. They think they are being really good, maybe having a savoury sandwich for lunch. But actually, it has got 20 grams of sugar. So, looking at the ingredients is massively important, as is realising when you are having sugar. You might say I am having a chocolate bar because I want a chocolate bar and it's got lots of sugar in but right now, I want it. But you also have to realise when you are having something savoury, like a sandwich, you have to realise this is sugar too. Personally, I used to think sushi was nice and healthy, but when you realise the white rice is actually full of sugar, then you have got the mirin which is poured all over it, again full of sugar, you start to have to really think about your choices. Even a hamburger, as long as it's without the bread, would have been healthier.

I am quite lucky as a dentist. I am the first one to see the damage that can happen. If you are having sugar and changing your diet, I can see the damage within just six months. Yet it might take three or four years for obesity, or five or six years for diabetes or heart disease to reveal themselves, but as dentists, we see the damage more quickly. The scary fact is that the number one cause of hospital admissions in the UK for children between the ages of 5 and 9, is tooth decay, and that is horrific. And it's because of our sugary diet, and yet it's 100% preventable.

Metabolic Syndrome

I believe the root cause of nearly all illnesses in our modern society, including diabetes, rheumatoid arthritis, Alzheimer's, Parkinson's, multiple sclerosis (MS), depression, asthma, obesity, heart disease, cancer, bipolar disorder, gout, high blood pressure, migraines, ADHD and many more, are mostly caused by metabolic syndrome. In addition, but to a lesser extent, there are six more common causes:

1. The poor state of our gut's microbiome
2. Toxins (not just eaten but absorbed through the skin or inhaled)
3. Lack of fasting
4. Sedentary or incorrect exercise
5. Stress and lack of sleep
6. Lack of sunshine

All seven of these are because we no longer live our lives in the way us Homo Sapiens have been programmed. We are no longer staying true to our primal design.

I believe we should not submit to illness. Some say that most of the modern diseases that finish us off are because we are simply living longer (even the fact that we are living longer is not true). Others say 'we have to die of something' and while, of course, they are right, wouldn't you rather, just like the centennials in places such as Ikaria and Okinawa, die just of old age?

Dr Aseem Malhotra

Let me explain what metabolic syndrome is. First, two-thirds of people now having heart attacks have metabolic syndrome. You have metabolic syndrome if you have any three of the following five. High blood pressure, pre-diabetes or type 2 diabetes, high blood triglycerides, low HDL and increased waist circumference. So think about those, metabolic being the biggest issue with heart disease, how quick can you reverse these risk factors? Within weeks, within 21 days. If you have got metabolic syndrome, you can get out of the definition of having metabolic syndrome within a few weeks of changing your lifestyle. Metabolic syndrome is a disease of modern civilisation. It's a cluster of risk factors, and I think there is very good evidence to say that it's not just about heart disease, but it's about cancer and dementia as well.

Professor Tim Noakes

Dr Gerald Reaven, now emeritus professor of medicine at Stanford University, has spent the past 60 years studying the condition that intellectually he now owns, insulin resistance. His greatest contribution was to suggest that insulin resistance and hyperinsulinemia (excess levels of insulin circulating in the blood) are the necessary biological precursors for at least four, but perhaps for all eight of the most prevalent chronic medical conditions of our day. The very eight that will bankrupt our medical services within the next two decades, unless we understand the crucial importance of his work and act without delay. The eight conditions most likely caused by high-carbohydrate diets in those with insulin resistance are:

1. Obesity
2. Arterial disease
3. Heart attack or stroke
4. Disseminated type 2 diabetes
5. High blood pressure
6. Non-alcoholic fatty liver disease (NAFLD)
7. Cancer
8. Dementia (Alzheimer's disease, also known as type 3 diabetes)

Reaven's metabolic syndrome refers to the combination of obesity, diabetes, abnormal blood lipid levels and high blood pressure existing in the same individual. It is this singular combination that best predicts heart attack risk. The key finding from Reaven's work is that these conditions are not separate; they are different expressions of the same underlying condition. So, patients should not be labelled as having high blood pressure or heart disease or diabetes or NAFLD instead, they should be diagnosed with the underlying condition, insulin resistance, with the understanding that high blood pressure, obesity, diabetes, NAFLD, heart attack, stroke, perhaps even cancer or dementia, are simply markers, symptoms if you will, of the basic condition. And that basic condition is insulin resistance, which, simply put, is the inability of the body to tolerate more than an absolute minimum amount of carbohydrates each day.

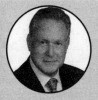

Dr Robert Lustig

Metabolic syndrome is the constellation of diseases that travel with obesity. Type 2 diabetes, hypertension, lipid problems, cardiovascular disease, cancer, dementia, fatty liver disease, polycystic ovarian disease; turns out this is now 75% of all healthcare costs, in both the US and the UK. So, people thought this was about obesity, turns out it is not about obesity. It is true that obesity travels with these diseases. I don't argue that. It is true that obesity is a risk factor for these diseases, but normal-weight people get all of these diseases as well. In fact, clinical depression causes weight loss but causes these diseases. Through the same mechanism, not just subcutaneous (just under the skin) fat you can see, it turns out to be the fat you can't see. It's the fat in your organs and the fat in your liver. And there are ways you get it. It turns out that sugar is the most potent way of getting fat in your liver, which in turn drives all of these diseases. And now we have demonstrated the mechanism. We even have the molecule, the intermediate, by which sugar is metabolised which causes all of these diseases. It is called methylglyoxal, it is an intermediary metabolite of the sugar fructose, and it poisons the liver cell, and in the process drives all of these chronic metabolic diseases. So we now have molecule to disease, disease to medical calamity, medical calamity to agricultural disaster, agricultural disaster to planetary immolation (later in the book, you will discover how Robert joins all of these dots).

Chapter 2 Highlights

- By eating a diet based on CARBS, sugar and packaged foods, deficient in essential nutrients, vitamins and minerals, many people trigger metabolic syndrome.
- Deadly fats to avoid include all trans-fats and vegetable oils, which are rarely derived from vegetables.
- Our hormones leptin and ghrelin control our satiety and hunger signals from the gut to the brain. To help them work properly, we should avoid CARBS and other sugars, exercise and take care of our microbiome.
- Insulin's role is to escort excess sugar out of the bloodstream and store it as body fat.
- Focus your mind and efforts only on the things you can change - and don't fear your genes.
- The government's obsession with levels of total cholesterol has led to the overmedication of millions of people with statins.
- Consuming 35g of fibre was associated with a lower risk of cardiovascular disease by as much as 54% and death from all causes by 37%.
- Fibre acts as fertiliser to out gut's bacteria.
- A low CARB diet in part works by removing hunger. Once you reduce your CARB intake, you no longer feel hungry, even when you are fasting.

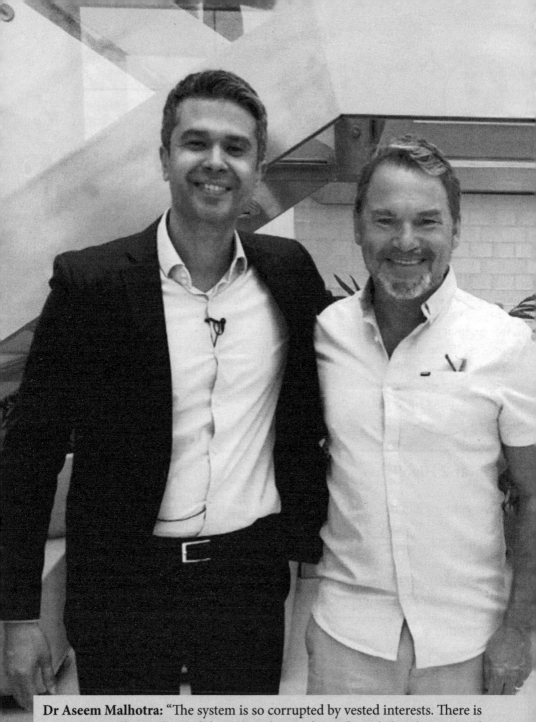

Dr Aseem Malhotra: "The system is so corrupted by vested interests. There is an epidemic of misinformed doctors and misinformed, misled and unwittingly harmed patients. There are a numbers of factors behind this, such as biased funding of research, funded because it's likely to be profitable and not because it benefits patients; biased reporting in medical journals, biased patient pamphlets, biased reporting in the media; commercial conflicts of interest, defensive medicine, and last but not least is a medical curriculum that failed to teach doctors how to comprehend and communicate health statistics."

CHAPTER 3

PUBLIC HEALTH NOT CORPORATE WEALTH

"There are three kinds of lies: lies, damned lies, and statistics."
MARK TWAIN

In this chapter I am going to explain how we have all been fed a big lie about the food we eat and how for the last 70 years, big corporations have been doctoring data.

In 1998, Labour's Gordon Brown was so convinced that diesel cars caused less pollution that he gave the people of the UK a lovely tax break for buying one. They made the fuel more affordable than petrol and did everything they could to move us all away from dirty petrol to their lovely clean diesel! Less than ten years later, they told us that they got it completely wrong and it is in fact diesel that is the devil in disguise, and that we are now going to emulate the Dutch and French by being offered incentives to scrap our diesel cars! The government screwed up on one source of energy and they are now screwing up on another – food. Or is it that they don't want us living beyond an age where we are a financial contributor to the wealth of the nation and therefore continue to recommend food that silently reduces the life expectancy of its citizens?

For many years, and against mounting evidence, the governments still did not take a stance against cigarettes. Even today, with full knowledge of the fact that one in two smokers die of a smoking related illness, they still allow them to be sold. Why? It is a well-known fact that governments make heaps of revenue by putting hefty taxes on cigarettes. But I believe there is an even bigger reason. Take the Russians. When I was there in 2016, it seemed that everyone smoked. I did some research and the life expectancy of a Russian male is only 64. Contrast that to Canada where very few smoke and men live on average to the age of 81. If that 17-year difference was the reality in the UK, it would cost the government hundreds of thousands of pounds per person in pensions. Now you could argue this idea is nonsense. Surely if someone suffers from cancer then the hospital bills will be huge? But they are still very small compared to supporting someone for another 17 years with a pension.

In 2015 pensions cost the taxman £74 billion in the UK and the number is set to grow rapidly over the next 30 years. In 2015 the NHS cost a little more than £100 billion to run, but when we consider that expense covers people of all ages, we realise that extending our lifespan might not be in the government's best interest. Maybe they are better off putting us up in hospital for a short period and demonstrating lots of care and compassion, while prescribing lots of tablets that often do more harm than good (plus the government gets considerable tax from the pharmaceutical companies) and then freeing up the hospital bed for the next unfortunate.

Put simply, governments that pay out pensions have little motivation to help us live beyond retirement age. Once we turn from an asset into a governmental liability – in other words from a taxpayer into a drain on resources – I am sure they would prefer for us to no longer be around. Even if in the short-term we become a burden on the healthcare system, it's more economical than us living for two or possibly three more decades. The same goes for food. If governments know CARBS and sugar cause obesity, cancer, Alzheimer's and many more life-shortening diseases, we can understand why they are not entirely motivated to let everyone know about it. Plus, just consider how huge the packaged food industry is and all that lovely tax it provides the government.

Imagine what would happen if the government forced manufacturers to put health warnings on all processed and ready meals. It would result in a huge drop in sales and lead to the closure of so many 'get fat quick' factories that the government would lose huge amounts of tax revenue. We can understand from their perspective why it's best to remain in denial and just keep quiet.

A question. Other than your family and friends, who else is really bothered about keeping you alive for longer? How about your life insurance company! While there are thousands of research papers out there, funded by interested parties peddling their foods and medicines that make their companies rich at the expense of our health and longevity, what do you think the motivation might be for a company that makes money by keeping you alive? Well, Credit Suisse might not immediately sound like the most likely people to conduct a huge medical research programme, but they did! They established, "Based on our medical research; we conclude that saturated fats pose no risk to our health in particular to the heart... saturated fat is actually a healthy source of energy".

Misrepresentation and Research
In 2012, Derren Brown flipped ten coins in a row and all were heads – everyone thought it was pure magic. However, it took thousands of coins to be flipped and nine hours for it to happen. On TV we saw only the final minute of Derren Brown's attempt

and not the previous nine hours of failure. Why is this relevant? Simply because much of the health and safety guidance we receive about the food we eat and the medicines we take is based on research funded by the food and pharmaceutical industry. And as we can see, if you take snippets of information in isolation, you can manipulate research to show only the results you want to show. If you want ten heads in a row, then just isolate and measure the last ten flips to prove your case. If you produce cereals and want to demonise fat and praise sugar, you can always twist research to support your case. If you can't, then keep on doing more and more research until a small selection can be isolated to back up your claim.

Still don't believe me? In the 1940s, cigarette manufacturers were still using research papers proving that smoking had health benefits! One advert even claimed, 'More doctors smoke Camels than any other cigarette', while another stated its product was 'for your throat's sake'. And in 1949, if you really wanted to be healthy and at the top of your game then you simply needed to 'smoke a Lucky to feel your level best'. Even though by this time there was lots of scientific evidence that smoking was harmful, the cigarette powerhouses kept on standing by their own research, which must have been conducted Derren Brown style.

In 2016, news broke that, 50 years previously, the sugar industry funded Harvard University scientists to conduct research that downplayed sugar's role in heart disease and to instead put the spotlight on dietary fat. Globally, the food industry spends millions of pounds on so-called nutritional research. One recent report in America suggested that as much as 90% of the studies that food giants fund result in outcomes that favour the sponsor's interests. Lobbyists, in-house laboratories and misguided research is both big business and it is rife.

I'm not normally a sceptical person, but when it comes to any nutritional or biological research, if it is in any way funded by someone with vested interests, I just don't believe it's of any substance. There is a great book by our good friend Dr Malcolm Kendrick called *Doctoring Data*, and it's a fascinating insight into how we - the general public of Great Britain - have been misled and misguided over recent decades. One of the things that Malcolm tries to stress is how, by linking correlation with causation, so many pieces of research arrive at the wrong conclusion. Maybe you read a newspaper headline that says something like, 'Eating Red Meat Causes Heart Disease', yet what the article doesn't state is that it reduces the chances of other diseases. Or another headline, 'Wine Increases Cancer Rates By 12%', yet what it doesn't tell you is that moderate consumption decreases the chances of heart disease and that in hotspots in the world where there are more centenarians than normal, red wine consumption seems an integral part of their longevity! Plus, these studies are nearly always anecdotal and based on surveys and questionnaires, not controlled trials. For example, there was one newspaper headline that read, 'Eating Bacon Kills'. What a load of rubbish. These types of negative headlines are just to sell newspapers and the research is often supplied by someone who is trying to sell the opposite of bacon, i.e. the cereal companies. One of two things might have occurred in this research: firstly, the correlation might be that people who eat bacon might be most likely to never fast, or might always have it with bread, or use it as a hangover cure, or are eating breakfast when others are exercising. Are you with me on this? Secondly, it might just be fake news!

Marci Angell, Editor of the *New England Journal of Medicine* (regarded as the number one medical journal in the world), wrote under the headline 'Drug Companies and Doctors, a story of corruption', "It is simply no longer possible to believe much of the clinical research that is published, or to rely on the judgement of trusted physicians or authoritative medical guidelines".

The only research you should ever listen to, is when thousands of very similar people are recruited for a trial, are then split into two random groups and the only thing that changes - and I mean the only variable, is the thing you are testing. Then, the trial must last many years and the rate of illness or death between the two groups measured. Then we need to know whether the outcomes are measured in relative numbers or absolute numbers (more on this in a moment). Do you really think, anyone will ever fund that type of research to see if bacon is unhealthy? Of course not. These types of properly researched studies are known as controlled, randomised and interventional, and surprisingly they rarely lead to any breaking news article. Please promise me one thing. If you ever read a newspaper headline linked with a medical study again, ask yourself six questions:

1. Was the study group properly *controlled*?
2. Was it *randomised*?
3. Was it truly *interventional*?
4. Was it *meaningful* (were thousands of similar people involved)?
5. Was one group's life *extended*?
6. What type of *statistical* measurements were used?

I have created an acronym to be used when you read a medical-related headline in a newspaper, and it is CRIMES. This stands for *Controlled – Randomised – Interventional – Meaningful – Extension – Statistics* (more on statistics shortly).

If you feel even just one of these six didn't happen, just take no notice of the article at all. It's just large corporates trying to manipulate your future spending habits using a Derren Brown type technique or newspaper companies using negative stories (sadly bad news still sells more papers than positive) to maximise profits. Oh, and one more thing. The Internet. Sadly, when one of these crazy stories breaks, it spreads like wildfire on the internet. Within days you do a search to see if there is any substance behind the headline and you get back thousands of results saying the same thing. So much so, you believe it must be right. The reality it is just that one bit of (probably fake) research that everyone is regurgitating and claiming as their own!

Here is something else I find bizarre. There is a number in the medical world called NNT, and it's the 'Numbers Needed to Treat', to get one, single positive outcome from taking a drug or medicine. You read that right, just one positive outcome. For example, if your doctor tells you to take statins to lower your cholesterol level, you would take them, right? Surely if they are recommending that you take them for the rest of your life, they must work? But according to medical research, independently confirmed by Bloomberg, the NNT for statins is 300. In other words, you need to treat 300 people with statins just to get one positive outcome! Yet, the negative side effects, which are sometimes severe, are believed to be 15 times higher. So, for every patient with a benefit, 15 people receive an adverse effect.

However, if you are a company selling statins, by mixing up the way the data is portrayed, you can create a headline that flips the risk and reward on its head. How so? You use both absolute risk and relative risk in the same report. Surprisingly, the difference between using absolute risk and relative risk is like the difference between addition and multiplication. A big pharmaceutical company, using the above statistics and NNT for statins, could create a newspaper headline that says 'you are 50% less likely to die if you take statins' (relative risk) and 'only 0.05% of people experience side effects' (absolute risk). How absolutely absurd and misleading is that?

Tim Noakes refers to statins as, "The single most ineffective drug ever invented". Dr Jeffry Gerber says, "Despite being the most prescribed drug on the planet, they will probably be gone in ten years".

Dr Malcolm Kendrick

Say you have a clinical study, and you have 200 people - 100 take a blood pressure-lowering tablet, and 100 take a placebo. At the end of the trial, imagine two people have died taking the placebo and only one taking the blood pressure-lowering tablet. So, the difference between two people dying and one person dying is a 50% reduction in death, that's the relative reduction. Whereas the absolute difference is just 1%. So, the pharmaceutical company is going to say 50% reduction rather than 1% reduction, and they are currently allowed to do this. There is no regulation on how you present the results of your trial. So, the benefits are nearly always portrayed using relative percentages and the downsides absolute. I have asked probably a hundred doctors the question of "What is the difference between absolute and relative risk?" and not one has ever been able to answer it to me.

Let me expand on what Dr Malcolm Kendrick is saying. A relative risk is relative only to itself. For example, if you buy two lottery tickets you increase your odds by 100%, yet the number is meaningless unless you know how many tickets there are in total. In medical terms, a 100% increase in baseline risk is irrelevant, if the risk is trivial.

Likewise, if your risk of a heart attack in the next year is, say, 1 in 1,000 and the drug reduces your risk by 100% (to 1 in 500), what about the 499 people that it does nothing for? Both relative and absolute benefits and risks are both pointless if you don't know the individual's baseline risk of developing a disease in the first place.

There should only be one measure of the success of a drug and that is if it helps people to live healthier for longer. There is no point saying a drug prevents heart attacks if everyone dies of cancer! How on earth does big pharma get away with using relative risk (the big number) to hype benefits and absolute risk to downplay side-effects? Simply because there are currently no rules to govern how they publish trial results. I no longer believe any newspaper headline derived from anecdotal and non-controlled research, which then gets portrayed using whichever type of mathematic equation best suits the interest of the company funding the research. I encourage you to do the same.

While I am on the subject of misrepresentation and research, I want to talk about the EAT-Lancet report. Firstly, it is important to know that the Lancet is one of the most influential medical publications on the planet. They recently published a paper suggesting that the entire human race should move to became virtually vegan. They suggested we could eat meat, but their recommendations effectively equate to a singular burger or a rasher of bacon per month.

The research was conducted by 37 authors, all experts in their field, who were bought together to answer one question, "Can we feed a future population of 10 billion people a healthy diet within planetary boundaries"? The report carried so much theoretical credibility, that shortly after the results were released, the recommendation of their near vegan diet became headline news on the BBC. Now what is surprising, is that 37 medical experts could recommend a near vegan diet, which does not provide sufficient magnesium, iron, choline, potassium, B12 and many other crucial vitamins and minerals. How could these 37 medical experts come to advocate a diet known to be deficient in nutrients?

Effectively what they proposed was an unhealthy diet full of CARBS. Not only did they claim that eating meat was bad for health, but they also claimed that all of these belching cows were extremely harmful to our planet too. Why would these 37 medical experts submit a document to possibly the most important health journal in the world, with these findings? Well, it turns out that most of the authors are either vegetarians, vegans or vegan activists. Now, does that sound like unbiased, unconflicted research? Leading the charge was Walter Willett. Reportedly he has received over $1 million in sponsorship from plant-based companies. Could that maybe cloud his judgement? Who funded the research? The Wellcome Trust. What industries is The Wellcome Trust associated with? How about the pharmaceutical industry, who of course are out of business without unhealthy people using their products?

I feel it's fundamentally important and only right that you know this stuff. You see, this bang up to date so-called scientific research paper, that all of the major newspapers are quoting and our beloved BBC too, is based (in my opinion) on completely inaccurate and debilitating health advice. Advice that will continue to further the movement towards vegetarianism and away from healthy natural fats. And literally, as I am writing this section, fortunately the World Health Organisation has just withdrawn their support of the report.

Dr Aseem Malhotra

To defend Ancel Keys a little, later in his life, even he realised his cholesterol hypothesis was flawed, and he was actually quoted in the New York Times in 1987 saying, "I have come to realise that cholesterol is not as important as I used to think it was". But by that time, the multi-billion-dollar industry had been established, and he couldn't get his new papers published. Which is actually what a good scientist does.

How did Ancel get it wrong? Can I not trust my doctor? One of the things I always tell my patients is that medicine is not an exact science; it is an art. And we use information and evidence to try and help people improve their health outcomes. But things change, and they evolve. One of the fathers of the what we call the Evidence-Based Medicine Movement, and I am also a professor of evidence-based medicine, which is basically analysing information to try and help people make truly informed choices about their health, was the late Professor David Sackett. He said, "50% of what you learn in medical school will turn out to be either outdated or dead wrong within five years of graduation. The trouble is nobody can tell you which half, and you have to learn to learn on your own".

It is really difficult for doctors to keep up to date, but that's why we have so-called guideline bodies that advise GPs, that GPs trust to be rigorous and independent with the evidence. But what I have learnt and one of the reasons why I changed my thinking, I thought this is not working. If we are doing everything right, why is the NHS in crisis, why have we got more chronic disease, we are doing something wrong here. So we have the guideline bodies, which I have now unfortunately learned, to put it politely, there is too much influence of industry. Whether it be the drug industry or the food industry, people who we as GPs rely on to give us independent advice.

The system is so corrupted by vested interests. There is an epidemic of misinformed doctors and misinformed, misled and unwittingly harmed patients. There are a numbers of factors behind this, such as biased funding of research, funded because it's likely to be profitable and not because it benefits patients; biased reporting in medical journals, biased patient pamphlets, biased reporting in the media; commercial conflicts of interest, defensive medicine, and last but not least is a medical curriculum that failed to teach doctors how to comprehend and communicate health statistics.

I recommend any parent or anyone who takes researching their health seriously, to read Dr Malcolm Kendrick's *Doctoring Data*. This book reveals how medical headlines are mostly inaccurate and how the root cause they promote are driven by lobbyists and researchers with a commercial interest in the results they publish. Other books shining a light on this shocking area and worthy of a read are *Over Diagnosed* by Dr H Gilbert Welch, *The Truth About The Drug Companies* by Dr Marcia Angell, *The Patient Paradox* by Margaret McCarthy, *$29 Billion Reasons to Lie About Cholesterol* by Justin Smith, *The Cancer Industry* by Mark Sloan, *Overdo$ed America* by Dr John Abramson,

Bad Pharma by Ben Goldacre, *The Great Cholesterol Myth* by Dr Jonny Bowde and Dr Stephen Sinatra and *Lies my Doctor Told Me* by Dr Ken Berry.

All that said, putting the lies and corporate deceit to one side, there is one type of company that benefits from us being healthy and living longer. And that is the insurance companies. In Zurich in June 2018, one of those companies, the $200 billion company Swiss Re, held an amazing conference on nutrition. The event very much focused on the benefits of eating a low carb, high fat diet. The corporation's Chief Medical Officer Dr John Schoonbee told delegates that, "The low-fat approach over the last 50 years was a failed human experiment".

Chapter 3 Highlights

- Professor Sackett once said, "50% of what you learn in medical school will turn out to be either outdated or dead wrong within five years of graduation.
- There should only be one measure of the success of a drug and that is if it helps people to live healthier for longer.
- You need to treat 300 people with statins just to get one positive outcome.
- If you ever read a newspaper headline linked with a medical study again, ask yourself six questions:
  1. Was the study group properly *controlled*?
  2. Was it *randomised*?
  3. Was it truly *interventional*?
  4. Was it *meaningful* (were thousands of similar people involved)?
  5. Was one group's life *extended*?
  6. What type of *statistical* measurements were used?

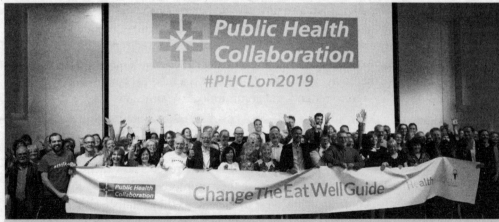

At the PHC Conference I enlisted the support of over 80 medical professionals to help me with my campaign to get the government to change their Eat Well guidelines. Please help support us by registering at *www.healthdaddy.com*.

CHAPTER 4

HOW TO OPTIMISE NUTRITION

"Let food be thy medicine and medicine be thy food."
HIPPOCRATES

In this chapter, we dive into more detail about which foods we are designed to eat, and which ones are responsible for our country's decline into ill health.

The DNA in our cells is principally still hard-wired to process the diet of our primal ancestors. They are still programmed to digest and derive benefit from a similar diet to that of our hunter-gatherer forefathers, and not the manufactured and highly processed foods that we consume today. Since the agricultural revolution around 10,000 BC, our food has steadily become less and less rich in nutrients, vitamins and minerals, and progressively manufactured with more and more starches, unhealthy sugars, hydrogenated oils and fake food ingredients that we are simply not designed to consume. While the quality of our food has been in a slow decline for circa 12,000 years, it's fallen off a cliff in the past 50 years. The food we consume en masse in Britain today is almost completely unrelated to that on which the human race has evolved.

If you are heavily overweight or obese, then there is no doubt about it – getting your weight under control is the most important step you can take to a healthier, longer and more enjoyable life. So let's get straight to one of the most important principles of living primally. Today, more people are going to gyms, jogging and cycling than at any point in the history of mankind, yet as a nation we are the fattest we have ever been. The same goes for most of Europe and America – in fact the whole modern world! Look at the statistics. In the UK, more than 9 million people are now paying for gym membership, and as a result there are now more than 6,500 gyms. Yet, even with our new gym obsession, according to the NHS, "Obesity levels in the UK have more than trebled in the last 30 years".

How is it that more and more people are going to the gym and yet we are getting fatter and fatter? Before you jump to the wrong conclusion, it is not the gym that is necessarily making us fatter, it's that more people are believing that getting fit is the best way to lose weight, when in reality we must first tackle what type of fuel we are putting in our tank. As Dr Aseem Malhotra says, 'You can't out exercise your fork!'

Dr Jason Fung

In the United Kingdom from 1997 to 2008, regular exercise increased from 32 per cent to 39 per cent in men and 21 per cent to 29 per cent in women. There's a problem, though. All this activity had no effect on obesity at all. Obesity increased relentlessly, even as we sweated to the oldies. The phenomenon is global. A recent eight-country survey revealed that Americans exercised the most - 135 days per year compared to a global average of 112 days. The Dutch came in last at 93 days. Weight loss was the main motivation for exercise in all countries. Did all this activity translate into lower rates of obesity? Glad you asked. The Dutch and Italians, with their low exercise rates, experienced less than one-third the obesity of those excessive exercising Americans.

We don't need to write too much about it in this chapter, because hopefully by now you realise that excess CARBS (other than fibre) are just terrible for our health. Just as we realised decades back that there was an undeniable link between smoking and cancer, in the same magnitude we are now aware that there is a direct link between CARBS and obesity. Recently the BBC ran an article on its website titled, "Obesity 'to be linked to more female cancers' than smoking", which went on to say, "Obesity is set to overtake smoking as the biggest preventable cause of cancer in UK women by 2043". Now I am going to repeat this probably 100 times throughout this book because it's the root cause to the vast majority of chronic diseases that are devastating so many families across our county. It doesn't matter which CARBS we are talking about, they all get entirely broken down into sugar in the body, and too much sugar causes a spike in insulin, and the health effects are cutting short millions of lives. I genuinely believe that the case against processed CARBS, sugary drinks, packaged foods, chemically grown crops, and so on, should be made as strongly as the case against cigarettes.

Eat Plenty Of Protein – But Not To Excess

Remember, it is protein that creates life. After a big session in the gym, if we don't consume sufficient protein (amino acids), then our muscles won't repair themselves. Plus, as we get older our ability to process proteins declines – meaning that we need to consume more to achieve the same results.

But it is important that we don't go all-out on protein consumption. While CARBS are quickly turned into sugar, excess protein can also be converted too. Therefore, if we overdose on protein there is a chance we might put on weight. Plus, a by-product of protein is nitrogen. When we consume too much protein, the nitrogen can cause problems for our liver and kidneys. However, when we get the balance right this nitrogen just passes through our system and exits in urine.

Consume Plenty of Good Fats, but Avoid the Ugly Ones

We have already discussed that it is not the consumption of fat that makes us fat, but CARBS and other sugars. However, while some fats are healthy for us, others are outright dangerous. At first the subject of fats can be overwhelming and appear difficult to comprehend, so I have decided to simplify the matter by breaking it down into a few subheadings and to only focus on the information that makes the biggest difference.

No wonder the subject of fats is so bewildering. For the past 50 years or so the government, backed by inaccurate research, has informed us that saturated fats are bad for us and we should eat polyunsaturated fats instead. That meant meat got a bad rap, as about half the fat found in cattle, sheep and pigs is saturated. The demonisation of saturated fats led to the decline of many breeds of British cattle such as the Hereford and Shorthorns and the import of leaner breeds of cattle from the continent.

And the poor pigs, who were once fat to keep them warm in winter, had their natural diet dramatically modified so that they are much leaner. If we look at photos of pigs from 50 years ago compared to those reared today, we will notice they are far skinnier in comparison. We have basically changed our breeds and reared them differently because we once thought saturated animal fats caused diseases. Today, other than in newspaper and BBC headlines, most leading doctors and I firmly believe that as long as the meat is organic, consuming the fat is actually healthy. It has to be, this is how our species developed. And what's more, as you will read later, organic meat actually protects the environment and helps in slowing down the advancement of global warming.

How did everyone get it so wrong? When the deadly trans-fats started to appear en masse, some misguided and ill-informed individuals lumped all fats under the same heading and deemed them all unhealthy. Yet, natural animal fats vs factory-created, chemically enhanced fats is like comparing chalk and cheese.

In the incredibly insightful book *Smart Fats*, written by Dr Steven Masley and Jonny Bowden PhD, CNS, they write, "We've been so concerned with 'saturated fats vs unsaturated' and 'animal vs vegetable', that we've lost sight of a far more important distinction: toxic vs non-toxic fat – or, as we call it, dumb fat vs smart fat".

Not only are most fats healthy for us, they are so much better at making us feel full. Unlike deadly CARBS, which spike our glucose and insulin levels, and then bring them crashing down shortly afterwards making us crave even more food, fat leaves us feeling full for longer – much longer. In fact, it is exclusively fat that has zero effect on our blood sugar levels. Remember, even our beloved protein can spike both blood glucose and insulin if over-consumed.

One of the reasons fats make us feel fuller for longer (satiety), is that it doesn't begin to get processed in the stomach, but instead has to wait until it reaches the intestines. Fat, just like a balloon, floats on water. The enzymes that break down fat are lipases. Lipases struggle to get at the fat in the stomach while it's floating on top of the watery mush being tumbled in our internal washing machine, and patiently wait for it to drop into the intestines. While the body is busy processing carbohydrates and protein, the side-lined fats make us feel fuller for longer.

Oils & Fats Are The Same Thing

While I mentioned earlier that trying to understand fats can be a little bit daunting, there are two fat facts that once known help put the rest of the more complicated stuff into perspective.

1. The only difference between oils and fats is that oils are liquid at room temperature.
2. All fats and oils fall into one of two categories – either saturated, or unsaturated.

The following chart shows the main groups of fats and oils and how they relate to one another. It's also important to understand that the overwhelming majority of the foods we eat, contain more than one type of these fats.

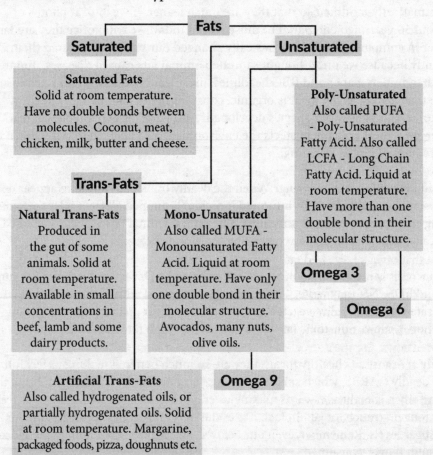

Fats

Saturated — **Unsaturated**

Saturated Fats
Solid at room temperature. Have no double bonds between molecules. Coconut, meat, chicken, milk, butter and cheese.

Poly-Unsaturated
Also called PUFA - Poly-Unsaturated Fatty Acid. Also called LCFA - Long Chain Fatty Acid. Liquid at room temperature. Have more than one double bond in their molecular structure.

Trans-Fats

Natural Trans-Fats
Produced in the gut of some animals. Solid at room temperature. Available in small concentrations in beef, lamb and some dairy products.

Mono-Unsaturated
Also called MUFA - Monounsaturated Fatty Acid. Liquid at room temperature. Have only one double bond in their molecular structure. Avocados, many nuts, olive oils.

Omega 3

Omega 6

Artificial Trans-Fats
Also called hydrogenated oils, or partially hydrogenated oils. Solid at room temperature. Margarine, packaged foods, pizza, doughnuts etc.

Omega 9

Omega 3

You need to fall in love with this fat, as it plays a leading role in being healthy. It is often the solution to so many problems and carries the key to health, happiness and longevity. We will discuss the merits later, but for now start eating plenty of nuts (especially macadamia nuts), organic oily fish, olives, dark chocolate, avocados or go out and source a quality omega 3 supplement, sourced from deep water fish. Or if you are vegetarian, be sure to consume plenty of flaxseed (also known as linseed) oil.

Why is omega 3 so beneficial? There are literally hundreds of reasons! For a start, it makes platelets, which are microscopic particles in our blood, less sticky. As a result, it reduces the likelihood of blood clots, which among other side effects can lead to heart attacks.

Omega 3 also reduces the risks of cancer, arthritis and makes our brains brighter too. And that's just for starters! If you're of my generation, your mother might have given you cod liver tablets as a child. Although they didn't have a nice taste, even 40 years ago our mums knew more about health than most people do today. I personally recommend omega 3 supplements to almost everyone I meet.

Omega 3 vs Omega 6

Firstly, although it's a little bit geeky, let me explain where the word 'omega' and how its bunch of numbers came about. Omega is the last letter in the Greek alphabet. The various numbers associated with them refer to how far from the end of the molecule chain the first double bond occurs. For example, in omega 6, the double bond occurs on the sixth carbon atom from the end (the omega).

Nature designed us to consume omega 3 and omega 6 in roughly the same quantities. Our body ideally needs this 1:1 balance for us to function properly. However today, it is estimated that those who consume a lot of fats via fast foods, packaged foods and vegetable oils actually consume a ratio closer to 1:20. That means the balance is out by a massive 2,000%. Is this a worry? You bet! Omega 6 causes inflammation and inflammation is a root cause of many deadly diseases.

It's not that omega 6 is a bad fat, it's just that it behaves like a reckless child in the absence of its sensible sibling omega 3. On a diet primarily based on CARBS the balance can be as far out as 25:1. That spells danger. Plus, if you love meat but always buy beef originating from corn-fed, hormone- and antibiotic-enabled cows, then you are probably consuming omega at about 7:1, rather than the 1:1 we get from organic, grass-fed cows. For the correct ratios of omega 3 to omega 6, look no further than some of the items in the Top 20 Superfoods on page 225.

Why all the talk about omega 3 and 6? Aren't there more omegas? Yes there are. They have some pretty special siblings that are quite advantageous for more niche health benefits, but as our body can create them naturally, they are not essential in our diet.

For completeness on the subject, scientifically omega 3, 5 and 6 are all poly-unsaturated fats, while omega 7 and 9 are mono-unsaturated.

Saturated Fats

Firstly, not all saturated fats are exclusively from animals. Coconut oils contain saturated fats too. While there is no need to take any precautions with the holy coconut, saturated animal fat is slightly different. With saturated animal fats, they are only truly healthy (and I am talking about all meat, dairy and poultry produce), if they are from an organic source. If we talk about meat from a cow forced to eat corn and pumped full of drugs, then the resulting fat is very bad indeed. If researchers and newspaper headlines were to separate organic saturated fats from saturated fats derived from factory reared animals, then I would then probably agree with their health warning for the latter. But sadly, they don't, they simply lump all meats together.

What Oils To Keep In Our Primal Pantry

Let's look in detail at some of the oils we will find on supermarket shelves, from the great through to the deadliest.

Coconut & Medium-Chain Triglycerides

Medium-chain triglycerides (MCTs) are the really good fat guys, and the king of the MCT jungle is the coconut. MCTs are the fats that just keep on giving! When consumed they turn almost immediately into fuel, kick start the body's process of converting body fat into energy and help suppress hunger. Because they have a shorter chain length than other fats, they travel rapidly from the digestive tract to the liver, where they are quickly converted to energy or morphed into ketones.

When we live primally, MCTs help increase our energy levels and, while I don't subscribe to endurance sport as part of a healthy lifestyle, on the odd occasion when playing a long game of tennis or if I do get roped into going for a run, I will consume a few serving spoons of coconut oil as my fuel. It provides energy just as fast as CARBS and other sugars, but without any of the negatives.

Although we don't count calories when living primally, it's interesting to know that MCTs have a lower caloric content than other fats. Not only are they low in calories and provide almost instant energy, they actually help the body burn its own fat stores in a process called thermogenesis. In the absence of sugar, MCTs encourage our body to create ketones (much more on ketones coming up).

Other than coconut oil, smaller concentrations of MCTs can also be found in other saturated fats including organic butter and full-fat yoghurt. However, virtually all other fats, whether they are derived from animals or plants, are what are known as 'long-chain fatty acids' (LCFA). MCTs are so good for our body that they are starting to be used in the treatment of cancer, obesity, Alzheimer's, Parkinson's and many other diseases.

Fat Facts

MCTs are a saturated fat. Let me explain something about their complicated name. Triglycerides are a type of fat (lipid) found in our blood and in certain foods. MCTs are beneficial triglycerides that have a reduced chain length, meaning that they are more able to quickly enter through the membrane of our mitochondria. This rapid absorption by our cells means they almost immediately become fuel for our organs and muscles.

Coconuts

Grant Petersen in his book *Eat Bacon, Don't Jog* preaches, "Olive Oil is good but not God: God is a coconut!" The mighty coconut is my favourite flexible friend in the kitchen. I use it as an oil, as milk to thicken curries, as a flour, as flakes in a salad… in fact I use it in every way I possibly can. I add it to smoothies, and I put it in my morning coffee. I use it as a moisturiser, sunscreen and even as a mouthwash.

Understanding The Types Of Coconut Oils

Sadly, unlike the labelling of olive oils, which are heavily regulated by the IOC (International Olive Council), there isn't currently a body that regulates the naming of coconut oils. For example, there is no official difference between extra virgin coconut oil and virgin coconut oil. It appears the 'extra' is just an invention of the marketing departments.

Virgin coconut oil, sometimes labelled as 'pure', means that the raw flesh (known as copra) of the coconut has been naturally dried and then cold pressed, maintaining the maximum amount of nutrients and beneficial oils. Virgin coconut oil should not be refined and should be processed without heat and exposure to sunlight. Regular coconut oil may have been dried artificially, boiled, bleached, deodorised or otherwise chemically treated.

Even though the labelling of coconut oil isn't strictly regulated, as long as you select a brand that you trust, don't let the lack of regulation put you off consuming it. Not only is it great to cook with, it is also fuel for the brain and medicine for the body. Here are just some of the benefits associated with coconut oil:

- May help to prevent Alzheimer's
- An instant source of energy that won't get stored as fat
- In the winter it helps to stop us feeling cold by boosting circulation
- Helps improve the quality of sleep
- Great as a mouthwash and whitens teeth
- Increases the absorption of magnesium and calcium
- Accelerates weight loss
- Boosts hormone production

Algae (a.k.a. Algal) Oil

A friend recently asked me about algae oil. My immediate reaction was that, although it would be great if we could buy it in a bottle, I hadn't yet seen it on a supermarket shelf or in a health store. So I did some research and lo and behold, we can now get algae oil in a bottle – and a glass bottle to boot! Double goodness! You will discover later why I love glass bottles, or more importantly why I loathe and discourage the use of plastic in their manufacture.

Why is this so exciting? Have you ever stopped to think why fish are such a rich source of omega 3? The reason is they eat algae, or if they don't eat algae, they eat other fish that eat algae. Or if they don't eat other fish that eat algae they… well, you get my point. Even when we eat fish towards the top of the food chain, such as tuna, we still get the benefit of some omega 3. Now algae oil is derived directly from algae, which is predominantly made up of omega 3 – docosahexaenoic acid (DHA). DHA is said to make up almost all of the omega 3 in our brains. Put simply, consuming algae oil (or the smaller fish in our oceans that eat algae) is going to give us a higher dosage of the fats that fuel our brain.

Butter and Ghee

Here is another health U-turn. For several decades, margarine had been masquerading as a healthy alternative to saturated butter. We now know that it is full of deadly hydrogenated fats. It might spread nicely on our toast (not that you will eat much toast after turning primal), but it is just not good for our health. Its smoothness might not put holes in our bread, but will put holes in the lining of our gut.

Butter, which has been demonised over recent decades, is in fact super-healthy as long as it originates from organic grass-fed cows. Yes, the fat is saturated, but we now know that saturated fat is no longer the enemy.

But even better than butter is ghee. Until recently, I never entertained having ghee in my primal pantry and assumed it was just for cooking Indian dishes. But then, while researching how to get my fitness back on track, I read an article singing the praises of its miraculous health benefits. To make ghee, water is evaporated (clarified) out of butter, leaving behind a higher concentration of fat and making it more suitable for cooking at higher temperature. As a by-product of the simmering process, the ghee often becomes more aromatic and can sometimes develop a pleasant, light nutty flavour. Many remote cultures around the planet use ghee as a natural medicine and some even make it from human breast milk.

Olive Oil

We all know that olive oil is good for us, and is said to make all those Mediterranean people healthy, but when you're standing in a supermarket aisle looking at a plethora of olive oil nomenclature on labels, no doubt you're wondering, 'which ones do those Mediterranean people actually consume'? To answer this, I studied the International Olive Council's (IOC) website and, whilst there was some confusion, I got some help from a lovely lady in their office. To class as a virgin olive oil, the IOC insist that, "Virgin olive oils are the oils obtained from the fruit of the olive tree solely by mechanical or other physical means under conditions, particularly thermal conditions, that do not lead to alterations in the oil, and which have not undergone any treatment other than washing, decantation, centrifugation and filtration". The following is to clarify the choices:

- Extra virgin olive oil – this is the Rolls-Royce of olive oils, as it is the richest in antioxidants and polyphenols. To achieve its 'extra' status, it has to have an oleic acid level of not more than 0.8g per 100g, and this provides it with a better taste and maximises its health benefits.
- Virgin olive oil – to achieve its 'virgin' status, it must have an oleic acid level of not more than 2g per 100g.
- Ordinary virgin olive oil – to have an 'ordinary virgin' status, it must have an oleic acid level of not more than 3.3g per 100g.
- Refined olive oil – this is obtained from virgin olive oils by refining methods that must not alter the initial glyceridic structure. It must have an oleic acid level of not more than 0.3g per 100g.
- It's important to note that refined oils often lack the antioxidants and anti-inflammatories that are found in virgin olive oil.
- Olive oil – a blend of refined olive oil and virgin olive that must have an oleic acid level of not more than 3.3g per 100g.

In addition to the above, you might come across olive pomace oil. These are second-class oils that can be produced with the use of solvents and can be blended with all sorts of other oils. With such stringent IOC governance over what constitutes the different grades, it's about finding a brand of oil that tantalises your taste buds and still fits your budget.

What about first cold pressed? Why is this not listed above? Simply put, it is not an IOC nomenclature. Many years ago, when they used mats to press olives, there was such a thing as first press and second press, but this is no longer the case these days. Today, it's just pure marketing hype. Speaking of marketing, don't be fooled by those who label their oils as 'light'. It's not an approved IOC description, and has nothing to do with calories. If anything, they tend to be lighter in flavour only.

Another useful thing to understand is that olive oil, unlike red wine, does not get better with age. Therefore, look at the labels and try to find those with the most recent harvesting dates. They should also be stored in cool, dark places - so even in the UK, during the summer, you might want to store it in the fridge. Once opened, really use it generously and try to consume it within a month or two. Regardless of the bottle's expiry date, regardless of how nice its aroma remains, the longer it's open and the more it's exposed to warm air and sunlight, the fewer health benefits you will receive from it. And, as always, go for a glass bottle so that it doesn't leech nasty chemicals into what should remain a bottle bustling full of pure healthfulness.

Sunflower, Safflower, Sesame, Cotton and Rapeseed Oils

They sound healthy, don't they? Sadly, they're often not. Their omega 3 to omega 6 ratios can be out-of-kilter by as much as 1:1,000. But an even larger danger lies in how the oils are extracted. The method is often less about nature and nurture, and more about science, technology and highly toxic processes.

While our body thrives on olive oil, coconut oil, and fats from meats, seed oils are often chemically extracted, bleached and deodorised in a way that just isn't fit for human consumption.

Soybean and Corn Oils

I am pretty sure you have already guessed that oils from soybeans and corn are not good for our health. Not only are they extracted from genetically modified crops, but they are extremely high in omega 6. When we heat these oils, they become easily damaged, and as a result can clog up our arteries.

Peanut Oil and Almond Oil

While nuts themselves are a primal Superfood, when their oils are extracted without all of the other nutrients and fibres, they become exposed to air and sadly oxidise – and oxidised oils are detrimental to our health. Plus, just like seed oils, the process used to extract nut oils is often extremely un-primal. Nut fans should look for cold-pressed and unroasted.

Trans-Fats (a.k.a. Hydrogenated Oils): Toxic, Ugly And Deadly

In the early 1900s, German chemist Wilhelm Normann discovered that you could add hydrogen to some cheap fats and make them even cheaper. Plus, when added to almost any packaged food, this deadly chemical cocktail massively extended the product's shelf life.

In *Smart Fats*, Dr Steven Masley and Jonny Bowden PhD, CNS, write, "Artery-clogging trans-fat, which we have likened to embalming fluid that turns our tissues to plastic, is a killer, pure and simple... great for shelf life, but not for your life". Why are they so unhealthy? Because before being hydrogenated or partially hydrogenated to solidify these nasty oils, they are often infused with chemicals. These cause havoc with our immune system, raise insulin levels and are most likely responsible for many types of cancer.

Where are these life-shortening oils used? Breads, cakes, junk food, fast food, fried food, biscuits, crackers, microwave meals, soups, doughnuts, microwave popcorn, margarine, coffee creamers, crisps and virtually every type of packaged or processed food we can buy in a supermarket. Hopefully, by the time you finish reading this book you will be put off purchasing packaged food and fast food for life. However, if occasionally you wander from the primal path, please read the labels carefully and make sure you avoid these poisonous oils at all times.

Vegetable Oil
It turns out, vegetable oils don't actually come from vegetables, but to differentiate them from fats derived from animals (and of course they are not minerals), they became known as vegetable oils. But be sure about one thing, they neither contain nor are derived from vegetables!

Even worse they are created from corn and soybeans, two ingredients that are in no way primally acceptable. The oil industry has misled us into believing that vegetable oil is made of vegetables and therefore must be healthy. Wrong! As in, really wrong!

Ever since the birth of the low-fat diet – a diet I sadly followed for more than two decades, the diet that kept me overweight and gave me a foggy brain – vegetable fats have been praised for being unsaturated, and therefore good for the heart. This is simply incorrect. It is just as wide of the mark as when the government told us to purchase diesel cars, as they were supposedly better for the environment.

Vegetable oils are rich in omega 6 which, on its own without the balance of omega 3, causes inflammation. And, as you will discover later, inflammation is the catalyst to nearly all Western diseases. In his book *Toxic Oil* (which on the cover states, 'Why vegetable oil will kill you & how to save yourself'), David Gillespie writes, "Vegetable oil makes you exceedingly vulnerable to cancer. Every mouthful of vegetable oil you consume takes you one step closer to a deadly (and irreversible) outcome. Every mouthful of vegetable oil you feed to your children is doing the same to them".

Maybe think about it like this. Around 100 years ago vegetable oils did not exist and cancer was very rare. Today one in two people living in Britain will develop cancer and it's almost impossible to avoid vegetable oils in packaged foods.

A Fat Summary
If all this talk on fats was a little too much, then here is quick guide. Be sure to only consume the good fats listed below.

The Good & The Ugly	
The Good	**The Ugly & Deadly**
Avocado	Trans-fats
Coconut	Hydrogenated oils
Coconut oil	Partially hydrogenated oils
Dark chocolate	Vegetable oils
Fatty fish	Oils from soybeans
Meat (only organic)	Oils from corn
Olives and olive oil	Hidden fat in packaged food
Organic butter	Hidden fat in fast food
Organic ghee	Fats from force-fed cows

The Smoking Point Of Fats

If we overheat certain fats and oils then, not only can we kill off their goodness, we turn them toxic. As a general rule of thumb, we don't want to make our fats and oils smoke. Therefore, depending on what we are cooking, we are going to need a few different healthy oils in our cupboard or fridge. And as oils are sensitive to light, make sure you keep them in the dark.

Fat/Oil	Smoke Point °C	Smoke Point °F	Good For
Avocado oil	271°C	570°F	Use for frying, searing and roasting or as a tasty salad dressing. 70% mono-unsaturated fat
Ghee (clarified butter)	252°C	485°F	62% saturated fat, has a distinctive flavour, excellent for frying, especially Asian dishes
Olive oil	242°C	468°F	Use for frying, searing and roasting or as a tasty salad dressing
Coconut oil (refined)	232°C	450°F	Great for everything! 86% healthy saturated fat, and a powerful antioxidant. Contains 66% MCTs
Macadamia oil	210°C	450°F	Can be expensive, but a great all-rounder for both cooking and applying to the skin
Olive oil (virgin)	199°C	391°F	Use for frying over medium-high heat or as a salad dressing. Rich in vitamin E and antioxidants
Olive oil (extra virgin)	191°C	375°F	Use for frying over medium heat. Or as a salad dressing. Rich in vitamin E and antioxidants
Lard	188°C	370°F	Made from the fat surrounding a pigs stomach, lard is most definitely a Primal fat. Makes the best fried chicken
Coconut oil (extra virgin)	177°C	350°F	86% saturated fat, a Superfood, use for everything except for frying
Butter	120-150°C	250-200°F	Use to add flavour in low temperature cooking
Flaxseed oil	107°C	225°F	With its low smoking point, not to be used for cooking. An excellent source of omega 3 (4:1 omega 3 to omega 6 ratio) and tastes great over salads or add to a smoothie

Meat

Let's start by reaffirming that living primally is not a diet - we're simply committing to eating as close to what primal man ate, and eat what our body has evolved to thrive on.

When it comes to animal produce, it is critically important to buy as natural as we can possibly afford. I am sure you have heard the saying 'we are what we eat' but, when it comes to animal produce, the saying should be extended to 'we are what our food eats'.

Free-range eggs, free-range chicken and grass-fed cows all provide us with heaps of benefits. They are rich in vital vitamins and have a really healthy omega 3 to omega 6 balance. Cows, pigs, chickens and lambs that are allowed to live naturally, in their natural habitat, feeding on their native primal diet, are really good for our health. But those that are forced to eat corn and grains, foodstuffs that we now understand turns to sugar in the gut, are nowhere near as healthy for us to consume. Remember, one of the core principles of living a primal life, is that we should only eat what we are designed to eat. It's exactly the same for cattle. They were designed to eat grass, not mass-produced cheap corn full of omega 6. The food is so unsuited to them that their stomachs bloat like a hot air balloon, and often the factory farmer has to stuff their feed full of antibiotics.

The antibiotics are not just used so that the cattle can digest food that they weren't designed to eat, but also to supersize them. The antibiotics kill off all of the bacteria that inform the cow that they are full, so it keeps on eating and becomes obese. As we are what we eat, there is a lot of research to suggest that if we eat meat or poultry that has been enhanced with antibiotics, a certain amount of it makes its way onto our dinner plate. So, if we are constantly eating meat produced in factories and not fields, we will undoubtedly damage the helpful bacteria in our gut and our hormones too.

We are not just talking the odd cow that is being stuffed full of drugs. In the USA, more than 75% of all antibiotics sold are consumed not by humans, but by factory-grown animals that make their way into the American diet. It's not just antibiotics, some cows are on hormones and steroids too! Add all of this to the immorally cramped conditions they live in, and we start to realise that factory meat has virtually nothing in common to the meat our primal ancestors once hunted.

In the excellent book written by Dr Mark Hyman, *Eat Fat Get Thin*, he informs us, "The ratio of omega 6 to omega 3 fats in grass-fed beef is about 1.5 to 1. In grain-fed beef it is about 7.5 to 1". Dr Hyman then further promotes the virtues of organic grass-fed meat, saying, "It also has two or three times as much conjugated linoleic acid (CLA) as grain-fed beef, a potent antioxidant that is protective against heart disease, diabetes and cancer and even helps with weight loss metabolism". So, next time we read a newspaper article saying meat is not good for us, it probably either stems from misinterpreted research or the article is just referring to chemically injected, industrialised factory-produced meat!

If you are still not convinced that we should go organic for everything we consume, then get hold of a copy of *Eat Your Heart Out* by Felicity Lawrence. The book's subtitle is, 'Why the food business is bad for the planet and your health'. Felicity goes behind the scenes of milk production, cattle and pig farming, and much more. It's a brilliantly insightful book, however the thing that took me most by surprise was SalmoFan. Felicity reveals, "I have personally never felt the same about farmed fish since discovering the SalmoFan – a little fan of colour charts that look for all the world like a sheaf of Dulux paint charts. The SalmoFan specify how much food dye a salmon farmer should administer with his feed depending on how strong a pink colour he wants his end product to be".

Avoid Grains

If it was a bit of a challenge to get you to realise that potatoes, pasta and bread make us fat and shorten our life, surely grains with all of their fibre can't be bad for us? Sadly, they are. Just like CARBS, grains get easily converted into sugar in our digestive tract. But aren't they full of healthy fibre? Yes they are, however, just like the strawberries in strawberry ice cream might be good for us, there are other ways of getting our strawberries without eating bucket-loads of sugary ice cream. We should get our fibre from nutritionally rich sources such as nuts, seeds and greens, but not from grains. Grains, just like CARBS, spike our insulin levels and turn to fat on our waistline faster than you could possibly imagine.

Hang on a minute, what about whole grain and brown rice – aren't these proven to be good for us? Sorry, no. They might be marginally less bad for us than their heavily processed brothers, but they still aren't primal and therefore our body is not designed to eat them. At the end of the day, while they might have a little more nutritional value, they are still just mutton dressing up as lamb.

One more thing. I hate to be the bearer of bad news, but corn isn't a vegetable – it's another form of grain. While corn on the cob might not be as unhealthy, as most of it normally passes straight through the body - popping perfect little yellow cubes out in our poo - just like other grains and CARBS, those pieces that do become digested are converted into sugar. In fact, stop and think about this for a moment. Since the mid 1960s, scientists in America have been able to genetically modify corn, so much so that it is now used across the globe as a sugar (high-fructose corn syrup) in packaged foods. Corn syrup will most likely one day in the future be regarded as an even bigger killer than cigarettes. High fructose corn syrup (HFCS), consumed en masse in packaged foods and sauces, ruins our healthy flora, fauna and colonises an army of deadly bacteria. In a recent report, the average American now eats 27kg (60lbs) of HFCS every year. This is simply way too much for the human body to absorb.

The Colour of Our Food

In the main, edible white stuff is not healthy. Bread, rice and wheat not only turn into sugar in the body, but also have most of their beneficial nutrients sucked out of them during their refining process.

So, with a broad-brush approach, if we avoid the white stuff then we are on our way to a healthy life. The only white foods we want to consume come in the form of vegetables, such as onions, garlic and cauliflower.

When you read through the list of primal foods in chapter 12, you will notice the appearance of some phytochemicals such as lutein, carotenoids and curcumin. A phytochemical (from the Greek word 'phyto' for 'plant') is a chemical compound normally produced by plants to help protect themselves. Several of these phytochemicals are associated with a colour, and when consumed in food, they will provide similar benefits to our health. All fruit and vegetables contain phytochemicals (which I tend to refer to as phytonutrients as it sounds nicer), and they are so beneficial to our wellbeing that many of them can now be bought as a supplement.

Orange & Yellow Fruit and Vegetables
These tend to contain carotenoids (I will let you figure out where this phytonutrient gets its name), which are known to slow down the ageing process and reduce the risk of various cancers. Foods such as carrots, apricots and bananas all get their colour from carotenoids. Yellow spices such as turmeric and mustard don't get their colour from carotenoids but from curcumin, which also has many health benefits, such as being a natural painkiller and a potent antioxidant.

Green Fruit and Vegetables
These normally contain the phytochemical chlorophyll, which is known to protect against cancer and to help heal wounds. Most dark green vegetables and seaweed contain high doses of chlorophyll.

Blue & Red Fruit and Vegetables
Blueberries, strawberries, cranberries and red onions contain quercetin. This gets to work in the body fighting off inflammation and battling with free radicals (more on these bad boys later). As inflammation is the root cause of many diseases, then consuming plenty of red and blue fruit and vegetables could be the most important colours to include in our daily diet.

Purple Fruit and Vegetables
These contain an antioxidant called anthocyanin. Blueberries are rich in anthocyanin, which has been linked to the prevention of neurological diseases such as Alzheimer's and Parkinson's. Other healthy purple foods include blackberries, plums and radishes.

Oxygen Radical Absorbance Capacity (ORAC)
The Oxygen Radical Absorbance Capacity (ORAC) database was compiled by scientists in 2007 working at the National Institute of Health and Aging (NIH) in the US, run by the Department of Agriculture. It measures the antioxidant capacity of different foods (foods that best absorb free radicals). Why don't more doctors talk about this? Because just like vitamins and minerals, as foods aren't patentable, big pharmaceuticals can't make money out of them. And if big pharma can't make

money, this type of research, even though it is hugely beneficial for our health, rarely makes it into medical journals. I also find it most interesting that the foods that are rich in antioxidants also seem to be rich in vitamins and minerals. This is particularly interesting if you are worried about dementia, Alzheimer's or Parkinson's, in fact any degenerative illness that relates to free radicals.

Dr Patrick Holford

If you can eat the equivalent of 6,000 ORAC a day, the more you will protect your memory. (While the Food and Drug Administration in America recommend 3,000 to 5,000 ORAC units per day for optimal health, I think Patrick's figure is much closer to where we need to be).

In the colour insert, I have listed the gram weight needed to achieve an ORAC score of 3,000. As long as we consume two or more of the listed foods each day, we will devour the necessary volume of antioxidants recommended by Dr Patrick Holford. But do bear in mind that the amount assumes the food is organic. If it is not, then to achieve the same antioxidant benefits, we will most likely need to consume considerably more.

Avoid Deadly Sugar

It is thought that primal man developed a bit of a sweet tooth by occasionally finding fruit, and in some regions, honey. When he did, he gorged on them. Remember, he didn't have a way of refrigerating food, so he just sat there and scoffed down as much as he could. It is therefore our early ancestors' fault, if you like, that we are programmed through our DNA to enjoy gorging on sweet things. But before you start thinking that it is therefore primal to eat loads and loads of sugar, remember that for our ancestral caveman, the fruit would only be available once a year! When we eat sugar, we are not consuming anything helpful. Sugar does not possess any of the vitamins or minerals our body requires. Zero! Although we don't count calories when living primally, l shall use them here to highlight a point. Let's say we have on average six cups of coffee a day, with two spoons of sugar in each. Chances are each spoon has 30 calories heaped upon it. So that's 60 calories per cup, multiplied by our six coffees a day and all of a sudden, we are consuming 360 empty calories a day.

Now, even the largest person who will ever read this book will have a limit to the amount of calories they can consume in a day, but to keep it simple, let's assume we consume above average and that we are currently ingesting around 2,880 calories a day. That means that one eighth of our intake is from empty calories. That means that one eighth of our intake, even if it wasn't doing us any harm (while of course by now we know it's wreaking havoc inside our body) isn't providing us with any of the vital stuff we need. Now let's add on the cakes, biscuits and fizzy drinks and before we know it, more than half of what we are eating and drinking is having zero positive effect. Plus, if you like the idea of intermittent fasting to lose weight (which we will discuss the merits of later), on the days where you are eating, you are going to need to bank some vital vitamins and good nutrients. We simply can't fast if on the days we eat normally we are eating empty calories.

Just like cigarettes and booze, sugar is addictive. Just like cigarette manufacturers stuff their cancer-causing products full of addictive nasties, food manufacturers put sugar into almost everything these days. From baked beans to canned meats, from sauces to even bottles of supposedly healthy water. Make no bones about it - food manufacturers attempt to get us addicted to their products by adding sugars.

While these food manufacturers are really clever and have all sorts of marketing spins, with a little knowledge we can spot the deadly white stuff even if it has been well hidden. On food packages, pretty much every word that ends in '-ose' is a sugar. Maybe it's a subliminal acronym for something like 'other sugar exposed', or buyer beware, 'obesity sugar exists'.

Dextrose, fructose, galactose, glucose, lactose, maltose and sucrose are all simply different types of sugar. As well as watching out for the deadly '-ose', treat all syrups with the same contempt. They are all high in sugar, with heaps of calories that offer minimal nutritional value.

How about this for an analogy. It is said that if a frog is put into a jar of boiling water, it will jump out immediately, but if the frog is put into cold water which is then brought to a boil slowly, it will not perceive any danger and will be cooked to death. It's the same with sugar. It doesn't kill you immediately, but both poisons and ages you, just a little bit every time you eat it.

Sugar Explained

Let's look at the three sugar groups. All the sugar groups are a type of 'saccharide' – the Latin word for 'sugar'.

- Monosaccharide (pronounced moh-no-sack-a-ride): a single molecule. These simple sugars include glucose – found in fruits and grains – and fructose (found in fruit).
- Disaccharide (die-sack-a-ride): a double molecule. These include sucrose, such as table sugar, and lactose which is found in milk.
- Polysaccharides (polly-sack-a-ride): including glycogen, which is how humans and animals store energy in the liver and muscles. Also, starch, which is how plants store energy. The indigestible form of polysaccharides is fibre, which the human body cannot break down and is therefore not detrimental to our health.

The Fizzy Equation

In 2016, the BBC reported that in the UK alone, we got through 14.8 billion litres of fizzy drinks the previous year, or 233 litres per person. To keep it simple, if we assume the average fizzy drink contains 10g per 100ml of sugar and therefore 100g per litre; that means the average person in the UK received 23,290g of sugar just from fizzy drinks. Grams are hard to visualise, so let's keep it simple. Most dieticians agree that there are 4g of sugar in an average teaspoon, so in the UK the average person is consuming 5,822 teaspoons full of sugar each year, just from fizzy drinks.

According to Coke's own website, they sell more than 1.9 billion drinks per day and, according to *www.coca-cola.co.uk* on the 19th November 2019, in a regular 330ml can of Coke Classic there are seven teaspoons (35g) of sugar. They also state, "Our original and iconic cola is still our top-seller. However, 43% of the cola we now sell is made up of Coca-Cola Zero Sugar, Diet Coke or Coca-Cola Life, which have less or no sugar". Interesting isn't it that they want to let us know that a lot of people are moving to the no- or low-sugar options?

Now for a little bit of maths. Let us assume that Coke drinkers around the world are similar to the UK and are consuming 57% Coke Classic. How much sugar is that? It works out as 1,080,000,000 drinks per day, which is approximately 37,800,000,000g of sugar. If you're struggling to visualise this number, here is a comparison: the amount of sugar consumed in Coke Classic around the world each day weighs far more than the weight of 1,000 London double-decker buses!

To keep it simple, I have created the following chart. It shows how many teaspoons of sugar we consume in each standard-sized 330ml can. Admittedly some of the brands don't actually produce a standard can, but I felt it the fairest comparison.

Drink (330ml)	Grams	Teaspoons of Sugar
Mountain Dew	46g	12
Cherry Coke	40g	10
Pepsi Cola	39g	10
Red Bull	39g	10
Monster Energy Drink	39g	10
7up	39g	10
Coca-Cola	35g	9
Vimto Regular	32g	8
Lucozade Energy Original	31g	8
Dr Pepper	26g	6
Fanta	24g	6
Sprite	23g	6
Schweppes Tonic Water	18g	5
Lilt	16g	4
Tango Orange	15g	4

Dr Dan Maggs

If you take just one thing away from this book, it would be don't drink sugary drinks!

Dr Jen Unwin

Is sugar addictive?
There is a lot of evidence and mechanisms to show that sugar is addictive. A lot of behaviours you see around food are indeed addictive behaviours. When we eat sugar, various things happen. Insulin goes up, and in the presence of insulin, other things happen. It's much easier for tryptophan to pass the blood-brain barrier, and tryptophan is a precursor to serotonin, which is the happy hormone. So if you have a lot of sugar, you get a temporary serotonin happy boost. Because you are going to want to have that feeling, it is something you are going to want to repeat. The receptors then make it habit-forming. It then becomes all about short term pleasure and rewards, often at the detriment of long-term happiness.

Dr Jason Fung

Talking about the big fizzy pop manufacturers.
Knowing that they were fighting a losing battle in much of North America and Europe, they took aim at Asia to make up for lost profits. Asian sugar consumption is rising at almost 5 per cent per year, even as it has stabilised or fallen in North America. The result has been a diabetes catastrophe. In 2013, an estimated 11.6 per cent of Chinese adults had type 2 diabetes, eclipsing even the long-time champion: the US, at 11.3 per cent. Things are even more shocking when you consider that only 1 per cent of Chinese had type 2 diabetes in 1980. In a single generation, the diabetes rate rose by a horrifying 1,160 per cent. Sugar, more than any other refined carbohydrate, seems to be particularly fattening and leads to type 2 diabetes.

Dr Joanne McCormack

I have a slide in my presentation that I share with my groups and it says, "You wouldn't feed your plants Coca-Cola, so why would you consume it yourself?".

Breakfast: The British Cereal Killer

Having breakfast regularly is not necessary and certainly not primal. Have you ever stopped and thought about where breakfast gets its name? It is named after its function – it breaks the fast. More marketing and advertising money is spent on breakfast cereals than any other type of food. Yet, they are one of the most rapidly digestible carbohydrates of all, rapidly turning into sugar once consumed.

For more than 25 years I got annoyed with myself if on a hectic day, with a busy schedule, I skipped breakfast. After all, we have been taught that breakfast is the most important meal of the day. We were taught that it sets us up properly for the day ahead; others told us that we can't function without a good breakfast; while marketers of cereals told us that it kicks starts our metabolism. And then there is the old saying 'breakfast like a king, lunch like a prince and dine like a pauper'. So, on days when I just couldn't fit in time for breakfast, I got angry with myself. Now, however, I have learnt that those days of skipping breakfast weren't doing me any harm - they were making me healthier. No longer are the low-fat yoghurts, cereals and large glass of orange juice the healthy breakfast option. They are in fact a recipe for disaster.

Now, while there are several reasons why breakfast is dangerous, I am only going to touch lightly on the subject. For a detailed explanation I highly recommend reading Terence Kealey's book, *Breakfast is a Dangerous Meal*.

First, it's important to say that I don't recommend that you stop eating breakfast until you have broken free from eating CARBS and other sugars. Don't start this principle until you have turned yourself into a fat-burning machine. You see the problem is this: when our body is used to eating lots of CARBS, after sleeping for seven to eight hours there is very little sugar left in our bloodstream (as it has all been sent to reside in our waistline and other fat stores) and we will wake up feeling hungry. Just like the smoker needs their next nicotine rush, the sugar eater desires their insulin spike.

What's more, as Terence Kealey demonstrates in his book, any sugar consumed within the first couple of hours of waking cause the body to create an even bigger insulin spike than normal, which of course is highly dangerous, especially for type 2 diabetes sufferers.

Breakfast really is a cereal killer. But, once you start to live more primally, your body will become used to burning its own excess body fat as energy (see ketosis - page 121), and therefore when you wake up you won't need to fill your face with stuff that quickly turns into sugar. Remember that the body treats sugar (or glucose as it is called once it is in the bloodstream) as a poison. It doesn't matter if it's sugar in our tea, fructose in our orange juice, a doughnut or a bagel, cereal or literally anything made of wheat or grain – it's all going to be turned into sugar before we reach our school or place of work.

But once you begin living primally, you rarely feel hungry in the morning and therefore simply don't need to eat. For me, since I started to eat this way I seldom have breakfast. I don't even miss it! Occasionally, when I want to get my children to try out something new (they actually like being my guinea pigs so please don't complain to the authorities), I might eat with them, but the rest of the time I just have a cup or two of coffee.

Pretty much the only other occasion I have anything else at this time of day is when I'm on holiday with my family, and I will join in with their ritual of blending fermented yogurt with lots of different berries. It's a brilliant way to get the healthy gut bacteria back on track, and the berries come loaded with amazing micronutrients.

You have already read in chapter 1 how corporations mislead us. If you want to learn more about how they screw up your breakfast, then read Felicity Lawrence's insightful book *Eat Your Heart Out*, which carries the subtitle on the cover, 'Why the food business is bad for the planet and your health'. In this book she reveals how Kellogg's went against government suggestions on labelling and instead pioneered a revolution with other food manufacturers, particularly those who formed part of the Association of Cereal Food Manufacturers (ACFM), to create labels that have misled us for decades.

Fibre

So if we are going to skip breakfast and cereals, are we not missing out on a source of fibre? Yes we are. But fear not, we can get plenty of fibre from shirataki, nuts, seeds, vegetables, fibre supplements and certain fruits.

For those who juice, stop right now! Juicing is one of the most ridiculous trends of the last 50 years. When we extract juice from our fruits and vegetables, we lose all of their great fibres, miss out on most of their nutrients (healthy nutrients are normally bound to the fibre) and often end up with a glass full of fructose (sugar). Orange juice is possibly the worst of them all. If you don't like fruit the way nature designed them, don't juice the goodness out of them, but instead retain all the benefits by liquefying or blending them. We need to throw the entire fruit into the blender, or we are missing out on the best bits. Sure, we will want to peel the skins off our oranges and bananas, but then it's essential to throw the whole fruit in our high-powered blending machine.

What is fibre? It's the rough guys who hang around with macronutrients. They can either be absorbed in water (soluble) or not (insoluble). Fibre is great at making us feel full without taking on lots of calories. In fact, insoluble fibre tends to pass through the system without leaving any calories behind, and even soluble fibre is extremely light in calories. For example, there are pastas, spaghetti and noodles that have been consumed in Japan for thousands of years that have zero calories and zero CARBS! How is that possible? Known as shirataki (meaning 'white waterfall') and made from glucomannan which is found in the root of the konjac plant, these transparent insoluble fibre noodles are edible, but not digestible. They absorb water so well that, while what is eaten might look identical to normal wheat noodles, they are actually made of 95% water temporarily suspended in fibre. The great news is they are now starting to become available in UK supermarkets.

Why tell you about glucomannan? Because it's a great example of what fibre does. It can fill up our stomach, and at the same time be used as a vehicle to transport micronutrients around our body. There are numerous health benefits for making sure we eat plenty of fibre in our diet, and I felt it right and proper to feature at least one quote from our amazing National Heath Service in this book. The NHS website states, "Fibre is an important part of a healthy balanced diet. It can help prevent heart disease, diabetes, weight gain and some cancers, and can also improve digestive health". Glucomannan is also the only ingredient recognized by the European Food Standards Agency (EFSA) to aid weight loss.

Water: The Miracle Cure

Different experts and different medical professionals all seem to have different perspectives on how much water we should drink, and even on what constitutes water! Some suggest we get enough of it in our sodas, coffee and tea to live a healthy life. But Dr Fereydoon Batmanghelidj's book, *Your Body's Many Cries for Water*, which has sold more than 1 million copies, suggests something very different: "Caffeine is a natural diuretic, forcing more water out of the body than is contained in the caffeinated beverage".

As someone who historically has been rubbish at drinking plain water, I have read many books and white papers on the subject and have come to the conclusion that we need between 1.5 to 2.5 litres of water a day. If you are petite and don't exercise much then 1.5 litres might be fine, but if you are well-built or exercise a lot you might need closer to 2.5 litres. Bear in mind that we shouldn't count water in coffee or alcohol towards our daily intake, as both actually dehydrate rather than hydrate. If you find water 'boring' try adding a slice of lemon, lime or ginger to improve the taste. Also, if you regularly have more than half a dozen cups of coffee or tea each day, you might find that it is the warm water that you are drawn to, rather than the coffee or tea itself. Try a glass of warm water with nothing added, then try it with blackberries, blueberries, strawberries, or lime to see if you prefer it.

I remember a good friend of mine called Edward, who was previously in the Royal Air Force, but whose career after leaving the military was that of a wine expert. He is someone whom you wouldn't naturally expect to believe in the virtues of water, but he always preached the following message to his colleagues. If your urine is clear then it is a healthy sign that you are well hydrated. If it is a pale yellow then you are reasonably hydrated, but if the colour is dark yellow to orange then you are seriously dehydrated. I remember him telling me that the brain is made up of 85% water and that it was important to keep it topped up, and to flush it regularly. Since then, I have read many books that say good hydration can help prevent Alzheimer's disease, and possibly even reduce its symptoms post-diagnosis.

There is growing evidence that water might cure far more conditions than many doctors and medical advisors currently realise. One problem is that our bodies are not very good at notifying us when we are dehydrated, and therefore we must not wait until we are thirsty before sipping water. I bet you're similar to me in that there are days when you get into the late afternoon and realise you haven't had a glass of water all day. Try to do everything you can to make consuming sufficient water part of your routine.

On the cover of Dr Batmanghelidj's book, *Your Body's Many Cries for Water*, there is the subtitle: 'You're not sick; you're thirsty, don't treat thirst with medication'. He goes on to say, "The simple truth is that dehydration can cause disease". In this brilliant book, full of insightful information about how the human body uses water, he explains how dehydration can be a cause of rheumatoid arthritis, lower back pain, neck pain, migraines, hypertension, Alzheimer's and much more, all backed by lots of scientific research. In fact, talking of Alzheimer's, Dr Batmanghelidj goes on to state: "The primary cause of Alzheimer's disease is chronic dehydration of the body". Later in the book he says, "People with Alzheimer's disease and children with learning disabilities should not drink anything but water". He delivers the message with great clarity and some great analogies: "In prolonged dehydration, brain cells begin to shrink. Imagine a plum gradually turning into a prune. Unfortunately, in a dehydrated state, many functions of the brain cells begin to get lost".

When it comes to exercise, keeping hydrated is really important as dehydrated muscles are weak muscles. During a one-hour workout we can easily lose a litre of water by sweating, and when it's hot it's possible to lose as much as three litres in just a single hour. Ever wondered why, if you jump on a pair of scales after a workout or a game of tennis, you are lighter than you expected to be? There is an old saying that goes, 'A pint's a pound the whole world round'. In a litre there is close to two pints, therefore in a normal one-hour workout we are going to temporarily lose around 0.9kg (2lbs) in weight - and if it's midsummer we could drop close to 2.7kg (6lbs) in water. By the way, if we lose around 2 to 3kg of water after an exercise session and don't promptly replace the fluids, then it can be extremely dangerous!

Exercising isn't the only time we will need to increase our intake of water. By the time you finish reading this book I am sure you will be consuming a lot more fibre with your meals. While fibre is hugely beneficial to our health, it acts like a sponge and absorbs lots of water. Therefore, as we increase our fibre intake, we must ensure to take on board more water.

Finally, I didn't know where to mention cellulite. I don't want to put it under diseases as it is not really a disease, so I thought I would put it under water, as keeping our skin hydrated helps to repair cellulite. There are two other major factors in having healthy skin and keeping the body's inbuilt 'cellulite criminal' at bay – they are getting our weight under control and exercising. When we are overweight, we have to distort our skin to cover the enlarged surface area. Sadly, yo-yo diets can leave us with excess amounts of skin. Interval training, both sprinting and weightlifting, produces hormones that enhance the levels of both collagen and elastin within the skin.

Is All Water Equal?
Sadly not. The best water is natural mineral water supplied in glass bottles, or filtered tap water. What is least healthy is bottled plastic water and unfiltered tap water. Let me explain why.

Tap Water
Don't get me wrong, in the UK tap water is extremely good for us, but it should be filtered to reduce the level of chlorine. While chlorine acts as a highly efficient disinfectant - killing off harmful bacteria that grows throughout the entire water supply system, from the reservoirs to the pipe network - it can also kill off healthy bacteria in our guts. Chlorine is a necessary evil in the supply of water to our homes, as without

it water could carry deadly diseases and harmful bacteria. Of course, all governments will tell us that chlorine in water is so low in concentration that it is totally harmless. However, as you will read throughout this book, it's critical that we look after the healthy gut bacteria in our microbiome and it's therefore just common sense that, no matter how low the concentration, we should do everything possible to filter out harmful chemicals.

If you want to know how harmful chlorine is, spill some bleach on your jeans (most household bleach is normally made of chlorine) and watch the colour disappear, quickly turning white and eventually burning holes in the material. Our delicate gut lining is only one cell thick, and therefore you can easily imagine what damage chlorine could potentially do to it. Don't fall for the 'concentration smokescreen' – poison is poison, regardless of its concentration.

Here is my tap water tip. Be sure to fit a water filter at home, or alternatively purchase a water filter jug. If you find yourself in a hotel room, and aren't sure if the water is filtered, be sure to boil it before you drink it.

Glass Bottled Water
There is so much plastic floating around, that if you gathered it all together, turned it into dust and covered the entire land mass of our planet – including the two currently frozen Poles – the dust would almost be up to our knees! Across all of the oceans there is an average of 46,000 pieces of man-made plastics per square mile, and it will take between 500 to 1,000 years for each piece to degrade. The effect of all of this is that we are unnecessarily killing millions and millions of fish and birds each month!

In the UK, it is estimated that every day we use more than 35 million plastic bottles, and more than half don't get recycled. That's right, what we drink in minutes, only use once and then throw away, takes the planet a millennium to get rid of!

Plastic bottles are not just harmful as waste, as the cost to the environment of their creation and transportation is equally as damaging. All in all, water in one-time use plastic bottles is just damn stupid. But this book is not primarily about saving the environment it's about saving you! So, let me stop my rant about plastic and its effect on our planet, and tell you why drinking water out of plastic bottles is bad for our health too.

Some of the toxins from the plastic can leech into the water and potentially harm our body. The main culprit is a compound called BPA (bisphenol A), which the European Food Standards Agency (EFSA) have already banned from being used in polycarbonate infant feeding bottles, but as yet neither the UK's Food Standards Agency nor the EFSA have banned it from being used in other products. Why not? I am sure you can guess by now. Could it be that preventing the death of babies before they can become taxpayers is bad news, but slowly and silently poisoning the rest of us, so that the effect is not felt until after we retire, is commercially and financially very efficient? If I am going a bit far with this let me apologise, but could BPA really be the industry's secret acronym for 'Bottles to Poison Adults'?!

I am sure in the coming years the government will have no choice but to ban the use of BPAs, which I am convinced leech poison into the water and cause damage to our gut's friendly bacteria. Studies have also shown that BPAs can mimic the hormone oestrogen, which is used in the female body to develop breasts, regulate periods and maintain pregnancies. Researcher Dr Jianying Hu of Peking University in Beijing says, "In recent years, BPA was shown to have [oestrogenic] activity, linking BPA to endocrine diseases and to an increased incidence of endocrine-related cancers".

Stop for a moment and think about how much of a nonsense this is! Something that is dressed up as a health product, often costing more than petrol, is anything but healthy due to it leeching BPA. Costing up to 10,000 times more than tap water, some of the biggest brands actually contain very much just that – glorified tap water! To me, branded bottled water is one of the cleverest marketing campaigns known to man and one of the most successful bluffs ever!

One last thought. To prove that British tap water tastes as good as branded water, we conducted a blind water taste experiment. The first time we took five leading branded bottled waters and chilled them to the same temperature as the filtered tap water. We served them in the same glasses as the tap water, and simply asked participants to say which one they preferred. We compiled the results and were completely blown away by the findings. The tap water came out joint first, scoring 11 times more preference as one of the leading supermarket brands. We then repeated the experiment, but without telling the participants we served the tap water at a slightly lower temperature than the bottled water. This time the tap water triumphed massively – 77% of all participants preferred the filtered tap water over five of the top water brands on sale in the UK.

The conclusion? Filtered tap water is not only 10,000 times cheaper than leading brands of bottled water, and it not only helps protect the environment for our children, but it tastes better too! Don't fall victim to bottled water advertising, further lining the pockets of corporations whose motives are driven by shareholder value and not our health.

The Pros and Cons of Being a Vegetarian

I have many wonderful colleagues who, due to their faith, are strict vegetarians. I also have other friends who are vegetarians for what they believe are ethical, moral, environmental and/or health reasons. While primal principles suggest that meat and poultry should be consumed as part of a healthy lifestyle, I have no intention of trying to convert any vegetarian into becoming a meat eater. While I do have many overweight and obese vegetarian friends, I also have several that are extremely fit. So, if you are vegetarian the two pieces of advice I would give are to try to pay even stricter adherence to all other primal principles, (as you are certainly missing out on some good healthy proteins, fats and micronutrients) and to take appropriate supplements.

If you are avoiding eating quality organic meat and animal produce for health reasons, then you have simply been misled. We are designed to eat meat. It has numerous health benefits and has been the staple diet of humankind since day one.

If you are avoiding eating meat on ethical or moral grounds, then I admire your restraint and motives, but before committing yourself to a life of abstaining, I would recommend you read a book by Lierre Keith called *The Vegetarian Myth*, where she explains why being vegetarian may not be as kind to animals and our planet as you might think. After spending 20 years as a vegan, she explains how she concluded that cultivating land is the biggest and worst effect man has made to the planet, and how the ploughing of fields destroys complete ecosystems, dislodging and killing many kinds of animals and birds. It appears that planting vegetables and other items of a conscientious vegetarian menu are mass killers in their own right.

Dr Robert Lustig

I am not against veganism, if vegans want to be vegan that's fine, if people want to go keto, that's fine too. The funny thing is both the vegans and the ketos are in agreement; they think they are in a war; the matter of the fact is that they are actually on the same side. They are on the side against the processed food industry. If they stopped battling against each other and worked together, we might solve this problem.

Dr Aseem Malhotra

We pick up the conversation after Aseem tells the sad story of his mother's ill health, which unfortunately lead to her dying prematurely. I wrote an article in the 'i', which got a lot of coverage. Basically, how the current movement at the moment towards people thinking that vegans or vegetarians are somehow healthier, there is no evidence really for that. I think you can have a healthy vegetarian diet. You can, in theory, have a healthy vegan diet, but the one thing I don't subscribe to, and for that reason I don't think you should do it, is because you are forced to take additional supplements just to survive as a vegetarian or vegan. Plus I see a lot of patients that have been vegan for a few years, and while it initially helped them, after a while they are getting sick and going back to eating meat, eggs and dairy again, and they feel better.

Now I am a very strong advocate to really fight that misinformation coming because there are lots of vested interests in the whole vegan movement. The vegan movement was initially supported by the likes of Coca-Cola and the sugar industry, and there are people in this space saying that people who advocate for low carbs are spreading dangerous advice. (Aseem lets out a big sigh.) I have no issue with people being vegetarian for their own personal ethical reasons. They don't want to eat animal flesh or animal products, and I understand that. My mum was like that, and I respected her and understood where it came from in a religious belief.

Professor Tim Noakes

If you look at humans, it's very clear that we are carnivorous. And anyone who tells you we aren't is not looking at the biology. The biology is so clear. We have a very acidic stomach; we have a very long small bowel and a very short large bowel, and we just don't have the bacteria to digest starchy foods. And by that, I mean the resistant starches, the cellulose, which is all done by anaerobic (without oxygen) bacteria. And the big guts of the chimpanzee and the gorilla is because they are full of these digestive bacteria that are changing the cellulose into saturated fatty acids. And that's the irony of it all. The cows and the sheep and other ruminants are converting grass, which is a carbohydrate into saturated fats. Why would they do that if it's going to kill us? And that's the issue. We are absolutely adapted for meat consumption and not for vegetables and grains. And it frightens me this push towards eating more vegetables. You simply can't get the nutrition. Humans would have to be eating like 12 to 14 hours a day. If you're a vegan or vegetarian if you are not eating 14 hours a day, what nutrition are you getting?

If you are vegetarian because you believe that animals are a huge contributor to global warming, then let me hand you over to Patrick Holden and Dr Robert Lustig, to explain a totally different viewpoint...

Patrick Holden CBE

The question of which sort of food should we eat to be sustainable, this whole plant-based thing over the past 5 to 10 years, where there is now a whole generation of young people who think it's the right thing to do to become vegan or vegetarian. When in fact you cannot produce healthy vegetables, without first building soil fertility with a crop rotation, which involves clover and grass. And the only way to turn that clover and grass into something we can eat is to graze it with cattle or sheep, ruminants; that means they have a stomach that can digest the cellulose material in the clover and grass. If we don't support those farmers by buying the livestock products from that system, they can't make this natural rotation work.

There are thousands of livestock farmers in the west of Britain right now thinking, what do we do? The price of beef and lamb is crashing, beef consumption has halved since the 1980s in the UK, and it appears no young people are eating lamb, they are all giving it up thinking it's the right thing to do. When in fact of all the meats we could eat, lamb is probably the healthiest and the most sustainable. Virtually all the lamb we produce in the UK is grass-fed, and even most of the beef is grass-fed. Now feed-lock beef, which is what characterises the American system, that is part of the problem, because all of those grains the animals are eating are grown in genetically modified soil, in an unsustainable way. So we need to become very educated and sophisticated and be able to differentiate between the livestock products that are part of the problem, which is intensively produced chicken, intensively produced pork and, yes, dairy products from these mega dairy herds; from those that are part of the solution, which means grass-fed lamb, grass-fed beef and dairy products only from grass-fed cattle.

It is true that cows emit methane, they always have and probably whatever we do, feeding them garlic or whatever, they still will. But that methane cycle is an ancient cycle that's been going on as long as there have been ruminants on the planet. But the methane which is critically responsible for climate change is that from burning fossil fuel. And if we use ruminants (cows and sheep) to build soil by grazing grassland or as part of a rotation, digesting the cellulose into food that we can eat, the soil carbon gain offsets the methane emissions. If cows and sheep are used to maintain the soil carbon bank, which is the second-largest carbon bank on the planet only after the oceans, then they are part of the solution, not the problem. If you look what's happened to the world now, we use to think that the rainforests and the primal wilderness was where we could hopefully keep the planet healthy, but now the planet is covered with farms, so the farms are the metabolism of the planet. And if the farming is wrong, then the planet is in an unhealthy condition, that is sadly where we are today. So if we want to address climate change and take CO2 out of the atmosphere and put it back in the soil, we need to change the way we farm and that will only happen when we change our buying habits.

When it comes to the EAT-Lancet report, not one of the 37 authors were a farmer! All these people are telling us what to eat without knowing about agriculture. How strange is that? Bless his heart, even David Attenborough, who is a national treasure, said on some program recently, "I am trying to cut down on red meat", I wanted to shout at the television and say no, please differentiate between the red meat which is part of the problem and that which is part of the solution. We should be eating real meats to support hard-pressed livestock farmers and the arable farmers who want to farm in a more sustainable way.

Dr Robert Lustig

Earlier in our interview, you mentioned that the food we eat has a big impact on greenhouse gasses. How do you see the link between eating well and solving the environmental issues?
People talk about greenhouse gasses as if they are all the same; they are not. It turns out there are three greenhouse gasses:

1. Carbon Dioxide. It has a heat-retaining capacity of 1. We need carbon dioxide, we would die without it, but there is too much.
2. Methane. It has a heat-retaining capacity of 25. And it is true that ruminants produce methane. But the point is that the amount of methane the ruminants make is only about 5% of the methane and most is coming from industry and cars etc.
3. Nitrous Oxide. It has a heat-retaining capacity of 210. Nine times greater than methane. This is the one that nobody gets. Where do you get nitrous oxide from?

Well, it's in every field, and the reason is because that is what happens to the nitrogen runoff, from the nitrogen fertiliser, that was needed to grow the crops. Because the animals who use to fertilise the crops, because of their manure, because that's nitrogen-fixing, now aren't there because the cattle are in Kansas and the corn is in Iowa. So you have to spray the corn with the nitrogen, which becomes nitrate oxide, which causes way more greenhouse gas emissions than the methane ever did and guess what, you have to do that for vegans too.

To fix the problem, we have to stop Washington and London from giving subsidies. So, this problem is real, but it is man-made. It's because we have made bad food cheap. Those bad foods not only cause metabolic syndrome but are bad for the planet too.

Dairy Produce

Part of the secret to avoiding many diseases lies in the maintenance of our healthy gut bacteria. Some 2,500 years ago Hippocrates, the father of modern medicine, taught, 'All diseases begin in the gut'. Okay, so that part of the secret is already in the public domain, but here is the bit – my hypothesis – to health, happiness and longevity that I believe governments know, but are keeping a lid on. Yes, all three – health, happiness and longevity – can be unlocked by understanding one secret!

I believe Hippocrates was in fact way ahead of his time, and that many diseases really do begin in the gut. There is something in our modern society that is causing mass murder of certain bacteria in our stomach. As you will discover later, our gut is one huge ecosystem. Our bodies contain more than 10,000 different species of microorganisms and together they and us exist in harmony. The fact is that we need them more than they need us. For every one human cell, there are nine non-human creatures living on or in our body! We are therefore only 10% human, as already noted! This isn't a new phenomenon; it has been that way ever since we descended from apes. More accurately, the harmony and balance has been mutually beneficial for more than 2.5 million years, but over the past 50 I believe it has started to fall apart. Just like the destruction of a glorious rainforest can happen when just one or two species become extinct, or a coral reef can become completely barren after a short period when sea temperatures rise too quickly, something is destroying the microbiomes of those of us living in Great Britain.

Whether it is diet, pollution, pesticides, starch, microwaves, fast food, fizzy drinks, ready meals, overly prescribed medicines, hydrogenated oils, continuous snacking, sugar or any one of the multitudes of modern world problems, something is upsetting the balance of our ecosystem at an alarming rate.

It might just be that nearly every disease and disorder we face in modern civilisation can be tracked back to the reduction or total elimination of just one or two varieties of necessary bacteria in our guts. Remember back in science lessons at school where we learnt Newton's third law (for every action there is an equal and opposite reaction)? I believe that while the action might be too many CARBS, or toxins entering our body from a plastic water bottle, it is actually the gut's reaction to these events that is causing us harm. While to live healthily and happily the key lies in preventing the negative actions in the first place, meaning that purely focusing on the gut is not necessary, the issue lies in the fact that we probably have already accidentally wiped out some species in our ecosystem.

This is where dairy enters the scene and where primal living takes a divergence from those following a strict Paleo diet. In order to defend and indeed rebuild the body's ecosystem – the microbiome – it's beneficial to eat a diet rich in fibre and fermented foods. While primal fibre is taken care of with choices such as nuts, seeds and lots of leafy greens, in the modern diet fermented foods are generally absent without leave! Later we will detail which fermented foods will help rebuild our gut's microbiome, but let's briefly just mention that three of the top five are derived from dairy – probiotic live yoghurts, fermented milk known as kefir and certain cheeses.

While yoghurts and cheeses start out as milk, milk itself is not necessarily as healthy as we were brought up to believe. The sugar it contains is known as lactose and it is estimated that, once we pass infancy, more than two-thirds of the world's population become lactose intolerant. What does this mean? It means that for two out of every three people it is not beneficial to drink milk. When we think about it logically, nature designed milk to help newborns grow rapidly. Whether it be human, cow, goat or dog, nature didn't intend us to rely on milk as we matured.

According to the US National Library of Medicine, "Lactose intolerance in adulthood is most prevalent in people of East Asian descent, affecting more than 90 percent of adults in some of these communities. The prevalence of lactose intolerance is lowest in populations with a long history of dependence on unfermented milk products as an important food source. For example, only about 5 percent of people of European descent are lactose intolerant". Lactose (a sugar) is normally broken down by cells found in the lining of the small intestine with the assistance of an enzyme called lactase. However, once past infancy there is normally a reduction of lactase in the gut and if the reduction is severe, the result is that we become lactose intolerant. If shortly after drinking milk you experience abdominal pain, flatulence, bloating, nausea or diarrhoea, then you are likely to be lactose intolerant.

Is drinking milk primal? Not really. Research suggests that civilisations only started drinking animal milk around 8000 BC. For the following millennia, consumption appears to have been sporadic and non-commercial. Then in the 1800s the calcium and phosphorus in milk became heavily promoted as good for our bones. As a result, a whole industry emerged and as demand grew, cattle started to get shoehorned into smaller and smaller milking sheds.

As overcrowding escalated these sheds became dirty and before long milk production became very unhygienic. In an attempt to make milk safer, dairy farmers responded by sterilising bottles and having doctors test cattle for disease. This did little to solve the problem and eventually lead to the heating of milk to 62°F (145°F) for around half an hour, killing off any viruses and bacteria in a process that became known as the pasteurisation of milk.

Understanding The Milk Label

- HTST – Created in the 1930s, High Temperature Short Time (HTST) pasteurisation is where milk is heated to 71°C (161°F) for 15 seconds, which provides a shelf life of several weeks. The process is often marketed as pasteurised.
- UHT – First used in the 1970s, Ultra High Temperature (UHT) pasteurisation is where milk is heated to 138°C (280°F) for just two seconds. This provides an extended shelf life of approximately nine months, and is often marketed as ultra-pasteurised.
- Homogenisation – After pasteurisation, some milk goes through a separate process called homogenisation. This process breaks the molecules down into tiny pieces and prevents a layer of cream from forming on the top of the milk.
- Semi-skimmed and skimmed milk – When milk is skimmed it means that the level of fat has been reduced through filtering. In the UK skimmed milk has around just 0.1% fat and semi-skimmed milk is typically around 2.5%.

When you consider whole milk is around just 4% fat and especially when we start to understand that natural fat has never been the real enemy, why would anybody use skimmed milk? Plus, when we remove the fat, we dramatically reduce the fat-soluble vitamins A, D, E and K. This has a double negative effect, because one of the health benefits of milk is its concentration of calcium, yet to truly absorb calcium you need vitamin D. In other words, if we skim the fat off milk, we remove most of the health benefits of drinking it in the first place.

As we can get all the beneficial vitamins and minerals that milk possesses through other means that are more in line with what we are designed to eat and drink, I personally avoid the white stuff. However, if you enjoy the odd glass of milk (and assuming you aren't lactose intolerant), let me offer a little advice. As with all meats and dairy product, going organic is crucial. Think about this for a moment – in America the number of dairy cows halved between 1960 and 2005, yet the total output grew by nearly 50%. How did they achieve this? Mainly via injecting cows with antibiotics, force feeding them grains and several other unnatural additives, all of which makes the end product very cheap to create yet unhealthy for human consumption. The safest milk to drink is whole organic pasteurised milk. There is an argument that suggests raw milk is more beneficial than pasteurised, but of course being raw it carries a slightly higher risk of carrying infection.

To conclude this chapter, let's get back to how I started this section on dairy by discussing our gut. While I am not a big fan of milk, I feel there are huge advantages in consuming yogurt and certain cheeses. While they both originate from dairy, these two products are super healthy. Yogurt achieves its creamy thickness as bacteria convert the lactose (sugar) to lactic acid. Cheese making follows a similar process, where the end result can be a product with various varieties of bacteria that are wildly beneficial for our guts. So much so, that by consuming just a small portion on a regular basis we might assemble a little army of helpful bacteria that help us lose weight! There is more to follow on this a bit later in the book.

Dr Patrick Holford

We do know that milk causes cancer cells to grow, obviously not a problem for the very young as they are meant to drink milk. What concerns me, and the logic is very strong, but the hard evidence is not quite there yet, but what milk does is it promotes a hormone called IGF-1, insulin-like growth factor. And if you look at that across the ages, it absolutely peaks in the mid-teenage years, when the breasts are fully formed and when the prostate is fully formed. The logic suggests that it is quite likely that overconsumption of dairy products in teenage years may produce a sort of over-growth of breast cells and prostate cells, that could set a background for a greater risk in later life.

But of course, everyone says what about the calcium? Milk has calcium, and bones have calcium, we have to have milk for bones. But it is very clear, in fact two of the top professors in America in the field of nutrition, professors Ludwig and Jenkins, both say this, there is absolutely no link at all between children's bone mass density and milk consumption. And no link for post-menopausal women's risk of osteoporosis and dairy consumption. No link at all. Absolutely none. It's a myth. Yes, we need calcium. If you are eating beans, nuts, veg and fish, you are going to get calcium. It's not a lack of calcium that is driving osteoporosis in later life. It's mainly a lack of vitamin D. If you go to the equator where there is a lot of sun, there is no osteoporosis. The further you go away from the equator, the greater the risk.

Got a Fat Pet?

Other than animals that are raised and nurtured to feed humans, when was the last time you saw any overweight or obese animal in the wild? In their natural habitat, it's a case of catching food or being caught as another creature's meal. Now, before you start to question me by saying what about whales and buffalo, let me counter that with a question – do you ever see skinny whales? The answer is no! The point is these species were designed by nature to carry excess fat to fight the cold when they migrate. Bears in the Arctic Circle are designed to store a huge amount of fat so they can draw on it during hibernation. As humans don't hibernate, we were not intended to be burdened with the amount of fat that so many of us lug around today, and nor were our pets! For those in Great Britain that have a cat or a dog that's overweight, suffering from poor joints and a weak immune system, the problem lies in the fact their owners are unintentionally making their pets sick. Cats and dogs are just not meant to be fat or obese. As very few of our pets go out and catch their own dinner in the manner they were designed too, we need to feed them proper nutrition, supplemented by vitamins and minerals. This is essential if we want to both cut down on our vets' bills and for our pets to live healthily and happily for longer.

Dr Joanne McCormack

A lot of pets are now getting diabetes, through the stuff in processed packets and tins. And there must be something in what we feed our pets that must be wrong for their bodies. There are now low carb vets as well as low carb doctors.

Chapter 4 Highlights

- Fats are either healthy, neutral or killers! Our longevity depends on us understanding the difference between the good and the ugly and following the right path.
- As our body can't produce omega 3, it's crucial that we get plenty from our diet.
- The balance between omega 3 and omega 6 plays a crucial role in our health and longevity.
- Organic grass-fed meat and dairy fats, plus coconut fats, are not demons and devils, but delightfully delicious and good for our health.
- Caveman ate organically and so should we. We were not designed to consume meat, poultry or dairy produce full of antibiotics and other dangerous toxins. The food in our fridge must be organic or outlawed!
- Despite what we previously believed about grains, they should be avoided like the plague. We must get our fibre elsewhere.
- Avoid most white foods and instead cook colourfully.
- Fibre is only found in plants. We don't acquire any dietary fibre from meat, poultry, fish, eggs, milk or cheese. That's why it's essential to add shirataki, nuts, seeds, vegetables, fibre supplements and certain fruits to our daily menu.
- According to *The American Journal of Clinical Nutrition*, a daily consumption of 35g of fibre is associated with a lower risk of cardiovascular disease by as much as 54% and death from all causes by 37%.
- For the sake of both your health and the planet, don't drink water from one-use plastic bottles. Instead, filter your water at home, put it in a glass or stainless-steel container and take it with you wherever you go.
- The health of our species depends above all on quality nutrition. Quality nutrition means growing foods in accordance with natures laws. All foods made in factories, by industrial processing, such as sugar, refined flour, packaged foods and vegetable oils, must be avoided.
- I have developed a simple acronym to help you avoid CRAP foods: Carbohydrates, Refined foods, Artificial colours and sweeteners and Processed foods.

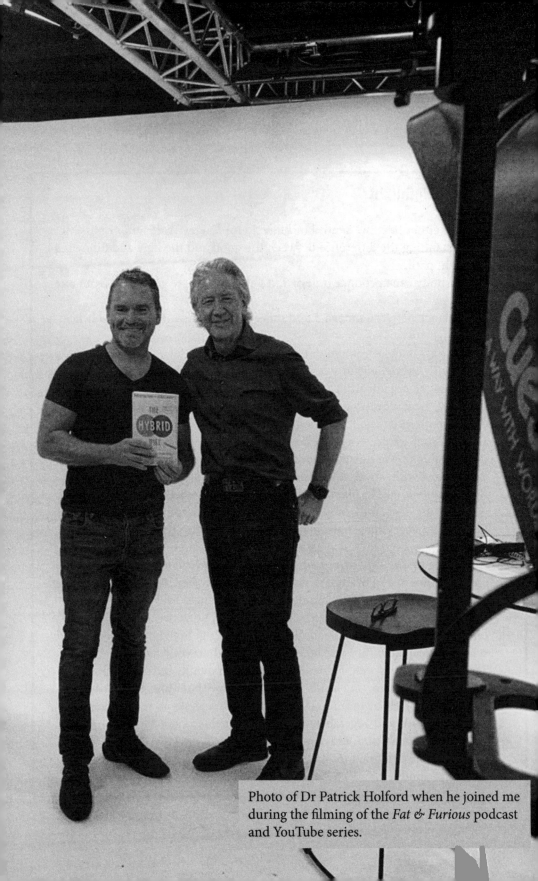

Photo of Dr Patrick Holford when he joined me during the filming of the *Fat & Furious* podcast and YouTube series.

CHAPTER 5

INTERMITTENT FASTING

"Don't graze unless you are a cow or want to be the size of one."
DR ZOE HARCOMBE

In this chapter we discover how having periods without food is something that the human body has developed to both endure and appreciate. And how, if we are to reverse Britain's decline into ill health, intermittent fasting is something that most people should partake in.

During the Second World War, when food was rationed, a common saying gained traction: 'eat little but often'. It might have been born out of necessity, but you still occasionally hear people saying it today. Sadly, from a medical perspective, it now appears to be very bad advice indeed. If you subscribe to our views on evolution – that we must both eat what we were designed to eat and eat at a frequency we have evolved to digest – then ask yourself whether caveman ate little but often! Of course not. He was constantly going from feast to famine. As it turns out, our body is not designed to eat little but often.

Dr Jason Fung

As a healing tradition, fasting has a long history. Hippocrates of Kos (c 460 – c 370 BC) is widely considered the father of modern medicine. Among the treatments that he prescribed and championed were the practice of fasting and the consumption of apple cider vinegar. Hippocrates wrote, "To eat when you are sick, is to feed your illness." The ancient Greek writer and historian Plutarch (c 46 – c 120 AD) also echoed these sentiments. He wrote, "Instead of using medicine, better fast today."

Eating Regularly is Not Normal

We aren't designed to eat regularly. Caveman and the hunter-gatherer didn't have fridges or freezers. They couldn't store an apple for a year like the oxygen-free warehouses the big supermarkets use today. They had no preservatives or tin cans. When they caught an animal, they had a feast, after which they might go days or even weeks without eating anything substantial.

It's not just our ancestors who fasted, various faiths and religions to this day still participate in different ceremonial fasts. Muslims celebrate Ramadan, the ninth month of the Islamic calendar, with a month-long fast known as Sawm. Christians participate in Lent and the Greek Orthodox Church asks that its followers fast for more than 180 days a year. Saint Nikolai Velimirović wrote, "Gluttony makes a man gloomy and fearful, but fasting makes him joyful and courageous. And, as gluttony calls forth greater and greater gluttony, so fasting stimulates greater and greater endurance. When a man realises the grace that comes through fasting, he desires to fast more and more. And the graces that come through fasting are countless".

What Happens To Our Metabolism When We Intermittently Fast?

Doesn't fasting mess with our metabolism and slow down our metabolic rate? Let me first explain metabolism and metabolic rate. *Dictionary.com* says, "In metabolism some substances are broken down to yield energy for vital processes while other substances, necessary for life, are synthesised". So metabolism is the breaking down of either our incoming food or our stored body fat to use as energy. But imagine what would have happened to our caveman ancestor if, on days when he couldn't catch anything, his metabolism slowed down. His energy levels would drop and his chances of catching his next meal would, just like his physique, get slimmer and slimmer. It would all be one huge downward spiral and before long he would starve and perish. When we fast our metabolism does not drop as many would have us believe, but in fact increases.

The idea of 'don't skip breakfast because you need to kick-start your metabolism' is fiction, probably started by marketers for some hugely profitable cereal-producing company. According to Dr Michael VanDerschelden in his wonderfully researched book, *The Scientific Approach to Intermittent Fasting*, "Studies conducted right after a fasting period have shown a metabolic rate increase of 3.6 – 14% for up to 48 hours". He then goes on to say that our body does not see a slowdown in metabolic rate for a period of three or four days after our last meal.

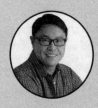

Dr Jason Fung

Most people expect that a period of fasting will leave them feeling tired and drained of energy. However, the vast majority of people experience the exact opposite. The increased adrenaline levels invigorate us and stimulate the metabolism. During a short-term fast, your body has enough glycogen available to function.

During a prolonged fast, your body can make new glucose from its fat stores - a process called gluconeogenesis (the 'making of new sugar'). Fat is burned to release energy, which is then sent out to the body. It is the fat-storage process in reverse.

Dr VanDerschelden also writes, "Think what it must have been like for humans in the hunter-gatherer days. These desirable traits of mind enhancement and energy would allow them to effectively search for food and kill prey, increasing survival. With that said, after several days of not eating, these intelligent adaptations would do more harm than good. We would not want our body to sustain a high metabolism and keep burning fuel three or four days after eating for fear of starvation".

So, there you have it – fasting doesn't decrease our metabolic rate but actually increases it. Therefore, let's assume we normally consume 2,500 calories a day spread across breakfast, lunch and dinner, but - if we fasted and ate them all in one meal we would start to lose weight because our metabolic rate would be marginally higher. Plus, what I experienced right from the very beginning with intermittent fasting is that we tend to eat way fewer calories in one meal than we would across three.

Let's also remember that the only reason humans carry fat is to feed the body when there is no food available. So, if we are overweight or obese, doesn't it make sense to use some of our existing fat reserves to power our body? Many times throughout this book you will read the statement, 'that's what we are designed to do', and put simply our body was designed to go through periodical cycles of feast and famine. Don't fear intermittent fasting – embrace it.

Dr Dan Maggs

I was never hungry in the mornings, but for many years I forced myself to eat breakfast because I thought it was the most important meal of the day. Would our primal ancestors have eaten when they weren't hungry? I don't think so!

Intermittent Fasting Prevents Numerous Diseases and Cures Others

The problem with eating little but often is that we constantly keep putting sugar back into our bloodstream. If we live constantly in feast mode, our liver and pancreas never get a break. As we read earlier, insulin is produced to carry poisonous sugar to our belly, bottom or thighs - and while it's active we simply cannot burn fat. But when we fast, insulin levels drop significantly and we turn into a fat-burning machine. The news gets better still. Our growth hormones (known as HGH) go through the roof when we fast. And as they are natural, they are far more powerful and beneficial than the synthetic ones that many athletes take to enhance performance.

What's more, our nervous system sends a little army of norepinephrines to our fat stores and they start breaking fat down into fatty acids that can be consumed as energy while we're fasting. It's kind of an either/or situation – either our body is focusing on creating insulin to deal with poisonous sugars or it is creating wonderfully beneficial

HGH. They are kind of mutually exclusive. They really don't get on together and hate being in the same room. For those who don't fast, it's one of the reasons why getting a good long sleep is important, as it's about the only time they can produce HGH. A report by the American College of Cardiology stated that fasting triggered a 1,300% increase in HGH secretion for women and a whopping 2,000% increase for men.

In periods of fasting our body goes into a mode of repairing, rebuilding and renewing our cells – virtually all of them. Plus, one of the biggest advantages is that we don't keep spiking our insulin levels, and as a result there is a greatly reduced risk of becoming diabetic, getting cancer or suffering from heart conditions. There is also growing evidence that it enhances several different brain functions and helps to prevent both Alzheimer's and Parkinson's disease. But there's also one factor that played a huge role in making intermittent fasting part of my lifestyle, and that is that fasting has now been scientifically proven to slow down the ageing process.

Dr Jason Fung

Regular fasting, by routinely lowering insulin levels, has been shown to significantly improve insulin sensitivity. This finding is the missing piece in the weight-loss puzzle. Most diets restrict the intake of foods that cause increased insulin secretion but don't address insulin resistance. You lose weight initially, but insulin resistance keeps your insulin levels and body set weight high. By fasting, you can efficiently reduce your body's insulin resistance since it requires both persistent and high levels. Insulin causes salt and water retention in the kidney, so lowering insulin levels rids the body of excess salt and water. Fasting is often accompanied by an early, rapid weight loss. For the first five days, weight loss averages 1.9 pounds (0.9 kilograms) per day, far exceeding the loss that could be expected from caloric restriction.

I think the most fascinating thing I read in Dr Michael VanDerschelden book *The Scientific Approach to Intermittent Fasting* was under the heading 'Top 10 Causes of Death' where he says, "Who would have thought that by doing an intervention like intermittent fasting, you could actually significantly go on to reduce your risk of the top two causes of death in the world, which are heart disease (cardiovascular disease) and cancer". Dr VanDerschelden then talks about how intermittent fasting can also prevent strokes (the fifth biggest killer) and of course we have already mentioned that it helps prevent Alzheimer's, which is the sixth largest cause of death. In addition, along with cutting out CARBS and other sugars, we know there is every chance we can avoid type 2 diabetes, which is the seventh biggest killer in the modern world.

There is another concept that I would like you to take to heart and it's called 'autophagy'. It is mentioned in many of the books I have researched, but one of the best and certainly simplest explanations I found was online, written by Nick English in July 2016: "It's a natural process called autophagy (literally 'self-eating'), and it's the body's system of cleaning house: Our cells create membranes that hunt out scraps of dead, diseased or worn-out cells; gobble them up; strip 'em for parts and use the resulting molecules for energy or to make new cell parts". Think of autophagy as our body's instinctive recycling programme. It sends faulty parts to the dustbin and at the same time stops cancerous growth.

The good news is that there are three ways to get our body to perform autophagy, and they are completely aligned to the principles of living primally:
1.   Consume a diet high in quality fats and low in carbohydrates.
2.   Embrace intermittent fasting.
3.   Do high impact intensity training (you will read about our approach to exercise in the next chapter).

While autophagy is the process, the actual garbage collectors are called lysosomes. They travel around the body constantly picking up the trash and performing a natural detox. But there is a small problem with lysosomes the older we get. They slow down and don't pick up the trash as efficiently as they did when we were younger. In our younger years, lysosomes are very much our heroes. But in our older years they become irresponsible and play a pivotal role in the ageing process. The single best solution in order to get them to do their detoxing job properly is intermittent fasting.

Why is this? My theory goes something like this. If a caveman was sitting in his cave constantly feasting, having all of his food brought to him on a plate and not having to go out to hunt or gather, then nature would be misled into thinking that everything was wonderful in his body and therefore there would be no need to deploy a task force to make repairs. However, the reality of a caveman's life was very different. He was constantly going from feast to famine. When he was eating, nature sat back and let him enjoy the spoils of his hard work, but when there was no food available and he started to feel hungry, nature began to get concerned. His body asked, 'Why has he not caught anything today? To ensure he catches dinner tomorrow, I better go and make sure I put everything into good working order'. The two main benefits of intermittent fasting are:

1.   It gives the body a break from food, allowing it time to enter a self-repair mode.
2.   It helps us to safely lose weight.

Dr Patrick Holford

There is a process of massive cellular repair, called autophagy, which means 'self-eating', which is triggered when you fast and switch to burning your own body fat. It can be triggered by low calories or also high fat, but it won't be triggered if you are doing a ketogenic diet with lots of meat and cheese and while you are building muscle. Because when you do weight training, you are telling your body to go into a growth phase and dairy products promotes a hormone called IGF-1, insulin-like growth factor, so while a high fat ketogenic diet with dairy products will help you lose weight, reverse diabetes and do all of these good things, it won't trigger autophagy. There is some great work by Professor Valter Longo in California. He has found that if you have five consecutive days, just five days of eating lower calories and a ketogenic diet; eat very low carbs and also low protein - there are certain things you can't eat because protein promotes growth - you can trigger cellular self-repair. Autophagy cleans up all our messed-up energy factories, called mitochondria, and it gobbles up cancer cells, and it gobbles up damaged proteins. It's like putting your car in for a service.

You don't have to do it forever, it's a short, sharp self-repair process. So maybe once a quarter or once a month if you are not well, do a five-day period, where you purposely trigger this self-repair process. It will be relatively high fat ketogenic, it will be very low carb, it can't have too much protein, it will be pretty much vegan, but you can have a little bit of fish. (I then asked Patrick what foods would keep us in autophagy and during the conversation, the following were mentioned: kale, seaweed, olives, cinnamon, coconut oil - specifically MCT C-8 - almond milk, almond butter, cacao powder, eggs, kimchi, asparagus, glucomannan, turmeric and vitamins).

But If I Intermittently Fast Won't I Lose Muscle Mass?

People considering fasting may ask themselves, 'Okay, so it doesn't slow down our metabolism, it reduces our chance of getting numerous diseases and is even considered by many as a way of curing type 2 diabetes, but don't those who intermittently fast lose muscle?'. Not true! If our caveman started to lose muscle on days when he couldn't catch lunch, then he would never catch an animal again. If it was true, the human race would likely be extinct, and you would not be reading this right now. After measuring my muscle mass after a 4-day fast, it had actually increased rather than decreased. According to research, for our body to consume our muscles as a source of energy when intermittent fasting, we would have to have less than 4% of our body as fat. Even elite sports people are rarely below 8%, so we most likely have quite a long way to go before burning up any muscle!

Remember that fat doesn't really consume much energy, but muscles do. So, we want to keep strong and healthy muscles because that way we burn more energy and the body finds it harder to put on weight. Have you noticed how most people who go on one of the many different diets that are based on restricting calories actually put on more weight after they quit? That's because when they diet, they lose muscle and when they stop dieting their reduced muscle mass burns fewer calories. Let me make it very clear that constantly going on diets is counterproductive, and it is detrimental to our health too. As I stated in the introduction, living primally is not a diet but a lifestyle. Because we don't have to count calories and instead work on understanding how different food types behave inside our body, it's simple to stick to and most importantly we get to eat lots of fantastic wholesome and tasty foods. Let's now look at the different ways of fasting. I recommend you read up on these and then just try whichever one you think fits in best with your daily routine.

The 5:2 Diet

The 5:2 Diet by Michael Mosley and Mimi Spencer is a great read for those who are sceptical about intermittent fasting. I fully recommend you purchase the 5:2 book before you start as it gives you both lots of tips on how to integrate fasting into your life, and more importantly will provide the motivation to keep you on the right track once you have started.

On the 5:2 diet, we eat normally for five days a week, and we get to choose which two days we restrict our calorie intake to just 600 calories for males and 500 calories for females. As long as we don't overeat on the other five days, then we have reduced our calorie intake by approximately 3,000 to 4,000 calories per week, and therefore mathematically should lose approximately a pound in weight each week. However, the authors are also believers in food with a low glycaemic index (GI) and high intensity training, so the likelihood is that if you follow the book closely, you will lose weight even faster. Remember I promised in the introduction of the book where I said that you wouldn't need to count calories? When it comes to fasting, for a short while you're going to need to. It's not that I lied in the beginning or that I forgot to mention this, it's just that it is going to take a few weeks into any of the above fasting programs for you to know what 500 or 600 calories looks like.

The 1:1 Diet or Alternate Day Fasting

The 1:1, or alternate day fasting, is similar to the 5:2 diet, but we alternate our fasting day with a normal day. This doesn't work for me because of my lifestyle, but thousands of people swear by it. Of course, what is great about this technique is that if we restrict our food intake to around 500 calories a day on our fasting days and managed to maintain it for a year (which believe it or not is easier than you might think once you get into it), 180 days of 500 calories a day sees us consuming around 360,000 calories less in a year, which equates to around 45kg or 100lb (more than seven stone). If you haven't got seven stone to lose, then once you have your body fat where you want it to be you can either slightly overeat on your non-fasting days, or move to the 5:2 method or even just fast once a week. Dr Krista Varady and Bill Gottlieb have written a great book promoting the merits of this approach called *The Every Other Day Diet*.

The 18-Hour Fast Diet

The 18-hour fast diet is where you commit to only eating in a six-hour timeframe each day, so that you are regularly fasting for 18 hours every day. This is very similar to the approach I use and it has now become a lifestyle that I find extremely easy to adhere too. I never feel hungry, I never feel like I am missing out, I always feel energised and my brain seems to be able to focus on things with much better clarity.

Dr Joanne McCormack

In my low carb groups, I suggest to people that they do time-restricted eating and intermittent fasting. One of my group leaders lost eight stone, and he does OMAD, which means he eats just One Meal a Day. I think when people say to you that's ridiculous, you do need to eat breakfast, you do need to eat several times a day, I think you should respond by saying something like, "Well yes you do, because you are a sugar burner and sugar burners need to eat more often than fat burners".

The Three- Or Four-Day Fast

With so many benefits of fasting, we might want to occasionally think about doing an extended fast. While there are many articles written and research done on fasting periods in excess of several weeks and in some cases even months, I haven't yet researched them sufficiently to entertain trying it for myself. And I would never recommend anything to others that I hadn't experimented with on myself.

I have tried and had wonderful experiences with three- and four-day fasts. While they may sound difficult to do, they actually get easier and easier the further into the fast we get. What's quite amazing is how the body reacts on a three- or four-day total fast. By day three, rather than feeling tired and sluggish like we might expect, we feel amazing and the body reaches peak performance. Research by the American Society for Clinical Nutrition carried out a study on people participating in elongated fasts and discovered that their basal metabolic rate (BMR) was at its highest on day three. Isn't that incredible? While most people believe our metabolism slows down if we even skip just one meal, it's actually at a peak on the third day of a fast! In fact, the same research showed that day three was also the day when those on the trial were at their maximum exercise capacity. So much for needing a sports gel and a bottle of sugar-loaded energy drink to be at our physical best.

Imagine the repair the body can do in three or four days without food. We really do starve all of those free radicals, especially those that like to kick-start cancer. We also stop or at least dramatically slow down any inflammation, and we give our guts time to complete a full spring clean of our entire digestive tract. I personally try to do a three- or four-day fast at least once every month. I recommend that once you have kicked the CARBS and experimented with either the 5:2, the alternate day fast or the 18-hour fast, that you pick a three or four day period where you know you have no dining commitments and give it a go. If in the unlikely, and I mean really unlikely event that it makes you feel ill, then you can always stop.

So as not to deplete the body's store of vitamins and minerals, one thing you might want to consider during a three or four day fast, is to increase the number of supplements that you take.

Dr Patrick Holford

When you fast, and you start to burn your body fat, your liver turns the fat into something called ketones. Ketones are a sort of new fuel. I got particularly interested when looking at brain cells, which is kind of my area of speciality, and if you feed a brain either glucose; sugar fuel, or ketones; fat fuel, the brain actually prefers ketones. Babies for their first six months of life are mainly running on ketones, and they are building up to 1 million connections in their brain per second. So, the brain loves ketones.

Starting Out

Let's say we have lots of weight to lose. We might start on the alternate day fasting method, and as we near our desired goal switch to the 5:2 diet. Then when we are happy with where we have arrived we move to the 18-hour fast. Here we get all the health benefits of fasting and our body gets to enter its repair mode every single day, but we are able to maintain our desired weight.

While fasting, we should of course continue to consume plenty of nutrients and minerals. And don't do what I did when I first started to fast and allow some of your calories to come from wine! During fast days we ideally shouldn't consume any alcohol, as we really want the body to fully maximise the benefit of its repairing mode.

Now, if on your first attempt you feel giddy, experience a headache or you really dislike the rumble in the stomach, then you have two options:

1. Just push on. Remember that this is how our body is designed to eat and you will soon get used to it. Personally, I have come to love the hungry feeling, because it's my body's way of sending me a message to say, "All is well boss, I am in repair mode and things are taking shape down here". But I confess it can take a bit of getting used too.
2. Don't give up, but instead for a few weeks don't drop straight to 500 calories but slowly start decreasing them on your fast day. Maybe try 1,200 calories for a few attempts, then when you have got used to it try 900 or 800.

But, whatever you do, no matter how hard you find it at first you must not give up. If you are on medication of any kind, then do check with your doctor before you try it. But try it you should, as it's crucial to our body to occasionally enter its natural repairing mode.

Professor Tim Noakes

Stephen Phinney talks about Europeans that went to live with the Inuits in the Arctic and ate a completely high-fat diet. For the first three or four days, they felt terrible and spent most of the time lying down. But after three weeks they had completely adapted, and they could do all of the activity that the Inuits could do. It just takes time to adapt.

Dr Jason Fung

Intermittent fasting tips:

1. Drink water: Start each morning with a full eight-ounce glass of water.
2. Stay busy: It'll keep your mind off food. It often helps to choose a busy day at work for a fast day.
3. Drink coffee: Coffee is a mild appetite suppressant. Green tea, black tea and bone broth may also help.
4. Ride the waves: Hunger comes in waves; it is not continuous. When it hits, slowly drink a glass of water or a hot cup of coffee. Often by the time you've finished, your hunger will have passed.

5. Don't tell everybody you are fasting: Most people will try to discourage you, as they do not understand the benefits. A close-knit support group is beneficial but telling everybody you know is not a good idea.
6. Give yourself one month: It takes time for your body to get used to fasting. The first few times you fast may be difficult, so be prepared. Don't be discouraged. It will get easier.
7. Follow a nutritious diet on non-fast days: Intermittent fasting is not an excuse to eat whatever you like. During non-fasting days, stick to a nutritious diet low in sugars and refined carbohydrates.
8. Don't binge: After fasting, pretend it never happened. Eat normally, as if you had never fasted.
9. The last and most important tip is to fit fasting into your own life! Do not limit yourself socially because you're fasting. Arrange your fasting schedule so that it fits in with your lifestyle.

Fasting Conclusion

It's important to experiment a little and find an intermittent fasting regime that works for you. But don't even think of trying to fast until you are on a low CARB diet as it will be too difficult and unpleasant. Once you have moved over to the colourful side of life and ditched all the starchy, sugary white and beige boring stuff, you will find intermittently fasting a breeze. One of the key things to try is to fit fasting into your life rather than your life around fasting. You don't need to do it in any type of rhythm. Because of social events and family holidays, you might find it harder in the summer months or at Christmas, but that's absolutely fine. When the time is right, just return to a method of fasting that suits your needs. I personally tend to mix it all up. Most weekdays ,if I am working, I don't eat anything all day and then just have an evening meal. At the weekends or on holiday, I might sit down and have a little breakfast with the kids. Then, once a month or so I will try to do a three- or four-day fast. I love them, I really do. By day three I feel on top of the world – full of energy, totally liberated and buzzing from consuming nothing but my own body fat. Regardless of which approach you finally settle into, let me summarise some of the potential benefits you might experience by becoming part of the intermittent fasting generation:

- Improved memory
- Slowing the ageing process
- Better concentration
- Reduced inflammation
- Lower heart rate
- Less fatty liver
- Reduced blood pressure
- Increase fat burning
- Decreased leptin
- Increased insulin sensitivity
- Decreased risk of cancer

Dr James DiNicolantonio

I like to take the concept of 'do what works best for you'. For me, skipping breakfast is so easy. I will say, though, for me if I worked out in the gym very hard say the evening before, I might not skip breakfast, I might eat three or four pastured eggs. When you want to build muscle, eat more protein, eat more food. When you want to start breaking down your body's old cells through autophagy, then fast. Fasting isn't like some weird voodoo thing. If our primal ancestors couldn't catch an animal or find any plants that day, then there were times where they would just fast. If you are a healthy person, you could fast for weeks, the body can do that, but you have to be careful because a lot of people aren't healthy. And you have got to be careful about the vitamins and minerals you are losing when fasting. So I like to think about it as doing periods of longer fasting, say a two day fast every couple of months, seems to provide additional benefit. Especially in people who have cancer, if you fast two or three days prior to chemotherapy, there are numerous studies showing that you get less radiation damage, less side effects and even improved outcomes.

When you restrict particularly protein but also sugar in the diet while fasting, you start activating longevity enzymes such as AMPK, FGF21 and these signals are not only improving insulin sensitivity, so when you get your next meal your body is going to absorb the nutrients better, but you are breaking down all the old and damaged cells.

Go Ketogenic Go Go

You have surely guessed by now that we believe that CARBS and other sugars are pretty much evil stuff. All wheat, grain, potatoes, rice, pasta etc gets turned into sugar in the body, then insulin comes to our rescue and caries the poisonous sugar off to our fat deposits and stores it as a future source of energy. However, the only time we can ever access this fat store is when there is virtually no insulin in our bloodstream. When insulin is limited and when we restrict the supply of new energy, we enter a state of what is known as ketosis. Here the body produces ketones (turning your fat into a usable energy source) to replace the sugar in our bloodstream. How do we get into a state of ketosis? Either we intermittently fast or our diet is very high in fat and very low in carbohydrates – preferably both!

Gary Taubes

If you are hypertensive, the evidence is pretty compelling that if you give up carbs, if you eat a ketogenic diet or you eat a low carb high-fat diet or Atkins, or whatever you want to call it, your blood pressure will come down significantly.

Ketosis, Ketones, Ketogenic and Ketoacidosis... What Are The Differences?

- Ketosis – when we eat very few CARBS and a diet high in fat, eventually we turn our body from running on sugar to running on fat. An analogy would be like knowing that diesel engines aren't any good for the environment, therefore we modify our car so it can run on electric. Ketosis is a metabolic state where we are burning ketones for fuel, not glucose. And by the way it's a truly wonderful free ride when we eventually get there.

- Ketones – is the name of the fuel. Simplifying it a little, glucose (sugar) is one type of fuel and ketones (fat) is another.
- Ketogenic Diet – a ketogenic diet is one whereby we eat very small amounts of CARBS (almost exclusively green ones), moderate protein and lots of organic, healthy and delicious fats.
- Ketoacidosis – even though its name sounds similar, this has nothing to do with any of the above. Ketoacidosis is a dangerous medical condition whereby there is a build-up of acid in the blood. It's a dangerous medical condition that mostly happens to people with type 1 diabetes who forget to take their insulin. The only reason I even mention it is that sometimes you will hear people saying that a ketogenic diet is dangerous. As they say, a little knowledge is often dangerous, and they are simply confusing two different things. Being in a ketosis metabolic state is what we were designed to do!

Where do ketones get produced? While insulin is created by the pancreas, ketones are produced by the liver. Just like a powerful motorbike that has been sat in the garage for too long, if we have been eating a diet high in CARBS and haven't intermittently fasted before, it might take a while to kick-start our ketone machine into order, but once it fires up we begin to feel like a completely different person. This period of firing up our ability to consume our own body fat as an energy source is known as the keto-adaptation period.

On a normal diet where we restrict calories, if we do manage to burn more than we consume then, while we might lose a little weight, we will most likely feel sluggish and irritable. If we are still eating CARBS but just fewer of them, our body will still be using the sugar as energy and only dipping into our fat store after its sugar supply becomes completely exhausted. I describe it as the body is in a state of confusion – it doesn't know which way to turn. To our body, using CARBS for energy is as simple as opening up the breadbin in our kitchen. It requires minimal effort. The food supply might not be the cleanest or the healthiest, but it is easily accessed. But to use our own fat, it's like going down into the basement to open the freezer. The food here is definitely safer, but it's a pain to keep going downstairs to get it. What we need to do is to tell our brain that the breadbin is not going to be filled up again. We need to tell it to stop looking there for fuel and to go and get all the food from the freezer downstairs and to put it in the fridge right next to the breadbin, which is going unfilled.

This conversion normally takes around two weeks of severely restricted CARB intake for the body to understand how to enter ketosis without any effort. It might take as long as six weeks if we have really damaged our metabolism through many years of CARB indulgence. The first days can leave us a little light on energy, but it soon passes and before we know it we will have more energy than ever. Once we have become keto-adaptive, rather than relying on the 2,000 to 2,500 maximum calories that our body can store in the form of glucose and glycogen, depending on our weight we will instead have access to more than 40,000 to 100,000 calories sitting there switched on and waiting for us to deploy as required! I know which fuel tank I would rather be able to access. But remember, it takes a while for the body to know where to look and this is the only time on the primal journey where patience is a virtue.

For over 20 years, while I didn't enjoy it, in an attempt to lose my big belly, I would endure several weekly jogs. But no matter how many miles I clocked up, I never did reduce the size of my gut. We can exercise as much as we like – we can run for miles or cycle for hours, but if we have sugar or insulin in our body we are not going to lose any weight. We can't burn fat in the presence of CARBS, sugar, insulin or starch. Period!

Nina Teicholz

One of the criticisms of going on a keto diet is some people say it's hard and it's not sustainable. But what is harder? It is harder to live as an obese person. It's harder to take four or five pills every day. It's harder to live with diabetes and inject yourself with insulin every day. And people say it's not sustainable. But there is plenty of research to show it is sustainable. But what is harder to sustain is to be sick. Not being able to walk up a flight of stairs. Feeling so bad, you can't go to work. Feeling depressed and lousy. And constantly being on medication and getting fatter and fatter. That is what is unsustainable. But it is a challenge. When I lived in the UK for a while, I used to love your huge Dairy Milk chocolate bars and all of your bread. And if you had said to me then that I had to give it all up, I would have said forget it. There is no way that I can live without it. But what actually happens is your palate, and your taste buds change. Your want, and desire, for sweetness completely goes away. It's amazing, and you wouldn't think that is possible. But it does. What tastes sweet to me now is that 90% dark chocolate. And now, sweeter than that and I don't like it. But I couldn't have imagined that before. But your palate does change.

Understanding Ketosis

Our body has two main sources of fuel: sugar/glucose produced from CARBS or burning fat through ketosis. Our body doesn't really differentiate between incoming fat or stored body fat, as it can produce ketones from either. Once we learn to switch on our ketosis metabolism, when we restrict incoming calories, losing weight becomes both a breeze and enjoyable.

Before we look at burning ketones, let's go back to what prevents us losing our fat. As we have discussed already, when we eat CARBS our body converts them to sugar, and, as our body regards sugar as both fuel and poison, our pancreas creates insulin that takes the glucose and either helps us burn it if we need the energy immediately or dispatches it to our fat stores.

While insulin is active, even if we are on a long run or cycle ride, it prevents us from using our body fat as fuel. This is where I personally went wrong for so many years. I could never understand why I wasn't losing weight even when I was running three or four mornings a week. I just didn't realise it was the pizza the night before, or the early morning orange juice and cereal, that was secretly ganging up on me and sending their by-product insulin to render all my good intentions and painstaking efforts worthless.

So, before we can even start burning our body fat and entering a state of ketosis, we must rid our body of as much sugar/CARBS/insulin as possible. Once we have insulin under control, our body will turn to our fat stores for energy. Then, when we open the door of our fat store, our body releases energy in the form of ketones. Ketones are effectively an alternative fuel source to sugar/glucose. Not just energy to drive our vital organs, but as fuel for our muscles and brain too. In fact ketones are the fuel of preference for our brain, heart, liver and muscles, yet many individuals haven't been able to supply this rich energy source since they were infants consuming their mother's breast milk!

Once we open the door and enter our fat stores we are said to be in 'ketosis'. Until we enter ketosis it is impossible to lose body weight. For decades, as I stood on my bathroom scales after my early morning runs, the scales always showed that I had duly lost weight as a result of my hard hour slogging my guts out. But I was misinterpreting the results. Because I always had sugar/insulin in my body, it was preventing me entering ketosis and therefore all I had really lost was water and not fat. It is so important to understand this that I am going to repeat myself one more time.

During that long jog or cycle, we will be putting stress on our joints and limbs while not really gaining any benefit, and most likely do more harm than good. Plus, as we will be burning lots of calories, we are sure to replace them with even more CARBS and other sugars as soon as we finish. Remember, just like nicotine makes a smoker want another cigarette as soon as it starts to exit the body, as insulin gets burnt it makes us crave more sugar and empty calories. I would like to blame the food corporations exclusively for this addiction. While it is true that in many cases, just like they do with cigarettes, manufacturers insert chemicals into food to make us crave them or even worse become addicted, Mother Nature had a hand in it too.

You see, at the end of the summer when she knew food was about to become scarce, she loaded her bushes and trees with sugar-rich fruit. To ensure that our caveman ancestors ate as much as they possibly could, stocking up their internal fat stores for the barren cold winter, she made it possible for us to consume CARBS, store them quickly and then fool our brain to eat even more. She effectively shut down the creation of the 'I am full hormone' leptin, so our caveman took on board and stored as much calories as possible.

While today the vast majority of adults in the Western world never enter a state of ketosis, primal man spent far more time in ketosis than out of it and if you were breastfed from birth you previously did too. In his brilliant book *Keto Clarity* author Jimmy Moore explains that within 12 hours of being delivered into the world we enter a state of ketosis, with ketones from our mother's milk providing around a quarter of our total energy. What I also found fascinating was that breast milk is rich in MCTs, which is what coconuts provide by the bucket-load. It is for this very same reason why much packaged baby milk contains either coconut oil or MCT oil. It is too early in the book to go off on a tangent and start talking about one of my favourite subjects, but for your health's sake please do everything possible from this point forward to fall in love with coconuts. They are simply one of nature's miracle foods and can actually accelerate the speed at which we enter the metabolic state of ketosis. So much so, that in order to bring forward the entry point into ketosis, many people now take MCT supplements.

Because our primal forefathers often went days without catching food, and during the winter ate very sparsely, they were constantly engaged in an intermittent fast orchestrated by nature. It's important to remember that when the supply of CARBS and protein is low, our body will run on fat. It doesn't distinguish from stored fat or free fat. Our stored fat, whether it is from our buttocks, love handles or waistline, results in exactly the same ketones as the fat we eat. So our caveman ancestors didn't have to worry about balancing their food, the fact that their bellies were often empty meant their ketosis metabolism kicked in automatically once their glucose and glycogen was depleted.

If we have a lot of weight to shed and really want to shift it, then one sure way to do so is to avoid as many CARBS as possible (even the good ones for a short while) and enter into a state of ketosis. If we can exercise as well and remain in ketosis for prolonged periods, then our weight should drop off. Warning: Don't drop the green CARBS (broccoli, spinach, etc) for long as we need to eat healthy CARBS such as leafy green vegetables and low-sugar fruits. The only time we should drop them from our diet might be for just a few weeks while we teach our body how to enter ketosis.

So how do we become keto-adaptive? We need to get our daily CARB intake to below 50g and ideally these should come from complex CARBS such as leafy greens. Jeff S. Volek, PhD, RD, and Stephen D. Phinney, MD, PhD in their book *The Art and Science of Low Carbohydrate Performance* sum it up brilliantly: "When it comes to cereals, breads, pasta, potatoes, pastry, candy, juices or other carb-dense foods we'll say it once… just don't go there. Because all of these are like the nuclear option in suppressing ketones, we've started calling them 'carbage'". They have created this wonderful word 'carbage' by combining CARB and garbage, and I think it should be added to the English dictionary!

Now you might wonder why I say low CARB, moderate protein and lots of quality fats. Why do we need to be careful of our protein intake? Aren't proteins the good guys? Yes, proteins are the good guys, and play a crucial role in our wellbeing. However, our body is really clever. It has the ability to turn protein into sugar. In the absence of CARBS, the body turns any excess protein into sugar and therefore while attempting to enter ketosis we need to be careful not to overdo the protein. If you remember back to chapter 1, I said that while the body must intake protein and fats to survive, it can function happily forever without a single CARB. Now we are getting into the detail, let me explain that the body does occasionally need glucose to function. If it can't locate it when it's needed, through a process called gluconeogenesis, it synthesises it from proteins. This is really important to understand if we want to either enter ketosis or lose weight, or more commonly both! While protein is undoubtedly vital to our survival and a critical macronutrient for our body's self-repair mechanisms, when we consume too much of it, in the absence of CARBS our body will convert any excess into the same by-product of CARBS – sugar.

Although we don't count calories, while we are training our body to enter ketosis it's ideal to aim for around 20% of our calories from green CARBS and protein and 80% from healthy fats. But remember these are just guidelines and every single one of us is different. For example, because I have damaged my metabolism so badly in the past, I only have to look at CARBS to put on weight. Seriously, it seems I am that sensitive to processed CARBS I only have to sniff a pizza and my waistline bulges! And the same happens when I consume too much protein. I seem fine with 30g of protein during or immediately after a workout, but on days when I am not exercising, I have to be just as strict about my protein intake as I am about CARBS.

As counting calories is not primal, a simple summary for ketosis is – virtually no CARBS, reduced protein and double our quality fat intake.

So, if we want to enter ketosis, it's all about maximising the amount of healthy fats we consume. But which fats I here you cry? We will learn about all of these little miracles of nature in detail later, but for now here is a snapshot of what can help us make up the 80% fat part of the diet:

- Organic grass-fed fatty meat (no need to trim the fat off)
- Oily fish
- Butter from organic grass-fed cows
- Extra virgin olive oil
- Coconut oil or coconut milk
- Coconut chunks
- Avocado or extra virgin avocado oil

Nina Teicholz

When you convert over to becoming a fat burner, it's a difficult process at first, because you have to develop all of these different enzymes to be able to run off fat. And why do you want to operate off of fat? What is the benefit of that? Well, I will tell you that the simplest benefit is that once you become a fat burner, you don't just operate off the fat you eat, when you are not eating, you operate off the fat of your body. Fat on your body is not just a curse that God gave you to mess up your teenage years, or whatever. It's a genius invention. It's like having granola bars strapped all over your body. To your body, it's like, well, while I don't have food right here on the table in front of me, I will just use this excess bit of fat here on my hips or my stomach for energy. Your stored fat is supposed to be your backup source of fuel. But you can't access that fat on your body unless you know how to be a fat burner. How do you do that? You have to reduce glucose.

Because glucose is an easier fuel to burn, while it's in your system, you will never consume your own body fat. And that is why, to lose weight, you have to reduce carbohydrates. Once you keep carbs low for a while, your body will automatically learn how to burn an alternative fuel source which is fat. And this process can take a while. That's why some diets such as Atkins, advise you go super low on carbs at the beginning, to speed up the transition time. It will make the switch happen faster. But for people who are metabolically unwell and have had poor metabolisms for a long time, it can take a month to six weeks, and it can be painful. You can have nausea, headaches etc. It's also why some people give up within a few weeks. They think something like, "I feel terrible, this can't be right, this can't be good for me". But people need to understand, that is just your body undergoing a huge transformation. Just like people giving up smoking or alcohol, it takes a while, but you have to get to the other side. When you arrive at the other side, you feel great. You feel better, lose weight, you recover from other illnesses, and symptoms that you didn't even know were diet-related. For example, I had no idea my own chronic sinus infections were related to my diet. I had taken antibiotics multiple times every winter, and yet since going low carb, I haven't had a single problem for years.

Is Ketosis Healthy?

My wife's first impression was no, it's not! A side effect of being in ketosis is that one of the three different kinds of ketones, acetone, is primarily detected in our breath. And boy does it sometimes smell very pungent! The first time I went into the blissful state of ketosis, my wife was so convinced that I had a stomach ulcer she pleaded with me to go to the doctor. However, I was feeling wonderful and healthy and knew that there was nothing wrong. It was only recently that I discovered that my initial bad breath was just the body learning how to burn its new clean fuel. If the same happens to you, then just chew on some fresh mint until it goes away. I believe that bad breath for a few days is a small price to pay for something that can slow down the ageing process, reduces the risk of such horrible diseases as cancer (remember cancer needs glucose to fuel its growth) and improves virtually all cognitive functions, so much so that many specialists are recommending ketogenic diets for Alzheimer's sufferers. In addition it:

- Helps accelerate weight loss
- Improves the quality of sleep
- Benefits the skin and can eradicate acne
- Helps hormones better control appetite
- Lowers blood pressure
- Makes it far easier to intermittently fast
- Provides the body with a superior amount of energy
- Increases testosterone for a better sex drive
- Improves moods and fights depression
- Increases the good cholesterol HDL

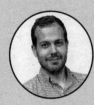

Dr Dan Maggs

I lost nearly five stone (31kg) on a ketogenic diet. It works by allowing your body to access all the energy you have stored as fat. Aside from that, the feeling of clarity and energy you get when your brain is mainly running on ketones is incredible.

Hannah Richards

Being hungry and having periods of fasting carry many health benefits for the body. We hear and say the phrase 'I'm hungry' quite a lot, but most of the time we don't actually mean it. However, when we do say it, all that has really happened is food has been completely emptied out of the stomach. Food passes out of your stomach into the duodenum and it can sometimes make a few gurgling noises which we associate with hunger, and of course you may well be hungry. However, hunger as we experience it will be vastly different from the way other cultures in history and in various places around the world today experience it. It is also something we will most likely be fortunate never to truly experience in our lifetime.

Having a juice day or a liquid day is an equally good thing to do to give your digestive system a rest. It is often overloaded, over-packed and overworked on a regular basis, which is why giving it a rest with a fast day can be beneficial and boost your microbiota, too!

Chapter 5 Highlights

- Fasting doesn't decrease our metabolic rate but actually increases it.
- The best diet is one that mirrors our 'feast and famine' history and gives the body sufficient resting periods in which to heal itself.
- Primal Alignment: Our caveman ancestors didn't plan their famine and feasts, their food supply always dictated it.
- If possible, vary your fasting styles just like our primal ancestors did. Without fridges or fast foods, the only eating routine they had was no routine.
- There is no such thing as losing body weight, we instead have to burn it. And we can only truly burn it when we have become keto-adaptive.
- Our body can only use one fuel source at a time, either glucose or ketones. Over time, on a very low CARB, medium protein and high fat diet, our brain acts primally and turns to our fat deposits as its primary source of fuel.

CHAPTER 6

OPTIMISE EXERCISE

"If I could give every individual the right amount of nourishment and exercise, not too little and not too much, we would have found the safest way to health."
HIPPOCRATES

In this chapter we discuss the basics of exercise and how we are designed to benefit from short, intense bursts of physical activity and how our obsession over the past 50 years with endurance sports has caused havoc with our body.

When it comes to exercise, we need to stop worrying about our chronological age and instead focus on our biological age. Our chronological age is just a number. I hate it when I hear someone claiming, "I'm too old to exercise". To my mind the term 'old' should be permanently replaced with 'older'. We're never old, we're only ever older. People in remote villages around the world, where they are living into their 120s, might have earned the right to claim they are old, but for the rest of us, we should just consider ourselves as older. Unless someone suffers from a physical disability, the vast majority of the following advice is applicable to everyone, regardless of age.

Here are the two most important and most fundamental principles of living primally:
1. We must eat what we are designed to eat.
2. We must exercise in a way that's as close to ancestral daily life as possible.

Dr Aseem Malhotra
A colleague and friend of mine, a truly inspirational man called Dr Tim Noakes, a professor of sports science, says that if you have to exercise to keep your weight down, your diet is wrong. And, the point is, you can't outrun a bad diet. You can't outrun your fork! I was

involved in exposing this in an article I wrote in the *British Journal of Sports Medicine* in 2015, where I wrote that it was time to bust the myth of physical inactivity and obesity, in that you cannot outrun a bad diet.

To capture in its entirety my primal approach to fitness, we are going to use an easily remembered acronym, MOMMS, for 'Max Out' – 'Move More' – 'Sprint'.

Max Out refers to our approach to weight training, where we use a specific type of routine that safely and efficiently pushes us to the max. We then focus on 'moving more' in our everyday life and eventually get to build a couple of extremely short 'sprints' into our weekly routine. These three separate areas of fitness build muscles and at the same time increase our flexibility and help us feel younger for longer.

The principle behind my MOMMS approach is to emulate what our primal ancestors did during daylight. It is about lifting heavy rocks (in our case weights), moving more and occasionally sprinting. It is not about laborious hours on a treadmill or exercise bike, nor is it about attending the latest craze in keep-fit classes. Caveman didn't jog for hours on end, nor did he take part in endurance cycle events. After all, the wheel hadn't been invented throughout most of human evolution!

What we desire is to be fit, but not at the expense of our health. What do I mean by that? Well there are lots of athletic people that put their body through hell on the running and cycling track, which in the short term might make them look fit, but in the long term potentially leads to an onslaught of health problems.

Research carried out by Dr James O'Keefe at the Mid America Heart Institute at St Luke's Hospital, suggests that people who exercise regularly live seven years longer than those who are physically inactive. No surprise there really. However, his latest research revealed something that will most likely astonish you and that is; 'Those individuals who participated in extreme endurance sports experienced significant heart damage'. More on this later.

Throughout this chapter, I will keep trying to highlight that MOMMS is the safest and most reliable way to achieve healthy longevity, and that the jogging fraternity and long-distance cyclists (and for three decades I wore both caps), run the risk of causing themselves a lot of long-term damage.

Let me start by introducing you to a highly relevant scientific concept: hormesis. It's a geeky word summarising the saying "a little of what doesn't kill you makes you stronger". An example of hormesis would be a vaccination, where we are injected with a small dose of the very thing the vaccination is trying to protect against. Stress is another example of hormesis. A small amount of stress is a good thing, while a large amount can kill you. Too much stress is linked to all sorts of horrible diseases, including cardiovascular and cancer. But a small amount of stress, as in the type caused by sprinting or by weightlifting, is a good thing. Sadly, we can't say the same about jogging long distances for hours on end, which can cause unhealthy damaging levels of stress. My exercise principles are geared around hormesis.

Move More

Caveman didn't jump in a car and sit in a two-hour traffic jam on the way to an office, where he sat for seven hours before going home to slump in front of the TV. Put simply, in Great Britain we don't move enough.

Even 40 years ago, I can remember my mother carrying half a dozen heavy grocery bags in each hand, the handles cutting into her fingers, half a mile from the nearest shop. Today what do we do? So that we don't have to push the shopping trolley too far, we drive around the supermarket car park multiple times trying to find a space as close to the entrance as possible! It's terrible to think how inactive we have become.

If you are overweight or obese and just beginning to live primally, then it is important to pay a little attention to that old saying, 'don't run before you can walk'. In fact, we don't want you to run at all, ever… well, unless a lion is chasing you. Looking at the three distinct areas of MOMMS – Max Out – Move More – Sprint – I am going to advise that you start moving more immediately, so depending on your current circumstances, potentially leave the weightlifting for a short while and only entertain sprinting when your weight is well under control.

In the Move More phase, it's crucial for our health, especially if currently you live a very sedentary lifestyle, that you start to move about a lot more on your feet. Get outdoors in the fresh air, walking, gardening, hiking, skiing, rowing, it really doesn't matter what it is, but get moving. Get involved with a swimming class or bowls or anything that gets you moving, but not so much that you're out of breath. Now there is a good reason I don't want you out of breath, because I want to have a clear distinction between movement and exercise. Both are vital for our health, but both perform very different functions.

I always tell my children to take the stairs and not the lift, but if this gets you out of breath, don't do it just yet, as that would be exercise and until our weight starts to fall off, we want to concentrate on just getting moving. Even 2,000 years ago, Hippocrates - the father of western medicine - told us, "Walking is man's best medicine".

If you live a few miles from work, try to walk there occasionally. If you live too far away, then park a mile or so from your destination and walk the last part. You will be amazed how you feel. Sir Richard Branson likes to get dropped off a mile or so from a meeting and walk. He will also often hold meetings with his directors while walking. Richard is patron of a charity my brother John and I started called The Colourful Life Foundation, and whenever we are with him it's interesting to see how he rarely sits still; he is on his feet at every opportunity.

Dr Shan Hussain

One foot in front of the other. A study presented at the European Society of Cardiology Congress in 2015, showed that 25 minutes of brisk walking a day could add up to seven years to your life and halve the risk of dying from a heart attack.

Max Out

While I truly believe that 80% of our health is shaped in the kitchen and only 10% in the gym, (with the other 10% being made up of combination of such things as sleep, stress and sunshine), I believe that, for numerous reasons, it is important to look after our muscles.

To understand the *Max Out* principle, which is a modified version of HIIT – High Intensity Interval Training – we need to go back and look at the daily activities of our primal ancestors. After a successful hunt, to get their catch back to their dwelling, they would carry small animals across their shoulders, or drag heavier ones by their hooves. While out gathering, without modern tools they would hack down trees and move heavy rocks looking for mushrooms and other fungi. None of these activities would take hours and hours, but our primal ancestors must have been able to muster great strength when required. Therefore, our body is designed, and in fact programmed, to do occasional bouts of heavy lifting.

But before you rush out and start lifting heavy weights, let's invest some time in planning what our workout should look like. To start, we need to understand the concept of homeostasis. Every cell and system in our body relies on a stable environment to function. Homeostasis refers to the internal balance the body must maintain to ensure health. When we exercise, we break down our muscles (catabolic process) and then ask our body to rebuild them (anabolic process) stronger and bigger than before.

Unless we lift heavy things, our body no longer engages in any meaningful level of catabolism, but for our primal ancestors the balance was perfect. They had to expend energy to catch and gather their food (catabolic) and then while feasting on their kill for several days their body had time to rebuild its muscles (anabolic). If the only exercise we do is opening the door to the grocery deliveryman or Deliveroo cyclist, then our homeostasis is going to be well out of whack.

Here are five reasons (and medically there are many more) why you need to maintain or build muscle:

1. It burns more energy than body fat.
2. It support our joints and bones.
3. It reduce the risk of injury.
4. It replicate the lifestyle of our primal ancestors.
5. It helps maintain homeostasis.

How Often Should I Max Out?

The good news is we are not talking about training every day and each session should not take more than 30 minutes! When we exercise too frequently, our muscles may actually shrink (atrophy) rather than grow (hypertrophy). The science behind the problems caused by over-training goes something like this: When we exercise our muscles but don't completely deplete them of glycogen, they actually can suffer atrophy. By leaving glycogen in the muscles each day while at the gym, it slowly begins to reduce the energy storage capacity in each cell in the muscle. To make matters worse, if during our gym session we do too many repetitions and sets, the exercise becomes more aerobic (with oxygen), which can cause a build-up of dangerous free radicals (more on this later).

We are all built differently. Our age, sex and current fitness level plays a big part in how quickly our muscles recover between sessions, and therefore what our recovery period should be. I know from personal experience that when I have completed a gym session where I have been truly in the zone, my body almost tells me not to train for at least a week. But then in other sessions, where I just couldn't motivate myself or push myself hard enough, I am itching to do another session, just two or three days later. Quality of sleep, diet, alcohol consumption, dehydration and even how stressed we are, can all play a big part in determining how quickly our muscles recover from exercise. And remember that all movement and exercise is accumulative. If we weight train on a Monday and then take in a game of golf or a yoga class on Tuesday or Wednesday, we might find we are not feeling ready for the next gym session for an extra day or two. My personal approach is that as long as I do at least one weight training session a week and walk plenty of miles, then the rest of the time I just listen to my body.

Age also plays a part in training frequency. In our late thirties or early forties, we start to lose muscles (known as sarcopenia). If we don't exercise, we lose as much as 5% of muscle every decade. Sarcopenia increases the older we get, and by our seventies shifts into top gear. But, as we age, because we often can't quite lift the same big weights as we did in our youth, ideally we need to increase the frequency of our exercise sessions. But once again, I can't emphasise enough that we are all built differently and that we should use the above as guidelines, while in the main listening to our body for when to hit the gym. One last thought on exercising as we age – in reality we should see more 70-year-olds bench pressing in the gym than we do those in their twenties! Brad Schoenfeld in his book *Science and Development of Muscle Hypertrophy* says, "After age 40, the body loses progressively more muscle mass each year. Regular resistance training can reduce this loss. Although the elderly do have a diminished hypertrophic response, they can gain muscle mass; however, a greater weekly training dose appears necessary to maintain the gains".

As we get older, losing muscles not only reduces our strength, but also leads to a serious decline in metabolic function. And that's really important, because keeping our metabolic system healthy by maintaining our muscle mass helps slow down the ageing process, fuels the brain and helps protect us against metabolic syndrome.

Time Under Load

Okay, so now we have a guideline on how often to hit the gym, let's state something quite obvious – do everything you can to avoid injury. I say this because I constantly meet people who injure themselves training and spend as much time laid-up as they actually do in the gym. Certainly, the older we get, as our recovery time gets longer and longer we really need to make avoiding injury a top priority.

My preferred method of exercise, which is also one of the safest, isn't to swing huge weights using momentum, but to keep each repetition nice and strict, really focusing the mind on the muscles we want to work on. Without the ability to isolate which muscle we want to work on, then the approach we are going to discuss will not prove as effective as it otherwise could be. This might sound a little vain but stand in front of a mirror and pose like a bodybuilder on stage. Try first without any weights to tense the muscle you intend to work on. This will send a signal to the brain and help focus its attention. Let's say we want to work our biceps. We should be able to tense them for about a minute and really feel a burning sensation without lifting any weights at all. This heightened awareness (known as kinesthesia – pronounced 'kenes-teez-ya') increases our ability to better target the muscle we want to exercise.

This *Max Out* method might sound a little strange to some readers at first, but I assure you, regardless of age, it works. Before you even lift your first weights, I would recommend that you take some measurements and store them in my Primal Living app. Once you have got all of your vital statistics noted, it's time to head off to the gym. It's really beneficial, especially in your first few sessions, to use the Primal Living app. It's totally free and really easy to use and give you advice, photos and videos on more than 100 different exercises. It also allows you to log your progress, which is great news because as you start to eat and exercise primally, you will be amazed at how quickly you will build strength.

Let me now explain what I mean by 'time under load'. Using a watch or a clock, or better still the Primal Living app, we are going to slowly and deliberately carry out each and every repetition (one complete motion of the exercise), whether it be a press-up or bicep curl, a pull-down or deadlift. These deliberately unhurried repetitions should take between six and 20 seconds depending both on our preference and the actual exercise we are doing. Our aim is to keep going until we reach complete failure. This is where we just can't move the weight any further without cheating. Once we hit this point, there are great gains to be made by not putting the weight down but continuing to push to the max for around ten more seconds.

Even without the weights moving, while we are holding for these last seconds, in a phase of exercise called 'isometric training' or 'static contraction', we should in most exercises find our muscles twitching or whole parts of our body shaking. Don't panic, hang in there. At this point, and this point only, do we class that we have reached *Max Out*. Unless we *Max Out*, we will still have spare glycogen in our muscles, and will most likely limit our growth.

Our ability to push to our true max, and the more microtrauma we can inflict on our muscles at a cellular level, combined with sufficient rest time, determines our success. Remember, weight training and sprinting are very different exercises to endurance jogging. They are polar opposites. Endurance sports are aerobic (with oxygen) and interval training is anaerobic (without oxygen). Effectively when we do short intense exercise, our muscles don't have time to take on board oxygen or fuel. Our body is forced to use an energy supply within our muscle cells called glycogen. When our muscles burn glycogen they produce lactic acid, which if I simplify it a little is what causes the burn we sometimes experience when weightlifting.

I want to explain a little further about what's happening inside our muscles as we exercise by using the analogy of a sponge. If we *Max Out* properly, we are effectively wringing out the sponge so that there is no water (or energy in our muscle's case) left inside. Once our glycogen has gone, our sponge will soak up everything it possibly can to replace it. Any sugars floating around the body will be quickly grabbed by our muscles before insulin has a chance to hand it over to our fat stores. What's more, we will be producing far less insulin as well, as our muscles will be hungry for any sugars and will temporarily make insulin semi-redundant. It's also why, when we eat straight after a training session, our muscles are said to grow. But be aware, this is not the same for aerobic exercises where the muscles aren't fully depleted.

Let's get back to *Maxing Out*. At that point, when the movement has stopped and you have held for roughly 10 seconds more, note down the time. For most exercises we are targeting the total time from starting to *Max Out* to be between 45 and 120 seconds. The total time is what we refer to as Time Under Load. If we didn't manage to last 45 seconds, then in our next session we must decrease the weight.

If we managed to do more than 120 seconds, then in our next session we are going to add more weight. Remember my earlier point 'we can't manage what we can't measure'? What we are looking for over a period of a few months is to be able to slowly increase the weight and still last for between 45 to 120 seconds. Once we start to increase the heaviness, we will have proven, beyond doubt that we have become stronger.

Primal Exercising Tips
1. Download the free Primal Living app. It will help you both measure your sessions and also motivate you to push just that little bit harder.
2. Remember that with some exercises, great things can be achieved even with very small weights or even static contraction exercises (just holding the muscle tense without movement).
3. With *Max Out* we achieve greater results by putting all of our effort into just one set per session. In other words, just performing each exercise once.
4. To ensure we *Max Out*, it is not possible to aim for a precise time or a nice round number of reps – we finish only when we have maxed out!
5. Make sure we don't hold our breath and breathe out during the hardest part of each repetition.

6. Don't screw up your face – it doesn't help lift anything and just makes you get wrinkles and lines!
7. We should remember that our sessions probably take up less than 1% of our week, but these short sessions are only effective if we are truly pushing our body hard.

Other Benefits Of Maxing Out
1. By lifting weights and Maxing Out, we increase our bone density and help increase our natural growth hormone.
2. We increase insulin sensitivity.
3. We become more metabolically efficient.
4. We limit inflammation, certainly when compared to endurance athletes.
5. When we *Max Out* primally, we get both a hormonal rush and heaps of mental simulation that slows down the ageing process.

Sprinting

If you remember back to chapter 1, we discussed how we have only been at the top of the food chain for around 100,000 years. When predators chased our primal ancestors, boy could they sprint. But can you ever imagine them going on a long jog? But shouldn't we include aerobic exercise like jogging or cycling in our exercise regime? No. In fact for the sake of your mid- to long-term health, you really shouldn't. Believe me when I say endurance training can be unhealthy! But when we replace log tedious jogs with extremely short quick sprints, we can experience huge health gains. Over the coming pages I am going to explain why we should say goodbye to those laborious long runs and hardcore cycle rides, and instead master the art of sprinting.

Back in chapter 2, we discussed the mitochondria, the powerhouse/ battery of our cells. It turns out that they love sprinting so much that they start to procreate, creating a greater and greater power source. When our hunter-gatherer ancestors experienced a close call with predators snapping at their heels, during the ensuing good night's sleep, nature decided to provide the cells with more power for the next encounter. The good news of course is the more mitochondria organelles we have in each cell, the more fat and glucose we can burn. However, our mitochondria don't reproduce when we're jogging or cycling because the last thing the body wants to do while undergoing endurance activities is to create something that burns more fuel!

Before we make sprinting part of our weekly routine, it is really important to get our weight down first. We will do more harm than good if our body fat is say above 25% and we start pounding the tarmac. Sprinting should be seen as pretty much the last thing on our list of lifestyle changes – in fact it's the primal icing on the cake.

What are the benefits of sprinting and why should we do it? Let's face it, even if there was no scientific reason it's kind of obvious that we are designed to sprint - as if our primal ancestors were not able to do so you wouldn't be around to read this book and I wouldn't be here to write it. Our species would not have lasted long if we could not sprint. As we have required the ability to sprint away from danger for more than 2 million years, you can bet your bottom dollar that nature has designed us to be good sprinters and to gain benefits from doing so.

In terms of return on investment, nothing gets close to sprint training. It burns fat while building muscle, increases the health of our heart and lungs, improves circulation and metabolism and provides us with better mental cognition. While long jogs and cycle rides rarely result in fat loss, sprinting is the king of fat burning. Even just sprinting for 10 to 20 seconds, three to six times a week, conducted over just one or two sessions can burn off heaps of fat. How is that possible? When we sprint properly, our muscles continue to burn up fat for days after the actual exercise. If you think sprinting only improves the muscles in our legs, think again. If we really want to find our six-pack, forget hundreds of sit-ups and ab-crunches – nothing beats flat-out sprinting.

Don't panic, when I say the word sprint, it doesn't normally mean on the road. You will most likely start with short sprints on an exercise bike in the gym or with a rowing machine, both of which are much safer for our body when we first start to sprint. However, once we have our body in shape and when we feel comfortable in giving it a go, then many people will naturally want to progress to sprinting on the road or track. Whether we are sitting on the bike or rower, or indeed running, the principles are all the same. Let's first look at the 'why' and then move to the 'how'.

When we sprint for short distances, it is done without the intake of much oxygen. It is therefore classed as an anaerobic exercise. This builds strength quickly, especially in our powerful, fast twitching muscle fibres. With our muscles' fast explosion of instant requirements, the heart has to pump really hard to deliver blood, which in return helps to strengthen the heart. And a stronger heart is a heart more resilient to disease. Plus, when we sprint, the body believes we are running for our lives and rewards us with extra mitochondria for our next dangerous encounter. This helps us burn calories faster and lose weight. And there is another benefit; the endorphins that are released act as a natural painkiller and provide us with a real feeling of wellbeing.

When it comes to achieving a return on investment, very little in life beats sprinting. In return for less than two minutes of significant discomfort (less than 1/5000th of utter exhaustion per week) we received all of the following benefits from our flat-out sprints:

- Lose weight (post-sprint we will experience an increased metabolic rate for several days)
- Build core strength, not just in our legs but our abs and bottom too
- Increased growth hormones
- Growth in our heart and arteries (a true cardiovascular workout)
- Lowered blood pressure
- Lower blood sugar levels
- Lower levels of insulin
- Improved cognitive skills (yes, we become smarter)

Personally, I normally try to do two lots of sprints each week. Sometimes it's one run and one exercise bike, other weeks if the weather is not so good, I might do one session on the bike and one on the rowing machine. I normally do them after I have finished a weight training session. In total I normally do just two or three sessions a week in the gym and never for more than just 45 minutes. So, my entire weight training and sprint sessions are on average just 8 or 9 hours per month. That's not a huge investment of time to ensure that the body is in good working order. If you don't want to go to a gym, you will probably need to spend around £200 to get a good exercise bike, a few dumbbells and some suspension cables and turn your garage or spare bedroom into your own fitness studio. It will most likely be the best financial outlay you will ever make.

One cautionary note on sprinting: while the legs are going to burn like crazy and our breathing becomes very loud and heavy, we should not feel any pain or tightening of the chest. If we do, we should immediately stop and let somebody in the gym know and once we recover go and see a doctor.

Endurance Sports Aren't All That Healthy

As I mentioned in the introduction to this book, I was a regular jogger for many years. I had completed three full marathons and several half marathons and all in respectable times. But throughout the entire period I was overweight and constantly injuring myself.

It wasn't until I read a book with the head-turning title *Eat Bacon Don't Jog* by Grant Peterson, that I realised how totally unnecessary - and in fact harmful to my wellbeing - all those painful miles I had accumulated had been. Grant writes, "Your body responds to too much running by releasing cortisol, a stress hormone. Cortisol triggers a process called gluconeogenesis, in which your muscles (made up of protein) break down into glucose". Grant then goes on to dig the knife in deeper to the committed jogger who suffers pain in the belief they are doing themselves good by revealing, "Jogging doesn't build strength or fitness – it just trains muscles to tolerate more jogging, and in the real world that's close to useless."

In Beyond Training, America's top personal trainer, Ben Greenfield cites lots of research detailing the long-term dangers awaiting those who undertake too many endurance sessions. For example, he writes, "The heart generally returns to normal within a week after completing a tough endurance workout or race. But for those who frequently compete in such events the results can be repetitive cardiac injury over days, months, even years". He goes on to describe a whole list of detrimental health conditions that can develop from undertaking endurance exercises, such as jogging and long-distance cycling.

Jogging and cycling carries an increased risk of cardiovascular disease and other causes of death. Yet sprinting, if we are able to motivate ourselves to really push hard, achieves the same positive results, is safer and takes up a lot less time. Sprinting achieves the same positive results as spending hours slogging our guts out endlessly jogging but is not a catalyst of cardiovascular diseases. You only get so many heartbeats, don't use them up too quickly!

For many reading this section, you will find it hard to believe that cardio isn't necessarily healthy. Don't get me wrong, it's not quite as dangerous as living a life glued to the sofa, but it's not that much better either. It certainly took me a lot of convincing to hang up my running shoes and cycling gear.

Let me be very clear, this is one of the biggest U-turns of opinion in the fitness world. I am personally full of admiration for people who realise that the advice they have been giving is flawed and are subsequently brave enough to explain how they got it wrong. Far too many people in life, especially medical and health professionals, never seem to admit to errors in judgement and spend their lives defending their flawed principles. So, with great pleasure, let me introduce Dr Kenneth Cooper who in 1968 became known as the Father of Aerobics (later creating The Cooper Institute for Aerobic Research) and who went on to sell more than 30 million fitness and health books worldwide.

Reporting on the success of *Aerobics*, the book that rocketed Dr Cooper to fame, Texas Monthly quoted, "The book was revolutionary, shaking up the sedentary sixties. Before its release only 100,000 eccentrics called themselves joggers, but by late 1968, the nation's trails were overflowing, and now more than 34 million people run regularly... and *Aerobics* brought instant fame to the unassuming Cooper – here and around the world. To this day, Brazilians call aerobic workouts 'Coopering'".

But here is the game changer. In a recent interview with a reporter, Dr Cooper reveals, "At the time, I knew scientific evidence had established that regular exercise was essential to good health and an effective life. But I erroneously assumed that more was better – that the longer you ran, cycled or swam, the healthier you would be".

He shares statistics about thousands of his clients – many of whom were rich and famous and even included President George Bush. He talked at length about how many Olympians had prematurely died of cancer and heart disease and goes on to speak about the effects of free radicals in our cells. Dr Cooper concludes, "Too much exercise can kill you". Today, The Cooper Institute for Aerobic Research instead recommends a new approach to aerobics for cardiovascular fitness that centres around strength training, muscle mass and increasing our flexibility. Yes, you read that correctly - the father of modern jogging, now believes it is dangerous and instead we should lift weights!

If you are a committed cyclist or runner, I am not suggesting you have to give up completely, but you need to either slow down to the most leisurely pace possible, ideally between 60 – 70% of your heart rate maximum, or use your equipment to perform extremely short sprints of less than 30 seconds duration.

Dr Aseem Malhotra

Steve, both you and I were avid obsessive exercisers. And a lot of people still think that if you do loads of exercise, you won't develop heart disease and it's completely false. In fact, one study published in 2017 showed that people who did seven and half hours per week of quite moderate to intense exercise, and there are still lots of people that do that, they are more likely to develop heart disease than people who just did moderate exercise, such as say just two and a half hours per week.

In fact, to maximise cardiovascular fitness doing light aerobic exercise for 30 minutes, say five times a week, is perfect. It also has the best evidence base when it comes to exercise impact on reducing heart disease, cancer and increasing longevity. We are not talking heavy exercise, but where your heart rate is between 50-70% of your maximum heart rate. To calculate this simply subtract your age from 220. They did a large observational study of ex-Olympic athletes, and they found that elite athletes don't live any longer than golfers or cricketers. So, what I say is a little goes a long way and know why you are exercising and listen to your body.

One of the problems with jogging, lots of my friends are orthopaedic surgeons, and they are saying to me that they are seeing more and more people in their 30s and 40s having knee and even hip replacements. One told me that it is because they are jogging on the road and that nobody should be jogging on the road. But there is this kind of mentality driven by, I don't know, maybe seeing it on the TV and as you know Steve, it's not the best way to get cardio anyway. It's much better to do high-intensity interval training and use compound movements. The question is, can you get cardio without damaging your joints and I think people need to think about that. Some people get properly crippled in older age because they have been doing lots of marathons and now, they can't walk, and that's not nice. I used to run 5k, slam it, every morning. Up at 6am, get on the treadmill, take a shower, straight into the operating theatre for ten hours or whatever, but then it started affecting my knees, so I stopped a few years ago. Now I do occasional sprints, very short sprints, but I don't do the long treadmill stuff anymore.

Still Not Ready To Hang Up Your Jogging Shoes?

Of course, people undertake endurance sports for a variety of reasons. It might be to lose weight, to build muscle and to look good in front of the mirror, to live healthier and longer or to appeal to a prospective partner. It might relax you or you might be one of the very few individuals who actually enjoy putting yourself through hell. I am sure there are a few other reasons as well, but let's look at each one of these in isolation and see how participating in endurance sports such as jogging and cycling aids or harms us in reaching our outcome.

"I jog because of the aerobic and cardiovascular benefits." Have you ever stopped to wonder what the two words 'aerobic' and 'cardiovascular' really mean? Aerobic simply means 'with oxygen'.

In other words, aerobic exercises are those where you take in more oxygen than normal. Is that good for us? Over the past 40 years that's what we have been led to believe, and it's probably the main reason we see more and more joggers on our streets. However, the reality is that forcing more oxygen into our body, beyond just normal breathing, is actually hazardous. It is the fuel needed to set lose free radicals within our cells, leading to the inflammation that itself is the root cause of many of today's modern diseases. So too much aerobic exercise is by and large a negative and not a positive.

But what about the cardiovascular system, doesn't that need to be exercised? It turns out that jogging and cycling for long periods of time at medium intensity does very little for our wellbeing above that of just walking and talking! The only way to really put excessive load on our cardiovascular system is to put excessive load on our muscles in other words sprinting and lifting heavy things.

"I jog/cycle to lose weight." We might lose water spending hours jogging and therefore jump on the scales and look like the run did us good, but we're not really burning fat. Remember, there is no such thing as losing weight. We can't just lose weight; we have to burn off our body fat.

It might be possible under a few specific circumstances to burn a little fat while jogging, but we are just as likely to burn off muscle and as muscle requires more energy than fat, when we eventually hang up our running shoes as our knees or joints give way, our metabolic rate decreases as we now have less muscle to consume energy. If we give away our muscles too cheaply to the jogging gods, in addition to those which we naturally lose as we age, then we are setting ourselves up to gain weight later in life. Every step taken forward while jogging or cycling might potentially make a minuscule gain right now but will actually result in a bigger backwards step later in life.

Plus, there is another huge problem. My good friend Glenn Lehrer, who is both an accomplished lapidarist and philosopher, taught me that everything in life is about seeking the most stable state of harmony and balance. In our body the pursuit of harmony is known as homeostasis. If, while we exercise, we are getting most of our energy from CARBS or other sugars, the moment the exercise is complete homeostasis kicks in and notifies our brain that we are starving and that we must be fed. It's not our fault that we reach for the sugar-loaded sports drink or CARB-loaded energy bar. Don't beat yourself up about it or try to take full responsibility – our desire for more energy is squarely the fault of homeostasis.

And there is another reason why so many of us struggle to lose those extra pounds through jogging. It is because we would have to run some serious miles to burn off lots of weight. Just look at the maths: one pound of fat = 3,500 calories, or for the younger generation one kilogram = 7,700 calories. Let's assume we're a fast and fit runner and we have the ability to burn 750 calories an hour. It therefore takes us more than four and a half hours to burn off one pound of fat. That's approximately the time it took me to complete each marathon! Plus, this assumes that we didn't intake any sports drinks, gels or bars on our way around and that we didn't stuff our face as a reward for our effort once we crossed the finish line. But we do! We all do – right?

In his book, *The IF Diet*, Robert Skinner refers to our caveman ancestors and says, "Your brain evolved a safety mechanism. If it sensed that you'd been moving for a long time, steadily depleting your blood sugar – and not replacing it – something was wrong. Either food was in short supply or you were a useless hunter. This is what your brain senses during traditional exercise". In the book *Primal Blueprint*, Mark Sisson says, "It's ironic that many in their 40s and 50s start engaging in marathon or triathlon training with hopes of improving health and delaying the ageing process when, quite often, it has the exact opposite effect".

Research has revealed that those who jog for more than 30 minutes continuously, with a heart rate of more than 85% of their maximum, are likely to damage their immune system and trigger inflammation for periods of up to three days post-exercise. Even at 75% of our maximum heart rate, joggers will experience raised cortisol levels (stress hormone) and reduced levels of both testosterone and growth hormones. Incidentally, both sprinting and weight training or any other form of high intensity intermittent training, actually increases both testosterone and growth hormones. These hormones are critical components of helping us to live more healthily and happily.

"I am an endurance jogger/cyclist because I love it." First of all, make sure it is the endurance aspect that you love, and not the fact that you are just exercising. Why not try the MOMMS method for a few weeks and see how it makes you feel.

The Conclusion On Jogging

I don't want you to think that I am advising you to either hang up your running shoes, or drop off your bike at the local tip, and return to a life on the sofa. Nothing could be further from the truth! If you love jogging or cycling, then I recommend that you purchase a heart rate monitor and still go outdoors and jog or cycle, but so slowly that your heart rate is only mildly elevated between 55 to 70% of your maximum heart rate. Then, just two or three times throughout your journey, try to sprint flat-out for around 10 to 20 seconds. This way, your workout will better reflect the type of exertion the heart has been designed to support and will not place it under excessive stress. With the primal way of slow cycling or jogging, leaving all the huffing and puffing to the wolf, the entire outing becomes more enjoyable, more sociable and much better for our long-term health.

Nina Teicholz

We currently have a problem with our military getting fatter while they are in service. Sadly, they follow the current government's food guidelines. Although they are getting plenty of exercise, both you and I know Steve, that you can't out-exercise a bad diet. Because they are feeding the military, for example, lots and lots of pasta, they are getting fatter. So, we are facing a situation where we don't have enough deployable troops, and that is a very scary thing.

Professor Tim Noakes

Tim, you have probably written more books and papers, and completed more scientific research on what the right diet for runners and athletes is than anyone else on the planet, please share with us your views.

Well, we have just published a new paper studying athlete's running 5k time trials, really good runners, running it in about 20 minutes. And, it made no difference to the results whether they had a high-carb or a high-fat diet. The performance was identical. My point is that the default diet for every marathon runner and recreational runner in the world is a high-fat diet. The communities we are talking to; European, North American and now Asia, where type 2 diabetes is quite high in the population, if you expose these populations to a high carb diet, you just promote diabetes. As a runner, I developed type 2 diabetes by eating a high carb diet. And I had a family history; my father died of the disease. So, with my genes and a high carbohydrate diet, you can run all you like, you are going to get diabetes. So that is the message we have to get out.

It's Under One Per Cent

With the exception of walking and moving more often, if we don't participate in un-primal endurance sports, we can become extremely strong and fit by just spending under 1% of our life exercising. All our sprinting and gym sessions needn't consume more than 1% of our week. Or if we find it hard to picture this, it accumulates to one full day of exercise in the spring, summer, autumn and winter! Yes – to both look and feel fit, we only cumulatively need to exercise for four days each year!

Chapter 6 Highlights

- MOMMS approach to exercise: Max Out - Move More - Sprint.
- Research suggests that just 25 minutes of brisk walking a day is associated with adding up to seven years to your life and halving the risk of dying from a heart attack.
- Don't participate in long cardio exercises as they can play havoc with our joints, damage our heart and wreck our metabolism.
- Both sprinting and weight training or any other form of high-intensity intermittent training actually increases both testosterone and growth hormones.
- A large observational study of ex-Olympic athletes found that elite athletes don't live any longer than golfers or cricketers.
- By lifting weights, we increase our bone density and help increase our natural growth hormone.
- Lifting weights increase both insulin sensitivity and metabolically efficient.
- When we *Max Out*, we get both a hormonal rush and heaps of mental simulation that slows down the ageing process.

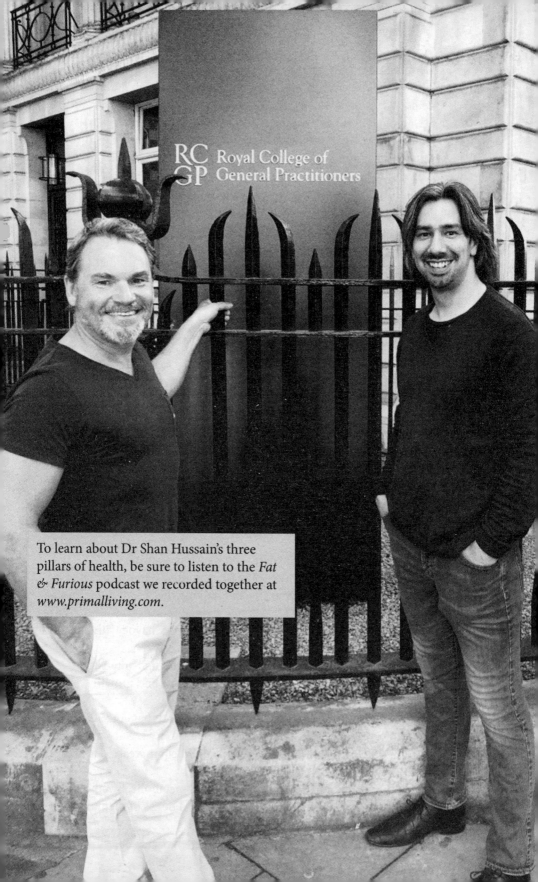

To learn about Dr Shan Hussain's three pillars of health, be sure to listen to the *Fat & Furious* podcast we recorded together at *www.primalliving.com*.

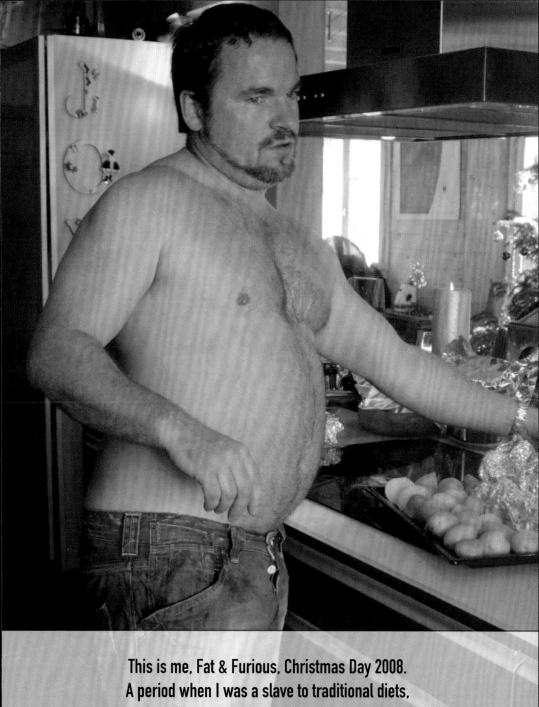

This is me, Fat & Furious, Christmas Day 2008.
A period when I was a slave to traditional diets,
keeping me imprisoned in my own body.

GLYCAEMIC INDEX

The chart below compares the GI and GL of most foods we find in the UK and the USA. I have tried to use portion sizes that are fairly conservative. So for example with white bread I have used just one slice, but if we were to eat two, then simply double the GL figure.

FOOD	GI	SERVING SIZE	GL PER SERVING
Lucozade, original	95	250ml	40
White rice, boiled	64	1 cup (186g)	33
Macaroni and cheese	64	1 serving (166g)	30
Baked potato	85	1 medium (173g)	28
Bagel, white, frozen	72	1 small bagel 70g	25
Rice Krispies	82	1.25 cups (33g)	23
Fanta, orange soft drink	68	250ml	23
Spaghetti, white, boiled, average	46	1 cup (180g)	22
Instant oatmeal, average	79	1 serving (250g)	21
Boiled white potato, average	82	150g	21
Raisins	64	1 small box (43g)	20
Coco Pops, average	77	1 serving (30g)	20
Corn Flakes, average	81	1 serving (30g)	20
Snickers bar, average	51	60g	18
Dates, dried, average	42	handful (60g)	18
Sponge cake, plain	46	1 serving (63g)	17
Rice cakes, average	82	1 piece (25g)	17
Spaghetti, whole-grain, boiled	42	1 cup (180g)	17
Instant mashed potato, average	87	1 serving (150g)	17
Spaghetti, white, boiled 20 mins	42	1 cup (140g)	16
Brown rice, steamed	50	1 serving (150g)	16
Coca Cola, (US formula)	63	250ml	16
Banana, plain, average	52	1 medium size	14
Sweet corn on the cob	48	1 piece (60g)	14
Orange juice, unsweetened	50	1 cup (248g)	14
Pizza	30	2 slices (260g)	13
Bran Flakes	74	3/4 cup (29g)	13
Oatmeal, average	55	1 serving (250g)	13
Quinoa, cooked	53	1 cup (150g)	13
Cheerios	74	1 cup (30g)	13
Sweet potato	54	1 cup (133g)	12

All brand name data was taken from www.health.harvard.edu on 12th April 2017

FOOD	GI	SERVING SIZE	GL PER SERVING
Potato crisps, average	56	1 bag (40g)	12
Apple juice, unsweetened	41	1 cup (248g)	12
Corn tortilla	52	1 erving (50g)	12
Hot chocolate	51	1 cup (28g)	12
White wheat flour bread	75	1 slice	11
Grapes, black	59	1 serving (120g)	11
Corn chips, plain, salted	42	1 serving (50g)	11
Pitta bread, white	68	1 piece (30g)	10
Muesli, average	56	1 serving (30g)	10
Ice cream, regular, average	62	1 cup (72g)	10
Kidney beans, average	34	1 cup (150g)	9
Graham cracker	74	2 pcs (14g)	8
Microwave popcorn, plain, average	65	1 serving (20g)	7
Chicken nuggets, frozen, reheated	46	4 pieces (100g)	7
Baked beans	40	1 serving (150g)	6
M&M's, peanut	33	1 handful (30g)	6
Apple, average	38	1 medium size	6
Oranges, raw, average	45	1 medium size	5
Milk, full fat, average	31	250ml	4
Milk, skim, average	31	250ml	4
Pear, raw, average	38	120g	4
Watermelon	72	1 serving (120g)	4
Green peas	54	1 cup (80g)	4
Parsnips	52	1 piece (80g)	4
Strawberries	40	1 cup (152g)	4
Tomato juice, no sugar added	38	1 cup (243g)	3
Grapefruit	25	1/2 slice	3
Chickpeas	10	1 cup (150g)	3
Cashews, salted	22	2 handfuls (50g)	3
Carrots, average	39	1 piece (80g)	2
Beansprouts	25	1 cup (104g)	1
Soy beans, average	15	1 cup (150g)	1
Peanuts	13	2 handfuls (50g)	1

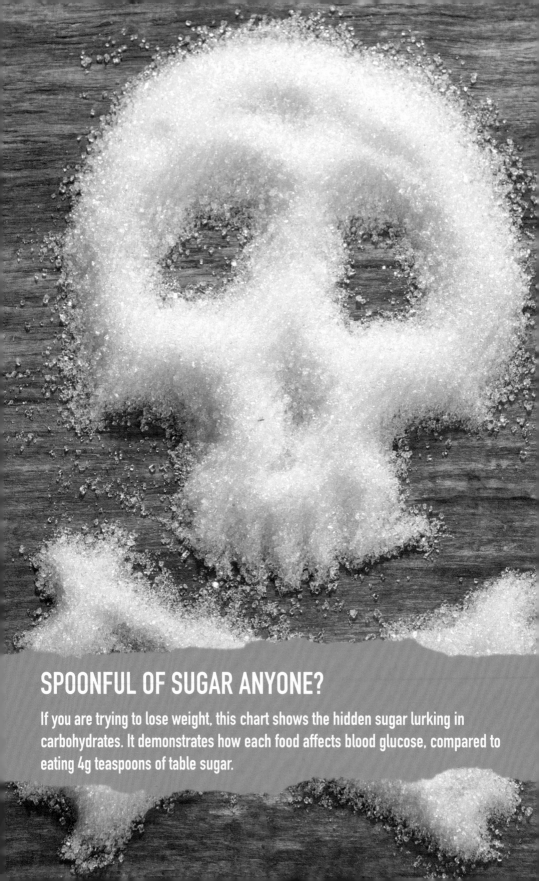

SPOONFUL OF SUGAR ANYONE?

If you are trying to lose weight, this chart shows the hidden sugar lurking in carbohydrates. It demonstrates how each food affects blood glucose, compared to eating 4g teaspoons of table sugar.

Breakfast	Serving	Sugar teaspoon equivalent
Pure Apple Juice	200ml	8.6
Cornflakes	30g	8.4
Coco Pops	30g	7.3
Shredded Wheat	30g	4.8
Bran Flakes	30g	4.8
Mini Wheats	30g	4.4
Oat porridge	150g	4.4
Special K	30g	4
Brown Toast	1 slice	3.3
Egg, Salmon, Bacon, Sausage, Tomato, Blueberries *	Eat as much as you like	0

Dinner	Serving	Sugar teaspoon equivalent
Jacket Potato *	Large	15
12" Subway (just bread)*	150g	15
Bagel *	Medium	11
Basmatic Rice	150g	10
Chocolate Muffin *	Medium	10
Potato White, boiled	150g	9.1
French Fries Baked	150g	7.5
Spaghetti White Boiled	180g	6.6
Sandwich (just the bread)	60g	7.4
Sweet Corn Boiled	80g	4
Frozen peas	80g	1.3
Broccoli, Cabbage, Celery, Cauliflower, Mushrooms, Spinach, Almonds, Hazel-nuts, Beef, Chicken, Eggs, Fish, Lamb, Pork, Veal, Shellfish, Turkey, Ham etc,	Eat as much as you like	0

Fruit	Serving	Sugar teaspoon equivalent
Raisins	60g	10.3
Banana	120g	5.7
Black Grapes	120g	4
Apple	120g	2.3
Watermelon, fresh	120g	1.8
Strawberries, fresh	120g	1.4

data courtesy of Dr David Unwin *calculated by Primal Living

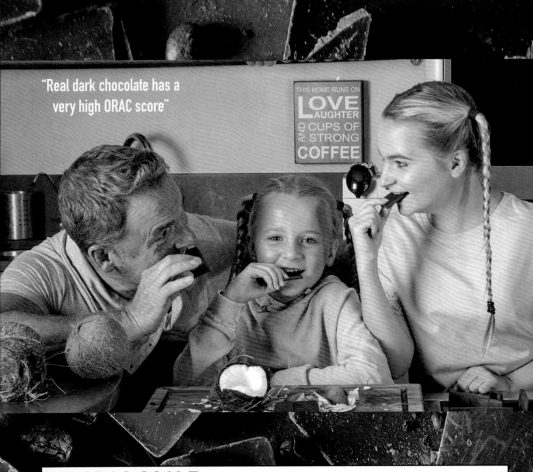

"Real dark chocolate has a very high ORAC score"

THE ORAC SCALE

	ORAC Score per 100g	Gram weight needed to achieve 3000 ORAC	Approximate serving size needed to achieve 3000 ORAC
Cinnamon	267,536	1	1 tsp
Oregano (dried)	200,129	1	1 tsp
Turmeric	159,277	2	1 tsp
Cocoa (dry powder)	80,933	4	1 or 2 tsp
Cumin seeds	76,800	4	1 or 2 tsp
Parsley (dried)	74,349	4	2 or 3 tsp
Basil (dried)	57,553	5	2 or 3 tsp
Dark Chocolate	49,926	6	2 or 3 squares
Curry Powder	48,504	6	3 or 4 tsp
Sage (fresh)	32,004	9	6 or 7tsp
Thyme (fresh)	27,426	11	8 or 9 tbs
Black Pepper	26,618	11	8 or 9 tbs

Goji Berries	25,300	12	Handful
Chili powder	23,636	13	10 or 11 tbs
Pecan nuts	17,940	17	Handful
Paprika	17,919	17	15 tbs
Ginger	14,840	20	15 tbs
Walnuts	13,541	22	Handful
Cranberries	9,584	31	Handful
Hazelnuts	9,454	32	Big handful
Artichokes	9,416	32	1/4 of the vegetable
Pistachio nuts.	7,983	38	Big handful
Blueberries	6,552	46	1/2 cup
Blackberries	5,347	56	1/2 cup
garlic	5,346	56	8 pr 9 cloves
Coriander leaves	5,141	58	Handful
Cabernet Suavignon	5,034	60	1/2 glass
Raspberries	4,882	61	1 cup
Almonds	4,454	67	2 handfulls
Granny Smith Apple with skin	3,898	77	1/2 apple
Red Wine	3,873	77	1/2 glass
Strawberries	3,577	84	1 cup
Peanut Butter smooth	3,432	87	5th of a jar
Cherries	3,365	89	1/2 cup
Peanuts	3,166	95	Handful
Cabbage (red)	3,145	95	1/2 cup
Brocolli	3,083	97	1 1/2 cups
Blueberry Juice	2,906	103	1 glass
Asparagus Raw	2,150	140	3
Pear	2,021	148	1
Cashew Nuts	1,948	154	3 handfulls
Avocado	1,922	156	1 Half
Radish	1,736	173	1 cup
Red Onion	1,521	197	1
Spinach	1,515	198	6 cups
Red Grapes	1,260	238	40 grapes
Tea (brewed)	1,253	239	3 or 4 cups
Onion	1,220	246	1
Olive Oil (Extra Virgin)	1,150	261	1 cup
Orange Bell Pepper	984	305	2

Here are foods that will help you optimise your nutrition and prevent the need to count calories. For the sake of your health, and that of our planet, try to ensure that the following are bought as natural and organic where possible. If not, some of the benefits listed below may be diminished.

ALMONDS

An excellent source of phytonutrients, fibre, copper (necessary for producing red blood cells), magnesium, calcium, zinc and selenium. Makes a fantastic flour for baking and a healthy alternative to milk.

ANCHOVIES

They are full of mineral goodness including calcium, selenium, iron and magnesium, plus they're loaded with Omega 3, riboflavin, niacin, folate, vitamin E, vitamin B6, vitamin B12, vitamin A and vitamin K.

APPLE CIDER VINEGAR

Full of friendly bacteria and acetic acid, apple cider vinegar aids weight loss, reduces LDL cholesterol and helps to lower blood sugar levels. Some studies suggest that vinegar can kill cancer cells and shrink tumours.

ASPARAGUS

It is believed to be the finest natural aphrodisiac. It contains aspartic acid, known to neutralise the excess ammonia in our body which is often a root cause of a drop in libido.

AUBERGINE

Also known as eggplant, they are actually a fruit and not a vegetable. They are a rich source of anthocyanins, a pigment with antioxidant properties that can protect against cellular damage and free radicals.

AVOCADO

It is a unique fruit in that it is primarily a fat. There are so many benefits of regularly consuming avocado, that if we had to take just one fruit on a desert island, it would win hands down.

BAKING SODA

Made from pure sodium bicarbonate. Helps maintain a healthy pH balance throughout the digestive system. Helps with digestion and promotes healthy bowel functions. Also helps to reduce acid reflux.

BEEF (ORGANIC)

Rich in Omega 3 and possibly the very best source of protein. Grass fed beef also contains a secret healing component called conjugated linoleic acid (CLA), which amongst other benefits assists in burning body fat.

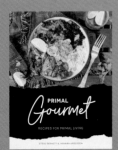

For delicious recipes that incorporate these Primal superfoods, and to help you optimise your nutrition, pick up a copy of Primal Gourmet, a Primal recipe book that I co-wrote with Hannah Anderson.

BELL PEPPER

Also known as capsicum. A yellow one contains roughly the same amount of vitamin C as five whole oranges! A red bell pepper equates to three oranges and the green bell pepper, contains twice that of an orange.

BLACKBERRIES

Just like strawberries, they are very sweet but don't contain many calories. Their nutritional value is tremendously high, with one cupful containing 30% of our fibre, and 50% of our vitamin C daily needs.

BLUEBERRIES

Possibly the most highly antioxidant substance you can swallow is the highly praised and delicious blueberry. They are rich in the flavonoid anthocyanin, which is responsible for their vivid colours.

BOK CHOY

Ranks as one of the highest sources of nutrients per calorie of all vegetables. It's stuffed full of antioxidants which studies have shown to lower the risk of developing lung, prostate, breast and colon cancer.

BONE BROTH

It contains an amino acid called glycine, which plays an important role in the health of our skin, our digestive system, circulatory and nervous system, muscle growth and repair and in managing our hormones.

BRAZIL NUTS

Offer an abundant source of selenium, which is a powerful antioxidant that protects the immune system.

BROCCOLI

Without doubt, broccoli is the ultimate vegetable and one that everyone needs to learn to love, especially raw. One portion has more vitamin C than an orange and more calcium than a glass of milk.

BRUSSELS SPROUTS

Sprouts increase the production of proteolytic enzymes. These make the digestion of both carbohydrates and proteins a lot easier. Sprouts are also known for boosting our metabolism, alkalising the body and helping to prevent both cancer and heart disease.

BUTTER

Has been demonised over recent decades but is in fact super-healthy as long as it originates from organic grass fed cows. Great for frying with as it has a high smoking point.

BUTTERNUT SQUASH

Technically a fruit and not a vegetable, butternut squash contains a huge amount of vitamin A which is good for the maintenance of the immune system and good vision, plus vitamin C, E, B6, thiamine and much more.

CABBAGE

Due to its high content of phytonutrients, cabbage has been shown to cure stomach ulcers. These compounds strengthen stomach muscles, which helps fight back against acid attacks. Rich in vitamins C and K.

CARROTS

They really do help us see in the dark! They are rich in beta-carotene that the liver converts into vitamin A, which when it reaches the retina, is converted to rhodopsin, a pigment that helps enhance night vision.

CASHEWS

Packed full of fibre, protein, antioxidants, minerals and vitamins. They are a rich source of vitamins including thiamin, riboflavin, pantothenic acid, pyridoxine, riboflavin, vitamin E and vitamin K.

CAULIFLOWER

Its wealth of phytonutrients and anti-inflammatory compounds fight off heart disease, ward off cancer and help us to lose weight. It is also rich in carotenoids, which help maintain healthy eyesight.

CAYENNE PEPPER

A type of chilli pepper that is closely related to jalapenos. It both helps to boost metabolism and reduces hunger. Making it great to add to dishes of you are trying to lose weight. Also believed to lower blood pressure.

CELERY

Used for centuries as a medicine, celery contains an array of phytonutrients that help lower blood pressure and prevent heart disease and inflammation. They're full of electrolytes that help prevent dehydration.

CHEESE

Those made from raw milk and haven't been pasteurised are a brilliant source of naturally fermented goodness. Soft cheeses are especially rich in helpful bacteria and can cure many smaller digestive issues.

CHIA SEED

One of the most popular superfoods in the world, chia seeds are extremely rich in fibre, Omega 3, protein and minerals. Gram for gram chia seeds contain more Omega 3 than salmon!

CHOCOLATE

Where the cacao content is higher than 70%, it increases insulin sensitivity, protects against type 2 diabetes, lower blood pressure, support brain functions such as memory and much more.

COCONUT

Coconuts are highly beneficial for our health as they contain vitamins B1, B3, B5, B6, C and E, and come jam-packed with healthy minerals such as calcium, selenium, sodium, magnesium and phosphorous.

SUPERFOODS FOR OPTIMAL NUTRITION

COD

From the same family as haddock and pollock, cod provides a rich source of iodine, selenium, phosphorus, vitamin B12, B3, B6 and a great source of protein. The fish is also rich in healthy omega 3 fatty acids.

COFFEE

A recent study suggests that regular coffee drinkers are less likely to fall victim to Alzheimer's disease. Its high concentration of polyphenols make it a great antioxidant too.

COURGETTE

Known as Zucchini in the USA, it is rich in vitamin C, vitamin B6, riboflavin, folate, magnesium and much more. It contains many antioxidants and anti-inflammatory phytonutrients.

CRANBERRIES

Full of vitamin C, manganese, vitamin E, vitamin K1 and copper. Contains a potent dosage of quercetin, which supports brain health, is anti-inflammatory and studies have linked it to the prevention of certain cancers.

CUCUMBER

Contains antioxidants that support our immune system and are excellent for balancing hormone levels. Its phytonutrients are said to reduce the risk of cardiovascular disease as well as several types of cancer.

EGGS

Contain everything needed to create life! They include all nine essential amino acids, vitamins A, B12, B2 and B5 as well as lots of minerals. They are full of good fats and many other traces of helpful nutrients.

FLAXSEED / LINSEED

Seen as the king of the plant world for its high levels of Omega 3. It also contains lots of fibre and protein as well as many other vital nutrients. Can be ground to make flaxseed flour (also known as flaxmeal).

GARLIC

Famed for its ability to lower blood pressure. There is also research that suggests its antioxidant power is one of the best at helping to prevent cancer. For acne sufferers, it cleanses the skin from the inside out.

GHEE

To make ghee, water is evaporated (clarified) out of butter, leaving behind a higher concentration of fat and making it more suitable for cooking at higher temperature.

GINGER

This miracle root is brilliant for curing sickness and digestive problems. Ginger is also known to reduce pain far more effectively than many pain killers. Very efficient at reducing discomfort during the menstrual cycle.

GOJI BERRIES

Regarded by many, as the most healthy fruit on the planet. Said to protect our eyes and immune system. Studies have shown that they protect against certain cancers and improves depression, anxiety and sleep.

GRAPEFRUIT

Its bitter taste is full of antioxidants and fibre, making it one of the healthiest citrus fruits we can eat. Several reports are emerging that suggest that it might help in preventing cells from becoming insulin resistant.

GREEN PEAS

Also known as garden peas, they are full of disease-fighting antioxidants, fibre and protein. Also a very good source of vitamin K, manganese, vitamin B1, copper, vitamin C, phosphorus and folate.

HADDOCK

A saltwater fish that is an extremely rich source of protein and packed full of essential vitamins and minerals. A great source of Omega 3, vitamin B6 and B12, magnesium, niacin, phosphorus, and selenium.

HAZELNUTS

Exceptionally rich in folate (vitamin B9), which is a unique feature for this essentially British nut. Helps to reduce the bad LDL cholesterol and increase the good HDL. If cold pressed properly, makes a great cooking oil.

HEMP SEED

Hemp seeds are known for having one of the most balanced nutritional profiles among all the seeds. They are an excellent source of Omega 3 and if cold pressed, makes for a great edible oil.

HOT PEPPERS

Also known as capsaicin, it is also used to treat various skin conditions. Today, its miracle cure is so widely acknowledged that we can purchase it as a supplement or a topical cream that we apply to our skin.

KALE

Stuffed full of sulphur, calcium and iron, kale is great for detoxifying our body and promoting a healthy liver. It protects our cardiovascular system, lowers our blood pressure and acts as a natural antidepressant.

LAMB

An excellent source of protein and Omega 3 fatty acids. It's rich in minerals such as zinc, iron, selenium, phosphorus, potassium, copper and magnesium, plus it's a great source of vitamin B12, B3, B6 and B5.

LEMON & LIMES

Their concentration of antioxidants helps prevent free radicals and therefore reduces the likelihood of many cancers. A phytonutrient called limonin, literally halts inflammation and many common illnesses.

SUPERFOODS FOR OPTIMAL NUTRITION

LENTILS

Whilst they do contain carbohydrates, they offer vegetarians a good source of fibre, folate, iron, manganese, potassium, zinc, phosphorus, magnesium, copper, vitamin B1 (thiamin) and vitamin B5.

LETTUCE

Romaine has 10 times more vitamin A than Iceberg. So to look after our skin or teeth, we should choose Romaine over Iceberg. It is also more concentrated in vitamin K, therefore helps to protects against cancer.

MACADAMIA NUTS

Provide a perfect Omega 3 to Omega 6 balance. They contain palmitoleic acid, which improves fat metabolism and therefore assists weight loss. They reduce the likelihood of heart disease and stroke.

MACKEREL

A typical 80g piece provides us with the following amount of our NRV. Vitamin D 201%, sodium 148%, vitamin B12 160%, vitamin B6 15%, magnesium 12%, potassium 11%, iron 6% and calcium 5%.

MANGO

Packed full of 20 different vitamins and minerals including, Helps to lower blood sugar levels and boost cognitive health. Its combination of magnesium, potassium and sodium, helps to naturally lower blood pressure.

MUSHROOMS

Rich in protein and fibre and an excellent source of vitamins D, B, C, calcium, selenium and potassium. They support our immune system and, amongst other things, are said to help prevent certain cancers.

OLIVES

Olives and their oil are a staple part of the Mediterranean diet, where their lifestyle and food choices dramatically reduces the occurrence of heart attacks, and leads to a disproportionate number of centenarians.

ONIONS

They are also full of phytonutrients which protect against many unhealthy strands of bacteria. They are thought to help prevent certain cancers and lower the risk of diabetes and neurodegenerative disorders.

PEANUTS

They have an amazing antioxidant we don't find in other nuts - resveratrol. It's an antioxidant believed to help prevent both heart disease and certain cancers. Don't eat too many though, as they are very calorific.

PECAN NUTS

An excellent source of protein, fibre and heart-healthy antioxidants. The nut supports bone development and can help protect the cardiovascular system.

PINEAPPLE

Rich in vitamin C and an excellent source of manganese. The richest source of bromelain, a mixture of enzymes that are anti-inflammatory and which studies suggest protects against tumours and cancer.

PISTACHIO NUTS

High in protein and fibre and a good source of phosphorus, copper and potassium. As they are rich in a specific amino acid called L-arginine, they can help improve blood flow in clogged arteries.

POMEGRANATES

Rich in vitamin C, vitamin K and potassium, studies have shown that they may help reduce the risk of cancer and all kinds of inflammation. They are also said to help treat high blood pressure and hyperglycemia.

POPPY SEED

The iron and phosphorus contained within the poppy seed is essential for muscle and bone maintenance. Regular consumption helps boost immunity, lowers bad cholesterol, fights anxiety and depression.

PORK

An excellent source of vitamins such as vitamin B3, B1, B2 and B6, plus minerals phosphorus, selenium, zinc, iron, potassium and magnesium. Pork offers a great source of protein without any carbohydrates.

POULTRY

All poultry, chicken, turkey, duck etc, are great sources of protein. They also provide lots of nutrients such as iodine, iron, zinc, vitamins (especially B12) and essential fatty acids.

PUMPKIN

A rich source of potassium which has a positive effect on blood pressure. Its antioxidants beta-carotene help to prevent degenerative damage to the eyes and may reduce the risk of developing certain types of cancer.

PUMPKIN SEED

Pumpkin seeds are rich in protein and B vitamins such as thiamin, riboflavin, niacin, pantothenic acid, B6 and folate. They also contain vitamins E, K and C as well as Omega 3 fatty acids.

RASPBERRIES

They are full to their capacity with cancer-fighting antioxidants. They are said to more concentrated in antioxidants than tomatoes and boost our mood and help us retain our memory as we age.

SALMON

Have you noticed how some fish becomes dry even if we just slightly overcook it, yet salmon always appears to remain moist? That's the huge amount of Omega 3 holding the fish nicely together in our frying pan.

SUPERFOODS FOR OPTIMAL NUTRITION

SARDINES

Also known as Pilchards, they help defend against depression, fight against cancers, improve our moods and memory, protect our heart, stave off Alzheimer's and Parkinson's disease and so much more.

SEAWEED

Full of calcium, folate, iodine, magnesium and a whole host of vitamin Bs. Recent research suggests that seaweed, which is also full of fibre, is great for our guts and helps slow down digestion.

SESAME SEED

Help in preventing diseases like arthritis, asthma, migraines, osteoporosis and certain cancers. Due to their high content of essential fatty acids, they are also extremely beneficial to the health of our skin. Great as a cooking oil.

SHELLFISH

Prawns, oysters, mussels, clams and shrimps have numerous benefits for our health, in particular they are a rich source of selenium and vitamin B12.

SHIRATAKI NOODLES

Comes from the konjac plant and is largely composed of glucomannan, which is a water-soluble fibre. It holds water so well, that when cooked it looks like pasta or noodles, but contains virtually zero calories.

SPINACH

A terrific source of antioxidants, full of minerals such as iron, potassium, zinc, as well as vitamin A, E, K and vitamin B9 (folate). Nitrate in its leaves is the secret behind its muscle-building properties.

SPRING ONIONS

Due to its highly beneficial sulphur content green onions have been used for centuries in Chinese traditional medicine. They provide a rich source of vitamin C, B2, thiamine vitamin A and vitamin K.

SQUID

Full of protein and healthy fats. Rich in niacin and vitamin B12 is important for red blood cell production and the health of the nervous system. Not so beneficial when bought as fried calamari!

STRAWBERRIES

Very British, and very good for our health. Full of flavour and fibre, it often surprises many people how truly healthy strawberries are. For some reason, many believe they are full of sugar. They aren't!

SUNFLOWER SEED

With vitamin E and copper found in abundance, as well as many other vitamins and minerals being very much present, sunflower seeds are extremely good for our health and longevity.

SWISS CHARD

Contains 12 different powerful polyphenols which can reduce the damage caused by free radicals, and slow down the ageing process. Contain syringic acid, which is known to regulate blood sugar levels.

TEA

Green tea especially is full of epigallocatechin gallate (ECGC), which speeds up our metabolism while at the same time suppresses hunger. It increases adrenaline, which in return produces heat and therefore burns calories.

TOMATOES

Believed to contain thousands of different phytonutrients, which suspended in their vividly coloured skin support a healthy heart, boost our immune system and may even reduce the risk of cancer.

TROUT

Evidence suggests that eating fish such as trout is associated with a lower risk of stroke and is possibly beneficial for mental health, for example to improve mood and help treat depression.

TUNA

Whether it is in a can or a fresh slice of raw tuna, this fish is full to the brim with goodness. When in a can we shouldn't buy it with added oil, as when we drain it we also drain away a lot of the Omega 3.

TURNIPS

Great for preventing colds and flu, as well as promoting healthy hair and skin. A rich source of zeaxanthin and lutein. Lutein has been nicknamed 'vitamin eye', as it promotes and protects healthy eyesight.

WALNUTS

As they are full of Omega 3, walnuts are good for the heart. They are also rich in L-arginine, they can help improve blood flow in clogged arteries. If cold pressed properly, makes a great cooking oil.

WATERCRESS

Used more than 2,000 years ago by Hippocrates to treat patients in hospital, it is an incredibly powerful natural medicine. It has more calcium than milk, more iron than spinach and more vitamin C than oranges!

WHEY PROTEIN

A great source of essential amino acids and other healthy nutrients. The benefit of consuming whey goes way beyond just building muscles and increasing strength. Studies show that it helps in reducing body fat.

YOGURT

Without doubt, a totally natural fermented yoghurt is full of millions of nature's tiny miracles, and adding just a small daily portion to our diet can do wonderful things for our gut flora.

CHAPTER 7

OPTIMISE LIFESTYLE

"Get busy living or get busy dying."
STEPHEN KING

Living primally isn't all about diet and exercise – it's a lifestyle change. In this chapter we find out how simple things like the amount of sleep we get, and the stress we have to deal with, can be optimised to help us beat the sick statistics.

Now we are eating the right things, intermittently fasting and participating in the right type of exercise. Excellent! We're almost there. Let's also look at other areas where our primal ancestors did things a little differently, and at some changes we might want to make to ensure we live as super healthily as possible.

Sunbathing - Sensible or Stupid?

Have you ever wondered why the further we live from the equator the paler our skins become? One of the most important vitamins to maintain good health is vitamin D, and what is the best source of vitamin D? The sun. Through evolution, as tribes migrated further and further from the equator, their skin became paler, so they could absorb as much vitamin D as possible from the diminishing sunrays. I find nature astoundingly resilient and, as a back-up plan to the fading of skin tones, the more north and south humans began to travel - receiving less and less benefit from the sun - nature provided an alternative source of vitamin D in cold-water oily fish.

There is a huge trick we can play on our body by being outdoors more often. Once out in the sun, our primally-designed body says, "Hey, spring must be around the corner, the days will be longer, and I will catch or gather more food". As a result, our metabolism gets a boost and we feel full of energy. In contrast, when we stay indoors and avoid the sun, hibernating on our sofas, the body predicts that winter must be coming – food will be become scarce - and therefore the body releases hormones that slow everything down. We feel lethargic, and as our metabolism becomes sluggish, we have neither the energy nor inclination to do anything remotely energetic. Isn't it remarkable that something as simple as being indoors or outdoors can have either a positive or negative spiralling effect on our wellbeing and energy levels?

Sadly, my mother refuses to come on many summer holidays with my wife, our children and me because she has been told by her doctors not to go out in the sun. She has missed out on so much over recent years, and even though many experts are now advising completely the opposite, it is proving difficult to get her to listen to recent research. Even when we explain that there is so much evidence that we are more likely to get cancer by avoiding the sun than going out in it, my mother just won't have it!

Of course, while turning lobster red is dangerous for all of us, getting an all-over light suntan is extremely beneficial. Not only does it make us feel great, it increases our body's ability to create vitamin D, which is one of the most essential vitamins of all.

Did caveman stay in his cave all day? Of course not, he was out and about trying to catch dinner. Did he smear factor 50 all over his body? Again, the point is our DNA expects us to be in the sun. Just as ancient hunter-gatherers would have done, we should shelter in the shade when it gets too hot, or after we have had enough exposure for our natural skin tone, but for those who avoid the sun altogether it's a huge health risk.

In March 2017, The Daily Telegraph newspaper reported, "Experts have overturned decades of advice by urging people to go out in the midday sun without sunblock – because the dangers of missing out on vitamin D can outweigh the risk of cancer". It goes on to say, "The definitive statement by seven leading health groups and charities, including Cancer Research UK, the National Osteoporosis Society and Multiple Sclerosis Society, is designed to clarify conflicting messages. It concluded that surrendering your body to the sun for 10 minutes should take place at midday during the summer months because that is when the sun is strong enough to trigger the body into making vitamin D". The research was also supported by the British Association of Dermatologists, the National Heart Forum and the Primary Care Dermatology Society – that's a pretty comprehensive bunch of leading authorities.

How Much Vitamin D Do I Need?

The US government recommends that children should receive 200IUs a day, those of us aged between 50 and 70, 400IUs and once we are more than 70 years old, 600IUs. But what is an IU? It stands for International Unit and it is used to measure the weight of how much of a vitamin we should consume daily, so 1,000IU = 1g. While the US government issue the above recommendations for vitamin D, many other specialists and nutritionists suggest we all benefit from substantially more. But how long does it take us to generate 1g of vitamin D by being in the sun? It is believed that if we stay out for just a few minutes each day, revealing most of our body to the light, then we will easily set the body up to create 1,000IUs. If we want to build up a reserve of vitamin D, then we should stay outside a little longer. However, to avoid burning, we shouldn't sit in the sun for more than 25 – 50% of the time that it would normally take us to turn a pinkish colour.

In 2002, scientists in Boston came to the conclusion that, "Small amounts of sunshine can greatly reduce the risk of breast, colon and prostate cancers". More recently, research released in March 2016 - after studying 29,518 women in Sweden over a 20-year period - suggested that those who avoided the sun were likely to die prematurely, with frighteningly similar statistics to those who smoked! They went on to say that, "Compared to the highest sun exposure group, life expectancy of avoiders of sun exposure was reduced by 0.6 – 2.1 years". Sunlight hitting the skin helps the body produce vitamin D, which in turn plays an important role in calcium metabolism, which in turn leads to healthier bones. The good news for those of us who live in the sun-deprived UK is that, as vitamin D is fat soluble, it can be stored in the body for fairly long periods of time.

Unfortunately, as we get older our body becomes less efficient at converting sun exposure into vitamin D. My poor mother. At the precise period in her life when she needs to be going out in the sun for longer periods, and uncovering more of her body to the healing benefits of the sun, on the odd occasion that she does venture outdoors on a sunny day, she dresses more like a teenager wearing a hoodie! Getting outdoors in the sun is not just about providing a much-needed boost to our vitamin D reserves. Exposure to sunlight tends to lift our mood and reduce stress. It's also good for reducing both blood pressure and acne!

In June 2016, The Mirror newspaper ran an article with the headline, 'Health benefits of sunbathing outweigh skin cancer risks'. The article goes on to say, "Sunbathing also reduces blood pressure, cuts the risk of heart attacks and is more likely to prolong life than shorten it. Sun worshippers worried by gloomy warnings [that] they risk getting skin cancer can start looking on the bright side". The same article goes further by stating, "The big discovery is that when skin is exposed to sunlight, a compound called nitric oxide is released in blood vessels that helps lower blood pressure". In a recent podcast I recorded with Dr Malcolm Kendrick, he confirmed this point and actually stated that because nitric oxide is so essential in maintaining the health of our endothelium (the inner lining of our artery walls), getting sufficient sunshine is one of the best protective measures you can take to avoid a heart attack.

Living in the UK, with our infrequent bouts of sunshine, what we need to know is how long after we return from our holidays abroad can our body store vitamin D? According to a 2010 article published by Paediatric Nephrology, vitamin D can be stored in the fat tissue for approximately two months. It's important to note the same article reveals that, once we have been in the sun, we shouldn't go and immediately have a soapy shower, as it apparently can take half an hour or so for the skin to complete the cycle of synthesising vitamin D.

What about sunbeds – are they a valid way to obtain a suntan? It appears that as long as they effectively balance UVA and UVB rays in a similar proportion to the sun, and that they are fitted with modern low-pressure lamps, then they are no different to sitting out in the sun and similar precautions, such as how long we should be exposed, therefore apply. If it's an older machine that only produces UVA rays, then other than getting a tan there is little medical benefit. This is because we need UVB rays to stimulate vitamin D production.

So, should we use a sunbed? It's obviously more primal to harness the sun's magic healing powers – not only is it free, it doesn't use expensive electricity, so therefore it's kinder to the planet. But if we don't have a chance to get out in the sun, then by all means use a sunbed. However, remain respectful of its powers and don't go getting burnt, as it still holds true that overexposure can lead to skin cancer. You may also have heard some people say that they like to build a base tan on a sunbed before going on their annual holiday. There is some logic in this, as it is possible to build-up melanin levels in our skin that can provide a little bit of natural protection against burning. But please do it in moderation and in short bursts.

If you want to learn more about the benefits of being in the sun, let me recommend you read Dr Michael Holick's book, *The UV Advantage*, in which he states, "Lack of sunlight is associated with a host of conditions from colon, breast, prostate and ovarian cancer to heart disease, high blood pressure, type 1 diabetes, multiple sclerosis and depression". Dr Holick is an endocrinologist, and he has some very sensible advice on sun cream too. He believes that the higher the SPF, the less vitamin D gets through, and once we get to SPF 15 or above, the benefit of the sun is reduced by 99.9%. Dr Holick says that when he goes out in the sun, he does 10 minutes without sun cream and then puts it on to prevent overdoing it. Later in his book, he goes on to say that he believes the correct exposure to sunlight has an equal benefit on the health of our heart to that of exercise! Then, in a section under the heading 'In the Beginning', Dr Holick talks of how ancient man understood the benefit of sunlight. From studying paintings in caves, he suggests that we can assume that even primal man understood the benefits of sun therapy.

Here's one final thought from Dr Holick, which fits with my belief that too many companies care more about their profit than they do people or the planet: "How did we reach a point in our history when sun became something to be feared instead of worshipped? Shunned instead of desired? The simple answer lies in the fact that there are many billions of dollars to be made in emphasising the only major medical downside of sun exposure (non-melanoma skin cancer) and not much money to be made in promoting the sun's many benefits".

American Dr William Grant believes, "An increase of sun exposure in the USA would result in 185,000 less cases of internal cancer". Compare that to the 1,200 people who sadly die of skin cancer, and I am sure you will draw the same conclusion as I have that sensible sunbathing is extremely beneficial for our health. However, let me repeat the sunburn warning. While we are after a light suntan, we don't want to burn. Remember, it takes approximately three or four hours after being in the sun for our sunburn to reveal itself. This is caused by extra blood flow to the burnt areas and doesn't normally reach its peak for around 18 hours after overexposure. So please, whatever you do, don't sit in the sun until you burn, otherwise it is going to be extremely detrimental to your health. Put simply, suntans are good for health on so many levels, and can prevent multiple cancers, yet sunburn caused by overexposure can cause skin cancer.

Let me explain the approach I take for my family and myself. We try on most school holidays to take the kids somewhere warm, where we can top up their vitamin D levels. We ensure each day that they go outside in the morning and play or swim without sunscreen. Jack, Tom, and even our little four-year-old Louie, go a lovely light-brown shade, and for them 50 minutes exposure is absolutely fine without any protection. I believe the girls would start going red after about 40 minutes, so I get them to go under the shade after about 20. (These are only approximations as it depends how close to the equator we have ventured.) Once they have hit about 50% of the exposure that would normally make them turn slightly red, they go in the shade and chill out for about half an hour, allowing their bodies sufficient time to maximise the gift they have received from nature. Then we slap on the sunscreen, allow it to soak in for 10 minutes or so, and let them go back out and play. What's more, we always make sure the lotions are as organic as possible, and when the kids or my wife and I are at a level where a SPF factor 8 is sufficient, we no longer use sun lotion and instead use coconut oil. Believe it or not, the very same oil that we recommend we cook food in, is Mother Nature's SPF level 8!

Depending on what you have been taught, you might feel that letting our four-year-old son out in the sun without any protection is irresponsible. But it really isn't. Sadly, we see too many misinformed parents who, with only the child's best interest at heart, slap on sun protection before the kid has had any chance to take in sufficient sunrays to convert to vitamin D. As long as we soak up plenty of sunshine in the summer, it will almost see us through the early part of the winter - especially if we can top it up by eating plenty of oily fish. If we feel we are running low on vitamin D, we can always ask our doctor to test our blood specifically for vitamin D levels - if he or she feels we are running low, then there are plenty of vitamin D supplements on the market. It's also likely that, if we are running low, our kids are too and therefore the whole family could do with eating more oily fish or taking vitamin D supplements. Better still, take a family holiday and boost your vitamin D levels through nature's natural source, sunshine.

If you still are not convinced about spending more time in the sun, then be sure to eat plenty of eggs, oily fish and consider taking a quality vitamin D supplement. Or get hold of Jeff T Bowles' book *The Vitamin D3 Miracle*. If I haven't convinced you, I am sure Jeff will. One of my favourite quotes from his brilliantly written work is, "Since the early 1980s, when doctors started warning us about too much sun, obesity rates in adult humans and many other diseases (including asthma and autism) have skyrocketed!"

During late autumn and winter, everyone in Great Britain needs to rely on dietary sources of vitamin D. The NHS states, "Since it is difficult for people to meet the 10 microgram recommendation from consuming foods naturally containing or fortified with vitamin D, people should consider taking a daily supplement containing 10 micrograms of vitamin D in autumn and winter". What I find very encouraging about this article, is that it is one of the first times I have seen the British government recommend the use of supplements. Let's hope this is a change of tide to one of prevention rather than cure.

A Good Night's Sleep

For someone who has run their own businesses for more than 30 years - burning the candle at both ends - researching how much sleep we require has had a profound effect on how I now live my life. Those who know me well will be astounded by what they read here.

There will always be periods in everyone's lives where - due to external factors such as work, having young children or even party season - getting a good night's sleep becomes a low priority. While the odd day or two of not getting enough sleep shouldn't cause any long-term health problems, sleep deprivation over a sustained period can be very harmful. I personally found the views I am about to share with you very hard to swallow. For the past quarter of a century I have preached that the early bird catches the worm; that while you rest you rust; that I will sleep enough when I'm dead - and a number of other one-liners that in the main suggest that life is just too short to sleep. What I have now learned from in-depth conversations with several of this book's contributors, is something very different indeed, and that the theory that 'life's too short to sleep' is incorrect. It should be restated as, 'life is cut short without sleep'.

It is really important that we don't confuse rest with sleep, as they are two very different things. While resting for a few hours on the sofa watching a movie might help us de-stress and unwind, it does not allow our body to go into repair mode. It does not allow the brain to process its learnings from the day or let our various hormones get themselves organised.

Dr Shan Hussain

One of the most common complaints I hear from patients is, "I'm tired all the time." On occasion, there may be medical causes for this, but the vast majority of the time the solution is very simple: sleep more, and then review your energy intake and expenditure.

Our Circadian Clock

In September 2017, American scientists Jeffrey C Hall, Michael Rosbash and Michael W Young won a Nobel Prize for their work on the internal clock of living organisms. Today, our internal biological timepiece is referred to as the circadian clock (pronounced 'sir-kay-dian').

We have already mentioned the stress hormone cortisol, and how it can wreak havoc in our body if it not controlled properly. It turns out that, if we don't get enough sleep at the right time of night, then as well as keeping ourselves awake we also rouse our cortisol monster. To explain why this happens we need to learn a little about our circadian clock.

Way before the British invented the grandfather clock and the Swiss perfected the wristwatch, Mother Nature beat them to it by creating the body's circadian clock. It doesn't need winding up or batteries but keeps time primarily by the rising and setting of the sun, which activates a hormone in our body called melatonin. Nature didn't create the circadian cycle (often referred to as the biological rhythm) exclusively for us humans, but for every living thing on the planet – from animals to fish, plants to microbes. Understanding the cycle is extremely important to our health, so much so that in the 1980s a whole new field of science was created to study it – chronobiology.

For those of us who live a distance from the equator, our body has to adapt to huge swings in the hours of sunlight that we receive throughout the different seasons. In the UK, during the darkest winter days, we get as little as eight hours of sunlight, but in the middle of the summer we receive a whopping 16. With our circadian clock being regulated by sunlight, it's a good thing that the change happens subtly, with sunrise and sunset changing by approximately just one minute each day.

Remember that what keeps our biological clock in sync is sunlight. The chart on the following page is based on the sun rising at 6am and then setting at 6pm, as it does mid-spring and mid-autumn in the UK - and pretty much all year round near the equator. At other times of the year, as the hours of sunlight move backwards or forwards by only a minute or so each day, our circadian clock is able to fairly reliably reset itself.

Let's look at our 24-hour clock, starting at midnight, give or take 30 minutes:

- 00:00 To make sure we feel tired, melatonin production reaches its peak around midnight. The thyroid gets to work and tells the mitochondria in our cells to burn energy to keep our inactive body warm. This is how we lose weight when we sleep properly.
- 01:00 Melatonin slows down our brain activity so that we can process what we have learnt in the day and form long-term memories.
- 02:00 Our deepest sleep, where the body starts to enter repair mode.
- 04:00 We are at our most relaxed at this time, and both our neurological and immune systems are hard at work.
- 05:00 It takes five or six hours of sleep for our body to reach its lowest temperature, this is why it's nonsense to get less than seven hours sleep.
- 06:00 We get a surge of cortisol and blood pressure rises in an attempt to wake us, and the brain mobilises our muscles.
- 07:00 The body stops producing our sleep hormone melatonin and switches on our hunger hormone ghrelin.

- 08:00 Our bowels become active and if we ate the day before they stir action downstairs.
- 09:00 The height of testosterone secretion for the day.
- 13:00 The most alert we will be all day.
- 14:00 Height of co-ordination (so we could track animals after the midday sun).
- 15:00 Fastest reaction times (so that we could catch said animals).
- 17:00 Maximum muscle strength and cardiovascular efficiency (in case we didn't catch an animal the first time).
- 18:00 Highest blood pressure of the day. As long as we are on a low CARB diet, in order to stop us eating too much, leptin will continue to rise until it's time for sleep. If for some reason it doesn't, then for goodness' sake don't eat CARBS, but try some coconut or avocado instead.
- 19:00 Peak of body temperature.
- 21:00 The body starts to produce melatonin to tell us we are tired and ready for sleep.
- 23:00 So that we are not going to the toilet all night, our gastrointestinal works start to go to sleep.

Until a few years ago, both of my two youngest daughters, Jessica and Lili - used to always sleep with their bedroom lights on. I tried everything to get them to sleep in the dark. I taught them about our biological clock and how, if they kept their lights on, or left their iPads and iPhones blinking all night, how they wouldn't produce enough melanin - and without it they wouldn't get smarter at school. But it all went in one ear and out the other. Then I remembered a two-word phrase that everyone has heard. I reminded them that, as well as feeling healthy and improving their intelligence, if they turned off their lights, they would become even more beautiful than they already were. I simply told them that it's called 'beauty sleep' for a very good reason, but it only becomes real beauty sleep when the room is totally dark. Any light in the room at all and the magic just doesn't happen!

The saying 'beauty sleep' is based on the fact that, while we sleep, our skin regenerates itself up to eight times faster than when we are awake. We all want to look more beautiful, but let's look at what happens on a less superficial level. While we are asleep:
- The body goes into repair mode and increases our growth hormones
- The brain assembles the jigsaw puzzle of knowledge that we learnt during the day
- The brain takes the daily knowledge and stores it neatly into our mental filing cabinets, so that we can more easily retrieve and recall it in the future
- The liver doesn't have to deal with incoming food (it's difficult to eat when we are asleep) so gets to work detoxifying our body
- The body increases the production of testosterone

Without Sufficient Sleep
- Knowledge and memories from the day's activities become scrambled
- The body struggles to regulate our body temperature, and becomes particularly inefficient at dealing with extreme cold or heat

- The body creates an excess of cortisol, and we become easily stressed. Have you noticed how short-tempered we become after a poor night's sleep? It's not our fault that we become irritable and ratty, it's an excess of the hormone cortisol
- Our immune system begins to fail
- Insulin struggles to regulate blood sugar levels, and a lack of sleep over time can lead to type 2 diabetes
- Leptin and ghrelin hormones don't function properly, leading to overeating
- Our body can lose control of its fight with inflammation

For years, I limited how much sleep I got because I thought it made me a better person, a smarter businessman, and because I believed it gave me more time to achieve things. Yet it turns out that, while I had a feeling of self-righteousness by getting out of bed at the crack of dawn, I was actually becoming a weakling by stopping my muscles from growing properly. I was becoming dumber by not allowing my brain to properly organise what it was learning, and I was killing my sex drive by not producing sufficient testosterone. Putting on my running shoes at 5am, feeling like the smarter martyr who was getting fitter than the rest of the population who were still in bed sleeping their life away, it was actually counterproductive - and rather than improving my overall health, it was actually impeding it.

How Much Sleep Do We Need?

There is no simple answer to this question as we are all different. The more active we are, the more sleep we potentially need. I also believe that it can vary a little from day to day. I personally sleep around six to eight hours during weekdays and get between eight and nine hours a night at the weekend. So, what do experts recommend? The National Sleep Foundation of America recently assembled 18 leading scientists and researchers and gave them the task of bringing their official recommendations up to date. As of June 2017, this is their suggestion:

Age	Hours Needed	May Be Appropriate
Newborn - 3 months	14 to 17	11 to 19
4 months - 11 months	12 to 15	10 to 18
1 - 2 years	11 to 14	9 to 16
3 - 5 years old	10 to 13	8 to 14
6 - 13 years old	9 to 11	7 to 12
14 -17 years old	8 to 10	7 to 11
18 - 25 years old	7 to 9	6 to 11
26 - 64 years old	7 to 9	6 to 10
65 years +	7 to 8	5 to 9

While we also have similar guidelines in the UK, the US study is so well researched that I personally prefer their findings.

It might be true that politicians such as Margaret Thatcher got by on four hours sleep each night, just as Donald Trump also claims to only need four to five hours, but is that actually good for our health? The simple answer is no! Researchers at the University of California in San Francisco discovered that 3% of people have a gene that enables them to perform well on just six hours sleep per night. But for the other 97% of us, in order to live a healthy, happy and long life we need to follow the above recommendations.

Dr Dan Maggs

You need as much sleep as you need! Don't try and cheat it else it will catch up with you eventually... somehow.

Deborah Colson MSc

If people are eating a diet which is high in sugar and refined carbohydrates, it can affect their ability to sleep, because the brain can be a bit wired. Magnesium is a really key nutrient for sleep; it really helps the mind to calm and prepare for sleep, and there's also an amino acid called taurine, which is really important to sleep. Taurine definitely has a very calming and relaxing effect. The main source of taurine is offal, for example heart, which of course most people don't eat.

Chilling Out and Cat Naps

There is definitely a place for taking time to relax when living primally, but that does not mean we are endorsing the couch potato way of life. Without doubt we are living in the laziest, fattest and most sedentary era ever. Think about the progression. We used to hunt for food, then we had to walk to stores to carry home food, then we could travel to restaurants – and even this burnt some calories. But today we can simply go online and order any takeaway we desire.

In the UK there is even a food portal called Just Eat, which can now deliver us almost any junk food meal we desire. We then sit down, turn on our TV and scoff down our food without even registering we're doing so. And remember 'scoffin' is only one letter away from 'coffin'!

It would be perhaps naive to think that our primal ancestors were on the go from sunrise to sunset. What we believe is that we should get around seven to nine hours of quality sleep each night. If we aren't able to do that during the dark hours, maybe because of work commitments or childcare, then we should try to make up our missing hours of sleep with a Spanish-like siesta in the afternoons.

Interestingly, on the Greek isle of Ikaria, where there is a high percentage of centenarians, afternoon naps are commonplace. Plus, the Harvard School of Public Health reported that just napping for 30 minutes, at least 3 times a week, lowered coronary mortality. Now I normally discard this type of research, as it is not derived from a controlled randomised, interventional study, but in this case the conclusion feels logical and it's certainly backed up by the longevity of people in regions where naps and siestas are regarded normal.

Dr Emer Macsweeney

I think people are increasingly recognising that sleep is very important for brain health. Actually, often people do say that when you've got a stressful day or a difficult day the next day, sleep is actually your best weapon.

There is now an increasing amount of evidence that sleep is not just important in terms of regeneration in the brain, but also the removal of potentially toxic compounds from the brain that we create during the day. Also, the quality of sleep is important. But if you can't get a good night's sleep, then even frequent 20-minute naps during the day are really excellent in terms of restorative influence on the brain. While we don't understand it all completely, I think it is now just incredibly well recognised that sleep is very important for the brain.

Flat Feet - Straight Back

Primal man didn't wear high heels or platform shoes. When he needed an elevation to view his prey, he climbed a tree. Constantly wearing high heels can cause all sorts of problems for our body. It's kind of obvious really, that the more time we can spend without shoes on, the better it must be for our posture and our body. And even for us gents, constantly wearing a half-inch heel shoe is not natural for the body either. That said, this is one of the smaller principles, and if wearing heels makes you feel more confident and less stressed, then continue to do so. However, whenever we find ourselves alone, we should try to go barefoot as often as possible.

There is also another reason for ditching the shoes and socks, and that is because it can reduce the chances of getting fungus under our toenails. My two big toes were a real mess and have been for many years. However, taking a leaf out of my own book, I have made a real effort to remain barefooted for as long as possible in the past two years and I frequently wear open-toe sandals in my office. The results have been fantastic. I think the combination of exposing my toes to fresh air - and also getting my vitamin D levels boosted - have both contributed to my nails returning to full health. I guess it shouldn't come as a surprise because, if you think about it logically, fungi grow in dark damp places - and that's exactly what my feet were experiencing while covered by socks and shoes. If you have to wear socks, then it's advisable to wear those made from bamboo fabric, as they contain both antifungal and antibacterial properties. When it comes to sitting down, we simply do too much of it! And what's worse is that we're not actually very good at it. Recent research has suggested that those of us who work in offices now spend more time sitting than those who are retired! On the NHS website it says, "Studies have linked excessive sitting with being overweight and obese, type 2 diabetes, some types of cancer and early death. Sitting for long periods is thought to slow the metabolism, which affects the body's ability to regulate blood sugar, blood pressure and break down body fat".

The Guardian newspaper ran an article in 2014 suggesting that, "We spend half our lives sitting down – and studies show it increases our risk of dying from practically any disease you can think of. But there is something we can do about it – we can simply stand up.

Research in the *British Journal of Sports Medicine* shows that reducing sitting time increases the length of your telomeres". What are telomeres? They turn out be a cap that sits at the end of each DNA strand that helps protect our chromosomes from fraying. Picture them like the little plastic tips (called 'aglets') that stop our shoelaces from fraying. If we spend too much time sitting then we apparently damage our telomeres, preventing our cells from doing their job properly.

In January 2017, The Daily Telegraph's website stated, "Elderly people who spend most of their time sitting down age significantly quicker than more active contemporaries, according to new research. A study of 1,500 pensioners found those who kept to a sedentary position for 10 hours or more a day and who did less than 40 minutes moderate physical activity had the body of people eight years older".

You would think that, because we practice the art of sitting for so many hours each day, we must be pretty good at it - but as you have just read, we're not. In fact, we're rubbish at it! We slouch, round the shoulders, and put all sorts of stress in the wrong areas. It must be something that we slowly develop, because I have noticed that my four-year-old son Louie sits with a perfectly straight back. I am certainly no physiotherapist, so I won't go into chapter and verse about how we should sit properly, other than recommend that when you get five minutes, you go to Google and type in 'how to sit properly' or 'good posture' and you will find lots of articles.

Alcohol

This is the hardest principle for me to write about, as I do like a drink. So here I am going to start by quoting an old proverb, 'do as I say, not as I do'. That said, if you like the odd drink you will be pleased to hear that I am not going to suggest you stop completely. Remember, this book is about happiness as much as it is about health - and if the occasional drink makes us happy, then we should go ahead and have one. If a couple of glasses of wine help us unwind after a hard day at work, our overall health will probably benefit from having a drink rather than going out of our way to avoid it. But we are talking about only one or two glasses. We aren't talking about drowning our sorrows, we're talking about a little relaxation. If we feel the need to get drunk to be happy, then it's important to seek help in getting to the root cause of our unhappiness.

Let's take a look at units. While we don't count calories when we live primally, we really do need to count our alcohol units. Firstly, where the British government got that '21 units a week for men and 14 for women' is a complete mystery. Only last week I read they are now saying men should only drink 14 units. Plus, in many books I have read about our gut, the common recommendation to keep our healthy bacteria in good working order is to suggest no more than one unit of alcohol per day. But here is my take on booze. First of all, we all know you can set fire to brandy, if you didn't then you have never lit a Christmas pudding! If something can catch fire it must be a really good fuel. Forget calorie counting, if something can easily ignite then the body must use it as a fuel. 'So what?', you might be asking. If we are eating and drinking too, it seems to make sense that the body is going to choose to burn the fuel that's easiest to burn first, i.e. the alcohol, before it even thinks of burning up that evening meal we just ate.

Virtually every time I step on my bathroom scales in the morning after consuming more than two units of alcohol the night before, I find that my weight has increased. During almost five years of charting my daily weight, almost every time where I have overindulged the night before, my weight is higher the next morning- even if I exercised and ate very primally.

At the end of the day, alcohol is full of empty calories – a whopping seven of them per gram. But it's not just the calories that are a problem, alcohol seems to disrupt our blood sugar control, makes our muscles less likely to take in the energy and instead deposits it all in our fat stores. The Drinkaware website sums it up very well, "While we can store nutrients, protein, carbohydrates and fat in our bodies, we can't store alcohol. So, our system wants to get rid of it, and doing so takes priority. All of the other processes that should be taking place (including absorbing nutrients and burning fat) are interrupted". One of the biggest sacrifices the body makes while dealing with too much alcohol is it fails to metabolise vitamin B. Among other things this can lead to depression, lack of concentration and damage to several cognitive functions.

I heard Olympic diver Tom Daley being interviewed on the Chris Evans radio show some time ago, and he said something along the lines of, a glass of wine has the same calories as a doughnut - and if he was going to have to choose one, he would rather have a doughnut! This made perfect sense to me. I had been eating strictly primal that week, but the night before hearing Tom, for no apparent reason, I had three glasses of wine. That's the equivalent of three doughnuts and on hearing what he had to say, I finally got the message.

The alcohol dilemma: undoubtedly a small amount of alcohol is good for us, but there is little margin for error, as over consumption is very unhealthy. Now, if we like the occasional drink, then all the research I have ever read points to our best bet being red wine. Tannins are a chemical found in the skin of the grape that helps protect it from bugs, and they are excellent antioxidants and in sensible quantity may help prevent cellular damage that leads to cancer. Also, resveratrol found in red grapes further adds to its healing benefits, although recent researchers have suggested that we would need to consume way too much wine for the benefit of resveratrol to be meaningful.

One final thought on alcohol, but this time it's aimed just at us men. Did you know when we consume lots of booze, our body converts the male sex hormone testosterone into the female hormone oestrogen? Yes gents, the more we drink the more feminine we become. Now that might explain a lot of the man boobs that we see in pubs!

Dr James DiNicolantonio
Red wine consumed with a meal can help reduce oxidative stress from the foods that you are consuming, it can help lower blood pressure if you consume it with food and it can help reduce post-meal spikes in blood sugar. Part of the reason why red wine over white wine is so beneficial is because it is fermented with the grape seeds and the skin. Therefore, you get more polyphenols, more of a substance called resveratrol and quercetin, and these plant polyphenols kind of help dilate the blood vessels and reduce blood platelet clotting.

Turn Off the Heat

When my son-in-law Jake and I decided to walk to the North Pole (you can watch the documentary on YouTube, it's called 'The Last Degree North Pole'), we were advised that, due to the extreme low temperatures, we would need to consume 9,000 calories each day of our week-long adventure. As it turns out, our clothing was so good that we only burnt 6,000 calories per day. But that's still a whooping 3,400 more than we would normally expend. What was really interesting was that, while we were walking and pulling our sledges, we took off our thick overcoats and even at -40°C we walked wearing very thin jackets. The point is this: when we are in cold conditions our body consumes a colossal amount of energy to keep us warm.

I once read that we actually burn more calories per hour standing in a cold sea on a British summer holiday than we do jogging for the same amount of time. Wow! Don't run a marathon but get into surfing! Apparently, when we are shivering, we burn around 100 calories every 15 minutes. Let me stress of course that we must not take it to the extreme or we might get hypothermia, which can be fatal. If we get too cold and can't keep heating our entire body, then it focuses on warming our core and horrible things begin to happen to our arms and legs. I witnessed this for myself when the doctor we took with us on our North Pole expedition got the insides of his gloves damp and suffered terrible frostbite.

What about cold showers? If you can, wow – what a great start to the day you are going to have. Actress Katharine Hepburn was said to have taken a cold bath or shower every day and swore by its benefits.

How does taking a cold shower contribute to our health? It makes us breathe deeply as we gasp so that we take in more oxygen. This leads to an increase in heart rate, releasing a rush of blood and energy throughout the body – that's why we should do it in the morning and not at bedtime.

Cold water is also great for our hair and skin too. It makes our hair shiny, stronger and generally healthier. It also closes our pores, which is why we should always use cold water after a shave. According to Dr Joseph Mercola, a natural health expert, "It can lower blood pressure, clear blocked arteries and improve our immune system".

On a scientific level, taking a cold shower, exposure to cold temperatures, cold-water swimming or cold baths, is referred to as cold thermogenesis (CT) and many elite athletes embed it into their weekly training. CT can:

- Help cure or reduce stress, and as we have already read stress is possibly the biggest cause of heart attacks
- Increase the strength of our immune system
- Increase metabolism
- Activate adiponectin hormones, which increase consumption of glucose and breaks down fatty acids

Hannah Richards

The best way by which we can take control of our health is to be more aware of the food we eat, the way we move, the thoughts we think and the hours we sleep. What you eat makes you who you are, what you absorb makes you able to be who you are, and how you eliminate waste products from the body allows you to be the best that you can be.

There are a few simple prerequisites to being a highly efficient, all-cylinders-firing, functional human being:
1. Optimum and intelligent food sourcing and selection
2. Optimum digestion and absorption and elimination
3. Optimum hydration levels
4. Optimum sleep
5. Optimum movement

Chapter 7 Highlights

- Health benefits of SENSIBLE sunbathing outweigh skin cancer risks.
- When it is sunny, go outside without sunscreen for up to 50% of the time that it would normally take you to turn slightly red. Then go under the shade, chill for half an hour and then slap on a mineral based, broad spectrum sunscreen.
- Aim for 7 to 9 hours sleep daily, if necessary, take afternoon naps.
- Sitting for long periods is thought to slow the metabolism, which affects the body's ability to regulate blood sugar.
- Undoubtedly a small amount of alcohol is good for us, but there is little margin for error.
- Taking a cold shower can help reduce stress and increase the strength of our immune system.
- Taking a cold shower or bath, can increase metabolism and help the body breaks down fatty acids.

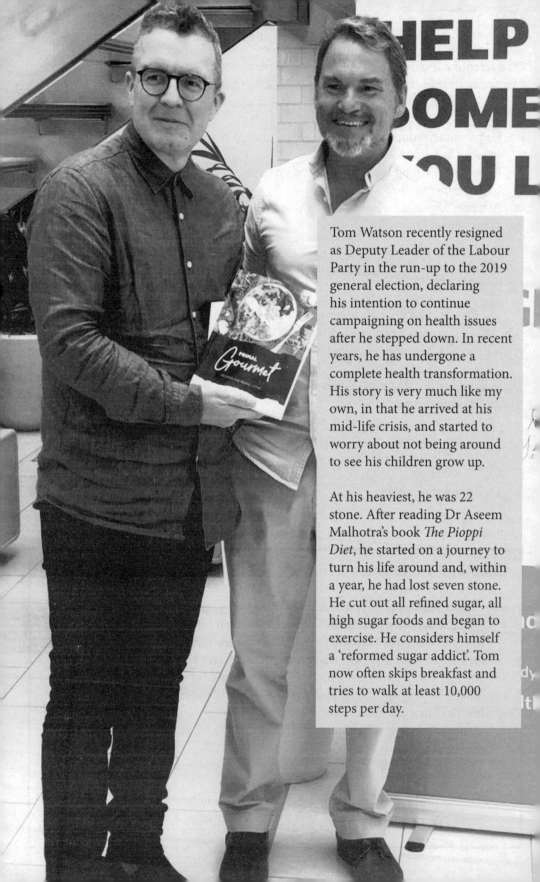

Tom Watson recently resigned as Deputy Leader of the Labour Party in the run-up to the 2019 general election, declaring his intention to continue campaigning on health issues after he stepped down. In recent years, he has undergone a complete health transformation. His story is very much like my own, in that he arrived at his mid-life crisis, and started to worry about not being around to see his children grow up.

At his heaviest, he was 22 stone. After reading Dr Aseem Malhotra's book *The Pioppi Diet*, he started on a journey to turn his life around and, within a year, he had lost seven stone. He cut out all refined sugar, all high sugar foods and began to exercise. He considers himself a 'reformed sugar addict'. Tom now often skips breakfast and tries to walk at least 10,000 steps per day.

CHAPTER 8

WHAT IS HAPPINESS?

*"Very little is needed to make a happy life; it is all
within yourself, in your way of thinking."*
MARCUS AURELIUS

In this chapter, we will look at how stress effects our happiness and discover that
pleasure and happiness are very different emotions.

Stress-related diseases are one of the biggest killers in the Western world. From cancer
to heart attacks, so many illnesses and early deaths can be attributed to it. While a little
bit of stress, such as that from exercise, is good for us, prolonged exposure – whether it
be conscious or subconscious – is really bad for our health.

Dr Shan Hussain
As a doctor, I regard stress as any physical, mental or emotional factor
that causes strain or tension on the body or mind. Mental or emotional
stress often results from adverse situations, such as family conflicts,
worries about work, or health issues, but it's important to remember
that stress is highly individual.

What's highly stressful for one person may be regarded as normal for another.
Whenever a patient tells me they feel ill or mentally exhausted or depressed from
stress, I take it seriously, even if the stress they describe doesn't seem that stressful.
After all, I believe physical, mental, or social stress may well be the fundamental basis
of most, if not all, disease.

Seven Steps to Happiness

I have spent years trying to uncover what makes people truly happy, and have come up with seven recurring traits of happy people:

1.   They don't worry much and therefore aren't stressed
2.   They have a close circle of friends or family and therefore a sense of belonging
3.   They challenge themselves frequently
4.   They have a purpose in life
5.   They have a high level of tolerance and can rationalise things
6.   They take everything and everyone less seriously
7.   They demonstrate gratitude and realise that comparison is the theft of happiness

Let me explain all 7 in a little more detail:

1. Minimise Worry

One of the best pieces of advice I have ever been given is to try everything possible to never waste time worrying about events that have happened, or those that we can't change. Instead, only invest time deliberating about things that we can influence.

Relax a little and try not to take everything to heart. If you can't change something or it has already happened, just whistle or hum to yourself Bobby McFerrin's 1988 song 'Don't Worry, Be Happy'. Adopt the more laid-back approach of the African tribes in Kenya and Tanzania, who in real life really do use the phrase from The Lion King, 'Hakuna matata' – the Swahili saying for 'no worries'.

If you hate your boss because he or she is unreasonable, have a chat with them to try to help them see the error of their ways - and if nothing changes, try to get them fired! I know this might sound like strange advice from someone who employs hundreds of managers, but bad managers are bad for both business and health. While work to a certain degree should be challenging, it should also be enjoyable and rewarding. Work must make you happy. If you hate your job, then leave and find something else that you enjoy. Life is too short to be stuck in a job you don't like. And never stay in a job just because the pay is good. Cash only buys pleasure, not happiness.

2. Family, Friends, Colleagues and Dogs

In the first edition of *Primal Cure* I told a story about the Greek island of Ikaria. Here is a snippet that highlights the importance of social interaction. On a small mountainous island, just a stone's throw from the Turkish coast, lives a small community of people who, when it comes to living healthily into old age, are breaking all sorts of records. Most evenings you find elders wandering into their neighbours' homes and sharing freshly prepared meals and several glasses of locally produced wine. Here they don't send parents into care homes; they remain together in strong family units. Their sense of community seems all but lost on the rest of the Westernised world. Interestingly, The World Health Organisation defines health as "a state of complete physical, mental and social wellbeing and not merely the absence of disease or infirmity".

There is a brilliant book written by Dan Buettner called *The Blue Zones*. Dan travels the world to regions with the highest concentration of centenarians (those that have lived to over 100 years), to discover the truth about living longer. One of the key similarities across all regions was a strong family bond, where people of old age still put their loved ones first.

In *The Art of Happiness* written by His Holiness the Dalai Lama, he talks about how having an intimate relationship with someone, whether it be a spouse, a friend or relative, someone to share your deepest feelings, fears and so on, plays a key role in making us truly happy.

Dr Shan Hussain

High-quality social interaction on a regular basis with your immediate peers is helpful for reducing and managing stress. In other words, make an effort to get together with your friends and family when you can. If your social circle is small, have you thought about getting a dog? A recent study in Sweden showed that dog owners were 23 per cent less likely to die of cardiovascular disease, and they also experienced a 20 per cent lower risk of mortality from all causes. The authors were unable to explain this link, but it was felt the additional physical activity and emotional connection between dogs and owners played the most critical roles.

3. Challenges

A challenge is something that stretches us physically or mentally. It might not give us pleasure at the time – it might be delayed until the activity has passed, such as the feeling of relaxation and achievement after a hard gym session or learning to play an instrument or speak a foreign language. Not only do these activities prevent stress, they also keep the brain functioning well.

4. Purpose

In addition to setting ourselves challenges, to be truly happy it's important to believe that our actions are making a contribution to something that we consider to be worthwhile.

It's been proven in several pieces of research that people who win huge amounts on the lottery usually become unhappy people. Why is this? Whilst everyone will have different opinions on what makes us happy, I am convinced truly happy people are those who have few worries, who enjoy sharing experiences with friends and family, but have a sense of purpose in their life.

Lottery winners tend to have lots of worries - perhaps about losing what they have quickly gained or guilt for having not earned it. They often become isolated from friends and have fewer challenges and less purpose in their lives! My advice is not to do the lottery. If you were to win, it could ruin your life and whilst you are sitting there waiting to win, you are not engaged in actions that will fulfil your purpose and enhance your self-worth.

5. Tolerance

In both our personal and work lives, the strongest relationships are the ones that give and take. There must be an element of tolerance in life, because without it we are likely to become very stressed indeed. Leading on from tolerance is the ability to rationalise. I recently walked passed two elderly ladies sitting on a bench, admiring the views across the river in Dartmouth, and heard one say to the other, "How do you always look so happy, I never see you depressed", the lady smiled back at her friend and said, "I am always able to rationalise things". From this I took it that she had a 'let it be' attitude, or as the French say 'laissez faire'.

Virginia Satir who was an American author and therapist, known especially for her approach to family therapy, famously said, "Life is not what it's supposed to be. It's what it is. The way you cope with it is what makes the difference".

6. Don't Be So Serious

One common trait I see in happy people, is they know when and when not to take things seriously. That includes themselves. There is a great saying, 'don't take yourself too seriously because nobody else does'. When things go wrong, as long as you can learn from it, don't hold on to the failure but let it go!

7. Be Grateful and Don't Compare

There might be a very famous advert that says 'go compare', but that's the very thing we should never do when it comes to our own lives, other than of course, to compare ourselves with those that are less fortunate. Gratitude is a lovely place to live!

One of the biggest problems with social media is that most people only post snapshots of their moments of happiness, and this is rarely a reflection of their true self. As A-ha once sang, 'The Sun Always Shines On TV'. Today's comparison culture on social media really is robbing happiness from the younger generations. Comparison, especially the comparison of others' apparent pleasure or monetary possessions, is the fundamental theft of happiness.

Pleasure vs Happiness

It is vitally important for our wellbeing to understand the difference between pleasure and happiness. Too much pleasure can often lead to reduced happiness. Chasing too much pleasure can lead to addictions, obesity, depression, ADHD, anxiety and even suicide. In fact, the search for pleasure can be associated with all chronic illnesses experienced in modern society.

Pleasure is often driven by rewards and usually is short-lived. Pleasure can often be achieved at the detriment of happiness. A few too many alcoholic drinks or a big tub of ice cream might deliver immediate gratification, but in the long run, make us less happy. And you won't be surprised to learn that reducing our CARB input and eating whole natural foods, helps to restore our natural balance of pleasure and happiness.

Technical Stuff

Chemical neurotransmitters are effectively chemical signal that effectively transmits a message from one brain neuron to the next. Neurotransmitters drive our feelings of pleasure or happiness; reward or contentment; enjoyment or gratitude. The neurotransmitter in the brain that drives reward is dopamine, while happiness is fuelled by serotonin.

This is such an important area and one that may be very new to you, as it was to me, that I want to hand the rest of this topic over to Robert Lustig who, as a paediatric endocrinologist (someone who diagnoses and treats hormonal disorders in children), has spent many years researching this.

Dr Robert Lustig

Today 4.4% of the entire world has been diagnosed with clinical depression, that is a 20% increase in a decade. I believe part of the cause is that us, as a society, have lost track of these two positive emotions; pleasure and happiness. We think they are the same. We have been told that they are the same. And I think we have been told they are the same by people who want us to buy stuff, I quote, 'to get happy'. Because they have something to sell. Hedonics sell. In fact, four out of the top ten exports out of the United States are hedonic substances. Oil, corn, soy and sugar. So, they tell us their products will make us happy. But pleasure and happiness are not the same. I would argue that they are diametrically opposite. They seem like they are related, they are both positive emotions, we like them both, so why should we care? Well, I am going to give you seven differences between pleasure and happiness that I outline in my book.

1. Pleasure is short-lived, like a meal. Happiness is long-lived, often for a lifetime.
2. Pleasure is visceral; you feel it in your body. Happiness is ethereal; you feel it above the neck.
3. Pleasure is taking; happiness is giving.
4. Pleasure is experienced alone; happiness is normally experienced in social groups.
5. Pleasure is achievable with substances; happiness is not achievable with substances.
6. The extremes of pleasure, whether it be substances or behaviours; nicotine, cocaine, tobacco, alcohol, street drugs, chocolate, sugar, or behaviours; shopping, gambling, social media, pornography; in the extreme, all of these lead to addiction. All of these can have a 'holic' at the end of the word, for example, shopaholic and alcoholic. But there is no such thing as being addicted to too much happiness.
7. And finally, the reason why I wrote the book. Pleasure is dopamine and happiness is serotonin. Two different neurotransmitters in the brain, two different sets of receptors, two different mechanisms of action, two different regulatory pathways and two different areas of the brain they work in. And the reason why we are in such a mess is because we lost track of this.

In this unregulated capitalist world that we have today, corporations try and generate as much profit as possible. And in the process what we have done is made everyone fat, sick, stupid, addicted and broke. Because we have peddled hedonics, because that is what sells and we made everyone miserable and sick. And we have basically destroyed economies all over the world by chronic disease.

Money can buy you pleasure, but it can't buy you happiness. People don't recognise the difference. And by seeking these short-term dopamine hits, they are actually doing themselves damage. It is all science. Dopamine is a neurotransmitter that neurons make to tell other neurons what to do. The next neuron has receptors, and dopamine binds to that neuron and causes it to fire. And in this process of firing, we get emotions, we get behaviours, and we get pleasure. It is the motivation neurotransmitter; it is the positive reinforcement neurotransmitter; it is basically the neurotransmitter that tells our brain this feels good; I want more. I want to do this again. Dopamine is the source of habit. It's not that dopamine isn't important, it is. Without it, we wouldn't have sex; therefore, there would be no human race. If we didn't have dopamine, we would be a sloth and never get out of bed.

But here is the problem with dopamine. It is excitatory. So, it always excites the next neuron. Now neurons like be excited, they like to be stimulated, that is why they have receptors in the first place. But they like to be tickled, not bludgeoned. Chronic over-stimulation of any neuron leads to neuronal cell death. But neurons don't want to die. So they have a plan B. They have a self-defence mechanism. What they do is down-regulate the number of receptors, which makes it less likely that any dopamine receptor will find a cell to bind to. So, more dopamine and fewer receptors mean less signal. Less signal means less benefit. So, you end up needing more and more to get less and less. And that is the phenomenon that we call tolerance. So next time you need a bigger hit and the receptors go down, you keep doing this repeatedly, with bigger and bigger hits, until you get nothing and eventually when the neurons do start to die, now you got addiction. And when they do die, they don't come back; they are gone for good.

When you kill those neurons in that reward centre, you are never going to get the same gain, you are never going to get the amplitude, of the response that you originally got. Which means you are never going to really get the same pleasure that you did before. This, of course, is the reason for recidivism from addiction and why people go back. You are trying to get back what you knew you once had. But you can't. And you are miserable.

Serotonin, on the other hand, the contentment neurotransmitter, the feel-good, the I don't need anymore, the relaxation, the zen neurotransmitter, it's not excitatory, it's inhibitory. It inhibits the next neuron; it keeps it from firing. So if you are inhibiting the next neuron, do you have to down-regulate the receptors? No, you don't need to, because there is nothing to protect it from. So, you can't overdose from too much happiness. But there is one thing that does down-regulate serotonin, and that is dopamine! SO THE MORE PLEASURE YOU SEEK, THE MORE UNHAPPY YOU GET. (I put that in capitals because it is so frigging important.)

Let me summarise the above. The more rewards we seek, whether they be alcohol, drugs, sex, shopping, gambling, possessions; the next like on Facebook or views on YouTube; snacks, sugar, bigger meals, chocolate - short term instant rewards, it actually down-regulates happiness in the long term.

Dr Robert Lustig

If you don't know the difference between pleasure and happiness, and if your pleasure is cheap, you are going to overload on that because you can, and make yourself extraordinary miserable. So, addiction and depression are actually two sides of the same coin, and they are driven by the same five changes in our environment, which have occurred over the past fifty years. They are; technology, processed food, sugar, sleep deprivation and drugs. All five of those are dopamine stimulators. All five of those drive reward. And all five of those lead to metabolic syndrome. Which then leads to low serotonin.

Then add some stress on top of these. And stress, by effecting an area right at the front of the brain, called the pre-frontal cortex; stress puts that pre-frontal cortex to sleep. It tells the executive function centre, your Jiminy Cricket part of the brain; the part of the brain that stops you from doing stupid things; the bit that tells you not to do something because you will pay for it tomorrow; stress basically puts the pre-frontal cortex to sleep. As your pre-frontal cortex goes offline, it revs up dopamine even more. And cortisol, the stress hormone, reduces the receptors for serotonin, thereby making you even more unhappy.

In order to turn this around, this global chronic disease, addiction, economic and climate-change debacle; because climate change is related to this as well. We need to tamp down our dopamine, not get rid of it, but tamp it down, we need to up our serotonin, and we need to reduce our cortisol. Those are the three goals:

1. Reduce our dopamine
2. Up our serotonin
3. Reduce our cortisol

If we do that, we will get healthy, we will enjoy our lives, and we will solve all of the biggest problems in our society. All at once. It is just one problem. So what can we do? Well, one thing we can't do is to rely on governments to help us, because governments are addicted to the money that these hedonic substances bring in for them. And they are all paid off by those industries anyway. So, don't expect anyone to help you out of this. You have to do it for yourself.

So, there are four things you can do, and they are free. But you really have to want to do them. This is what is needed to achieve the three goals of reducing dopamine, upping serotonin and reducing cortisol. I call them the 4 Cs. And they are:

1. Connect. Face-to-face human interaction. Social interaction. Not online or on the phone. This is because, in the back of the head, there are some neurons called mirror neurons and these only work face to face. It's the only way to transmit empathy. And this drives up serotonin. (Robert talks a lot more on this on my podcast and in his book.)

2. Contribute. Contribute to others creates serotonin. Giving not taking. Help others.

3. Cope. Three things will help you cope with things; sleep, mindfulness and exercise. With mindfulness, for example, we need to stop trying to multitask, because every time we do, we get a cortisol bump and it takes 23 minutes to refocus. All of these reduce cortisol. If you couple mindfulness and exercise, you can basically reverse depression.

4. Cook. There are three things in food that matter. Tryptophan, which is an amino acid, it's the rarest amino acid, and it is in short supply. Yet it is the precursor for serotonin. So, if you are not getting enough tryptophan, you are not making enough serotonin. So, where do you get tryptophan; by far the number one is in eggs. Next poultry and salmon, but in vegetables not very much. So, you need those things. But the world is going vegan, which is not necessarily good. You also need omega 3's. They are heart-healthy, anti-inflammatory, anti-Alzheimer's. They are membrane stabilisers; especially in the neurons in your brain. And finally, we are consuming too much sugar; fructose, because it drives dopamine and lowers serotonin.

Hope

Dr Jen Unwin

Where there is hope, there is happiness, and where there is happiness, there is longevity. I think modern medicine has been stripped back of its ability to help people to be more hopeful and yet positive phycology, often makes more difference than all of the clever medicines and things they can do today. The placebo effect of positive phycology can be very powerful.

Switch Off The TV and Read A Book

Dr Shan Hussain

Common sense tells us that too much TV is bad for our health. But is this really true, and how much is too much? Aside from working and sleeping, watching TV is the most commonly reported daily activity in many developed countries. A large 40-year meta-analysis in 2011 confirmed that prolonged TV viewing is associated with increased risk of type 2 diabetes, cardiovascular disease and all-cause mortality. The association was linear and strongest among people watching TV for over three hours per day.

But reading books, well that's a whole different matter. According to a 12-year study performed at Yale University and published in Social Science and Medicine, book readers experienced a 20 per cent reduction in mortality compared to non-book readers. Reading for only 30 minutes each day helped people live an average of 23 months longer compared with non-book readers, regardless of gender, wealth, education or health.

Avoid Those Selling Happiness

Have you ever noticed how the big food and fizzy pop corporations are always trying to sell us happiness? They all realise that happiness is the ultimate human goal. Happy meals, happy hours and Coca-Cola's 'Open Happiness' advert that ran for more than seven years, all promise to deliver the holy grail of life. McDonald's actually deliver a double dose of happiness. Firstly they sell you 'Happy Meals' and then tell you 'I'm Lovin' It'. But the reality is what they are really selling is short term pleasure, short term reward and the reality is that if we consume too much of their 'happiness' produce. The long-term effect isn't happiness but a life of misery. For full disclosure, creating happiness has always been part of my own companies' positioning; it even forms part of our jewellery company's logo, all be it in Latin. But luckily our marketing team fully understand the difference between pleasure and happiness and are hell-bent on delivering genuine happiness.

Eating Rubbish Leaves Us Stressed and Depressed

During the world wars, you would assume Britain was a pretty depressing place to live, and therefore, depression must have been rife. But according to data, depression rates in our country have only started to sky-rocket since junk processed foods became our staple diet. There seems to be so much correlation between sugar/processed CARBS and depression that the two must be linked.

Good food equals a great mood! You will read throughout *Fat & Furious* various ways to avoid stress and other brain-related disorders by eating the right food. The main culprits, of course, are CARBS and other sugars, which become deadly poisons that stress out the body when over-consumed. For now, let's keep it as simple as possible - out of all the courses at the dinner table that we eat, which are the most laden with sugar and most damaging to our health? Desserts, of course! And if we write desserts backwards, what does it spell? STRESSED. Enough said!

Hangry

Professor Tim Noakes

As both a scientist and an athlete, what was life like for you before you went low carb? Towards the end, I was often angry at times, without any understanding of it at all. And that's the 'hangry' (anger that is bought on by being hungry) expression. I was perpetually hungry, yet I was always eating. I would come home at night, and my wife would ask me why I was eating so much. And of course, it was things like bread, and

I was always drinking sports drinks and back then I could never run without my sports drink. And of course, when you finish, you had to have more sports drinks. My tea was loaded with sugar. So, I had all of the features of sugar addiction. I was starting to put on weight, so I started snoring. Then I had all the other symptoms, not of insulin resistance but of intolerance to carbohydrates, particularly to cereals and grains. I had four or five different conditions. Which I now know were an allergy to cereals and grains. And as soon as I removed them, they cleared within weeks. I won't go through all of them, but I think it's important to know that if you have rhinitis, your nose is always running, I promise you that is an allergy to cereals and grains. I also had mild asthma, and it disappeared without the cereals and grains. Your concentration goes down, and your energy goes down, you get angrier and more hostile, those are some of the key characteristics.

Chapter 8 Highlights

- Stress-related diseases are one of the biggest killers in the Western world.
- Having an intimate relationship with someone, plays a key role in making us truly happy.
- Life is not what it's supposed to be. It's what it is. The way you cope with it is what makes the difference.
- Gratitude is a lovely place to live!
- Comparison, especially the comparison of others' apparent pleasure or monetary possessions, is the fundamental theft of happiness.
- Pleasure and happiness are not the same, normally they are diametrically opposite.
- Two different neurotransmitters in the brain, two different sets of receptors. Pleasure is dopamine and happiness is serotonin.
- One of the things that down-regulate serotonin, is dopamine! So, the more pleasure we seek, the more unhappy we get.
- Where there is hope, there is happiness, and where there is happiness, there is longevity.
- Good food equals a great mood!

CHAPTER 9

OPTIMISE YOUR ENVIRONMENT

"Never doubt that a small group of thoughtful, committed citizens
can change the world; indeed, it is the only thing that ever has."
MARGARET MEAD

It's time to retreat back to our cave. In this chapter, we look at how toxins are affecting our health and how to best avoid them.

Avoid Murder by Toxin

In 2006, ex-Russian spy Alexander Litvinenko was killed in London, when apparently someone slipped polonium-210 – a radioactive substance – into his cup of tea. Then, in February 2017, the estranged older brother of North Korean leader, Kim Jong Nam, was attacked at Kuala Lumpur Airport. Two women wiped a highly toxic nerve agent called VX on his face, and he died within just 30 minutes.

Why mention these two high-profile cases? To highlight, without any uncertainty, that toxins can kill. Do I honestly believe that toxins kill more people than they are held responsible for? Yes, without a doubt. Pretty much the only toxins our primal ancestors were exposed to were the odd poisonous mushroom or venomous bite. But fast-forward to today and we are exposed to a mass of toxins. These can be in the form of:

1. What we eat and drink
2. What we inhale
3. What we apply to the skin
4. Electromagnetic fields

Toxins in What We Eat and Drink

There is not much to cover here that we haven't already mentioned. If we are avoiding packaged food and only buying organic produce, then we are doing pretty much everything we possibly can do to be safe. On the odd occasion, when we unknowingly digest something that might be slightly toxic, as long as it's in a small dose then our clever gut and liver will likely be able to deal with it.

As well as being very careful about our food choices, we should be equally careful in how we store and cook our foods. For example, don't store any food in plastic, unless you are 100% sure that they don't contain bisphenol A (BPAs). This is especially crucial if you are going to microwave your food. Also, avoid using Teflon-coated pans if they are scratched or chipped as they can potentially leak dangerous chemicals into food. Another metal that should be avoided for cooking is aluminium. There have been several studies where they have found a link between the regular use of cooking in aluminium and Alzheimer's. Food grade stainless steel is always the best choice for your health, as well as the longevity of your cooking utensils. When food burns it also becomes toxic, but we will cover this subject later when we discuss cancer.

Toxins In What We Inhale

Don't smoke, period. Hold your breath momentarily as you race past the smokers huddled together outside the airport or office. When it comes to traffic fumes, try to avoid busy roads and instead learn to walk along the quieter back streets. We should be really careful in city centres, especially where there are lots of traffic jams: the densely packed buildings and skyscrapers lock in fumes, creating what some are calling urban canyons. A recent report compiled on behalf of the EU by the University of the West of England listed some very interesting findings. To measure air pollution, they fitted car drivers, cyclists and pedestrians with a carbon monoxide monitors. On studying their research, what I found most interesting was that, on open roads, the level of pollution falls off quite quickly the further we are from traffic. For example, cyclists at 2.5 metres from the middle of the road were on average exposed to 0.5 toxic parts per million, while pedestrians at six metres from the middle of the road were exposed to 0.1 toxic parts per million. So, when we can't avoid going into highly congested cities or towns, it's important to try to get as far away from traffic as possible.

Toxins In What We Apply To The Skin

For full disclosure, let me first tell you that a company that I am involved with, Primal Living, do sell a range of natural skincare products. Therefore in this section, I have deliberately not updated it from my first health book *Primal Cure*, which was written a long time before we decided there was a genuine need to create a complete range of healthcare products.

Have you ever wondered what is in the shampoos and shower gels that we lather all over our body? Have you ever stopped and thought about how that antiperspirant stops us sweating all day? Do you know what's in the creams and makeup that we apply to our skin?

In Canada, some people decided to find out the answer to these questions. You can read the full report at *www.environmentaldefence.ca*. They trawled through the handbags of six ladies and conducted tests on items including foundations, concealers, powders, blushes, mascaras, eye-liners, eye shadows, lipsticks and glosses. In total, they tested 49 different products, and the results were alarming. All 49 contained nickel, all but two contained lead, half contained cadmium and ten contained the poison arsenic. And, before you start to think that Canadians use inferior cosmetics, nearly all of the products were brand names that you would recognise and most women in the UK use regularly.

One of the people who had their makeup scrutinised was Erin Charter. On hearing the findings, she said, "The product that I spend the most money on, because I believed it was better for me, ended up being the worst out of everything tested! I'd like to have some indication of these ingredients on the label, so I could make informed choices. Or, better still, I'd like there to be rules to protect me from these chemicals, so I don't need to worry so much".

While there are numerous white papers and continual scientific debates as to what constitutes 'safe' levels of heavy metal exposure, I find it hard to comprehend how anyone could ever tell. How is it possible to truly measure what is the safe level of covering your body in known poisons over a sustained period of many years? Imagine going to one of the many uncontacted tribes in Peru or Indonesia and saying, "Hey, would you like to make yourself look more attractive by putting on modern makeup? But before you do, we have to warn you that they contain at least nine different elements that are known to be poisonous". What do you think they would say? Would it be, "Hey, that sounds like a good idea, let's stop using the natural herbs and colourings that we have used for generations and go for your scary cocktail of prettily labelled toxins?"

Is it really that bad to put poisonous things on our skin and to spray them in our hair and under our arms? Think back to chapter 2 (page 44) where we discussed how, when the small intestine has done its job, it sends blood to the liver for a safety check before it is then allowed to be pumped around the body. The problem with what we put on our skin is that, without a safety check, it is free to be absorbed directly into the bloodstream. Am I really implying that we would therefore be safer swallowing our shampoo, deodorant and makeup than we are applying it to the skin? Yes, I am. If we were to swallow them, our inbuilt safety mechanism would kick in and we would normally vomit. If we did somehow manage to swallow them, then our liver would give the thumbs down and send them to our back door for a quick and timely departure.

I have a simple piece of advice on choosing any skincare products, and that is always to read the ingredients. If you would not be happy to eat it, then don't apply or spray it!

Think about it this way: for 2 million years we have had to build a defence mechanism for poisonous things that we might consume. Every single month, our primal ancestors had a varied diet of hundreds of different plants and bugs. This diversified diet meant that they would occasionally eat a berry, a mushroom or plant that was not healthy for them. Therefore, through evolution, Mother Nature has built in a fairly robust safety mechanism against things that we might accidentally consume.

But, as we have only been smearing our body in poisonous creams, makeup and cleansing products for just over 100 years, nature hasn't yet had chance to evolve and create either a natural defence or a warning mechanism. When I told my wife this, her immediate reaction was that I was wrong; to be honest that's not an unusual response! She reminded me of how our daughter Lili had come out in a huge rash after having her face painted and how our sister-in-law Paula's eyes had become swollen from a reaction to sun cream. Of course, as always, my wife was right. However, these were reactions to highly concentrated poisons in just one application. The body was smart enough to detect this and react immediately, therefore alerting them not to use those products again. But what I am talking about here isn't huge concentrations of poisonous things in just one application, but a lifelong drip-feed of them into our systems.

Think about it another way. We know that toxins attack the immune system. We also know that underactive thyroids are related to the immune system, and it is a fact that this condition is much more prevalent in females. Why is this the case? Could it be because females apply far more products on the skin than males? In her insightful book, *Hashimoto's Protocol*, Dr Izabella Wentz makes a very similar point, "When we swallow a substance, our gut and liver process it first before it goes into the circulation system. When you apply substances through the skin, the substances skip the gatekeepers of the digestive tract and liver". In an article in The Huffington Post titled, 'Why Your Makeup is More Harmful than You Think,' it says, "When it comes to antiperspirant, you may want to consider going for the less potent, natural options. When you shave your armpits, you're scraping off a layer of skin – and then you apply the carcinogenic-filled deodorant right onto the vulnerable area right near your lymph nodes. Yikes!"

It's not just the creams, makeup and sprays that can cause us harm, but the clothes that we wear too. We should try to avoid synthetic material, instead dressing in clothes made from natural fibres such as cotton or bamboo. While we are talking about clothes... There was a recent news clip on the BBC, where the fire brigade conducted an experiment to show the dangers of using skin creams containing paraffin. They set alight six identical ladies tops, one that hadn't been worn and the rest that had been worn for different periods of time. Amongst the points they were trying to highlight, it was frightening to see how quickly the clothes caught fire if they had been in contact with skin creams containing paraffin (of which sadly there are many on the market), even if the clothes had been washed. The conclusion was that tragically 44 women in Britain have died since 2010 due the paraffin in their clothes catching fire. Now while that is very frightening, what is more concerning to those of us living in Britain, is the toxic effects that same paraffin might be having on the health of our bodies.

Embrace The Coconut and Avoid Toxic Hygiene

We have already talked about the huge health benefits of coconut oil and, in chapter 12, we will look at other ways to make the coconut a staple in our diet. But here, I would like to discuss several other ways in which coconuts can help us avoid toxic substances and thereby improve our health and wellbeing. As well as being one of the only Superfoods that we should consider for our skin, hair and teeth, I highlight it here in an attempt to try and get everyone to start thinking about natural, non-toxic and non-poisonous solutions to personal hygiene.

Teeth and Gums

If we swirl coconut oil around our mouth for five to ten minutes, not only do our teeth become whiter, we will be providing our entire mouth with a full detox. Known as oil pulling, you can create your own pulls or there are several brands available in health stores. As there are no added chemicals or other nasties, coconut pulling is extremely healthy and an additional benefit it makes our breath smell great too. No wonder so many celebrities, including the lovely Gwyneth Paltrow, are said to be now pulling with coconut.

By simply mixing it with baking soda, you can even use coconut as a toothpaste. If we miss the minty taste of chemical-laden commercial products, then we can always add a little bit of mint to it.

Coconut and Our Skin

In the gemstone world, experts often liken the outer layers of a pearl to that of a woman's skin. If skin looks youthful and translucent it is sometimes described as pearlescent. When we are young, the fat in our skin can hold plenty of water, but as we age our fat breaks down and our skin dries out. To avoid wrinkling, it's important to keep skin moist. Obviously, water is not the answer, as it doesn't penetrate the surface of the skin – if it did, we would never get out of the bath! The primal answer to a pearlescent vibrant skin is, of course, the application of quality organic oils. Coconut is the king of all oils, and pretty much the only oil that has a medium-chain fatty acid (MCFA). Applying coconut oil directly to the skin helps maintain a youthful look. Don't just take my word for it. When Nicole Scherzinger was asked what the one skin product was she couldn't live without, she didn't name one of the beauty products that she was an ambassador for, but coconut oil! If you suffer from acne or spots, one of the best solutions is to apply a cream or lotion containing lauric acid. This has rich antibacterial, antiviral and antifungal properties and roughly half of the oil found in coconut is lauric acid, so it is great for applying to spots too.

Coconut as an Organic Shampoo

For healthy hair, it's important to keep our entire body hydrated, so drinking plenty of water is extremely important. For a full, bouncy and shiny head of hair, coconut oil is simply the best primal shampoo you will ever use. In fact, without realising it you probably inadvertently use a little already!

Many brands of shampoo and skin products blend coconut oils into their formulas, the only problem is, to make their product feel and foam like regular shampoos, they often blend it with chemicals that are toxic and potentially very dangerous to our health. According to leading nutritionist Dr Josh Axe, "It is the protein loss in hair that leads to dryness and breakage. The lauric acid has a low molecular weight, and can actually penetrate the hair shaft, nourishing the hair with vitamins, minerals and the medium-chain fatty acids".

Toxins in Electromagnetic Fields (EMF)

While not a toxin as described above, I couldn't leave out the dangers we face from putting our mobile phones to our ears too frequently. As a parent, I am concerned – or should I say frightened – by the fact that current claims that low frequency electromagnetic field exposure are safe is based on very little conclusive research. The World Health Organisation (WHO) currently state on their website, "The electromagnetic fields produced by mobile phones are classified by the International Agency for Research on Cancer as possibly carcinogenic to humans". Does that sound frightening? It does to me. Especially when you consider how big and powerful the telecommunication giants are, I doubt we will find out the truth for several more decades.

WHO's website goes on to say, "The power (and hence the radiofrequency exposure to a user) falls off rapidly with increasing distance from the handset. A person using a mobile phone 30 to 40cm away from their body – for example when text messaging, accessing the internet or using a 'hands-free' device – will therefore have a much lower exposure to radio frequency fields than someone holding the handset against their head. In addition to using hands-free devices, which keep mobile phones away from the head and body during phone calls, exposure is also reduced by limiting the number and length of calls. Using the phone in areas of good reception also decreases exposure as it allows the phone to transmit at reduced power".

My advice is going hands-free or don't use your mobile phone at all. However, it's not just your phone that produces a toxic electromagnetic field. The modern kitchen and bedroom are hotspots too. In the kitchen the microwave is the most harmful. While the food is fine once cooked, don't stand too close to it while it is cooking. Other appliances such as washing machines and blenders also generate an EMF, but they are far weaker. In the bedroom, try not to overuse your hairdryer and let your hair dry naturally where possible, just as our primal ancestors once did.

Dr Robert Lustig

My colleague Chris Madsen at UC Berkley did a study, that shows that kids who charge their mobile in the room at night, get 28 minutes less sleep than those who charge them outside of the room. And what we all need to do is to stop using screens one hour before bedtime. No screens. Books fine, but not screens as they are detrimental to the production of serotonin. Technology damages the pre-frontal cortex, and you need it for creativity.

The problem is, with digital, we are seeing everything, rather than imagining it, and this is why kids are getting stupid. And it's been going on since TV, but it has revved up since the digital revolution.

Dr Patrick Holford

About ten years ago, and this is a bit controversial, there was a survey that showed that left-handed people had more left-sided brain tumours and right-handed people had more right-sided brain tumours. We are talking about mobile phone use. And there is this rather aggressive brain cancer that is on the increase; it's gone up tenfold in the last twenty or so years, called glioblastoma. Two years ago, a very big study in a top journal said that ten years of mobile phone use more than doubles your risk of getting glioblastoma. So, we have an association. Then last year, there was a very good study that took these glioblastoma cells and exposed them to the amount that would be normal in a mobile call and found that the DNA fragmented, and bad things happen. So, we have a mechanism. But we will never have proof because it takes ten years to develop. So, you would have to have two groups for ten years, all doing the same things, but one group using mobiles and one not. But we are in the age of technology, so we are not all going to stop, but it's better to use it on speaker away from your head and always try and get a good signal.

Primal Detox

Every now and again, I believe there are huge gains to be made by undertaking a week-long detox. In the modern world, our immune system, which is controlled by our gut, really benefits from a deep clean. While detoxing has become something of a cult over recent years, I believe the type of detox most people take part in reaches nowhere near its full potential. You see, to really cleanse the body it's not just our food we need to clean up, but our environment too. For me, a true detox should consist of:

- Only consuming clean organic foods.
- Eating just the Top 20 Superfoods that you will read about later.
- All meals to include cruciferous vegetables whose glucosinolates supercharge detoxification.
- Eating foods high in sulphur, such as eggs, onions, garlic and chicken.
- Take curcumin supplements to aid detoxification.
- Consuming plenty of vitamin C as it helps flush toxins out of the body.
- Undertaking several fast days during the detox period.
- Consuming supplements to replace missing vitamins and nutrients.
- Not using a mobile phone or if we have to, ensuring its either on speaker mode or use headphones.
- Only drinking water that is filtered.
- Completely avoiding BPAs and plastic bottles.
- Avoiding antiperspirants, perfumes or aftershaves.
- Avoiding toxic shampoos or toothpaste.
- Wearing underwear made only of natural fibres.
- Drinking lots of green tea, which contains catechins that aids detoxification.

Flushing Toxins by Sweating

It's important to stop poisoning ourselves with unhealthy sprays, creams and shampoos, but we can also use our skin to clear toxins. One of the best ways to get our skin working for us is by sweating. When we sweat, our body naturally detoxes from the inside out.

As those living primally are not big on long jogs and epic bicycle rides - both activities where you would definitely sweat a lot - we need to look for alternative ways to detoxify. This is where taking a regular sauna can help. If you can't get to your local sauna, then when you do your gym routine try turning up the heat. If your gym owner won't let you do that, then put on lots of layers during your workout. It is really important that, on a regular basis, we find a way to sweat out our toxins. On a biological level, when we sweat it helps remove bacteria from our epidermal layer of skin and increases the rate at which dead skin cells are replaced.

Chapter 9 Highlights

- Avoid toxic creams, potions and lotions.
- Technology damages the pre-frontal cortex, and we need it for creativity.
- Do not use digital screens or watch TV an hour before bedtime as they are detrimental to the production of serotonin.
- The World Health Organisation recommends that those using a 'hands-free' device will have a much lower exposure to radio frequency fields than someone holding the handset against their head.
- When choosing any skincare products, always read the ingredients. If you would not be happy to eat it, then don't apply or spray it!
- Completely avoid BPAs and single-use plastic bottles.

CHAPTER 10

OPTIMAL GUT HEALTH

"The gut is the seat of all feeling. Polluting the gut not only cripples your immune system, but also destroys your sense of empathy, the ability to identify with other humans."
SUZY KASSEM

In this chapter we look at how the British diet causes havoc with the natural flora and fauna of our gut and what we can do to fix it.

Hippocrates taught us that, 'All diseases begin in the gut'. As I believe this to be so true, I am not going to apologise for already quoting this twice. I know there is a lot to comprehend in this book, so if I was asked to draw your attention to just one statistic, it is the following: scientific research now suggests that up to 90% of all known illnesses can be traced back to an unhealthy gut.

Wow! Doesn't that suggest we need to knuckle down and learn a little more about this extremely complex organ? Grab a black coffee or a cup of green tea and let's begin…

Our bodies are not just single living individuals, but thriving ecosystems comprised of 100 trillion microscopic creatures living and working in and on us. As we discovered in chapter 1, we are less likely to inherit diseases or illnesses that runs in our family than we probably fear, and one of the reasons for this is that only 10% of our cells contain any human DNA! The other 90% is made up of bacteria, fungi and microflora, all of which can't pass on anything genetically.

In *10% Human: How Your Body's Microbes Hold the Key to Health and Happiness*, author Dr Alanna Collen writes, "Over your lifetime, you will play host to bugs the equivalent weight of five African elephants. Your skin is crawling with them. There are more on your fingertip than there are people in Britain". Our 100 trillion microbes can be divided into more than 10,000 different species. This array of vastly different creatures living on and in our body are collectively referred to as our microbiome.

As Dr Martin J. Blaser explains in *Missing Microbes*, "In ecology, biome refers to the set of plants and animals in a community such as a jungle, forest or coral reef. An enormous diversity of species, large and small, interact to form complex webs of mutual support. When a keystone species disappears or goes extinct the ecology suffers. It can even collapse".

A lot of today's research into the human body and how it functions is now focusing on the importance of our microbiome. While these tiny creatures exist all over our body, inside and out, it is primarily their accumulation in our gut that has the biggest impact on our health. Getting the varieties of microbes in our gut balanced is now believed by cutting-edge science to have positive effects on all aspects of our health. From weight control to a healthy heart, food metabolism to a good memory, these creatures need to be respected and controlled.

They say a picture paints a thousand words, and when I am trying to create an image of what's happening in my gut - where many creatures are so tiny you wouldn't even see them under a normal microscope - I close my eyes and visualise ants! Just like ants working in a colony to perform tasks beyond our imagination, the bacterial army in our gut affect not just our health, but also our mood, emotions and behaviour. In *10% Human*, Dr Collen writes, "Imagine, for example, one strain of bacterium that feeds on a particular compound found in our food. If we eat that food, thus feeding these bacteria, and they are able to 'reward' us with a dose of happiness through the chemicals they produce, so much better for them. The chemicals they produce could cause us to crave the food they feed on, and even to remember where we found it".

Dr Aseem Malhotra

We are now beginning to understand that these microbes are essential for brain development, as well as being heavily involved in the regulation of the immune system and metabolism. The microbiota are also involved in the production of the hormone serotonin, which, when depleted, can lead to depression. Environmental and processed food chemicals that wipe out the good bacteria from our gut and reduce diversity have been linked to the development of many disorders including obesity, depression, allergies, autoimmune diseases and the metabolic syndrome. Artificial sweeteners, antibiotics and the lack of fibre appear to have a negative effect on the gut microbiome.

It will come as no surprise to you that one of the best ways to get our microbiome under control is to follow the principles laid out in this book– avoiding CARBS and other sugars, eating protein, fibre and lots of berries and nuts. If possible, we should try to avoid taking any antibiotics and, if we do take a course, then make sure we immediately rebuild our microbiome by taking a quality course of probiotics.

Our guts are a bit like a coral reef. While coral reefs can be devastated by a rapid rise in sea temperature, the colonies living in our microbiome can be eradicated by either a strong virus or antibiotics, and of course sometimes both. Just like the physical coral is still intact after bleaching, our intestines remain in place too, but they become barren. For months, maybe years afterwards, the gut's environment rests on a knife-edge. While some species are completely wiped out, one strand (firmicutes) seems to feed on disaster - and either avoid being exterminated or are very quick to regroup after a big environmental event.

Firmicutes are the bacteria that make us fat by rinsing every last calorie out of the food we eat. While firmicutes survive, overall diversity is greatly reduced, and some species never return. This imbalance is known as dysbiosis (sometimes referred to as dysbacteriosis). While antibiotics and major infections can cause complete wipe-outs, medicines, poor diets and mild illnesses can all knock our microbiome ecosystem off balance.

While there are several things we can do to reconstruct our microbiome, the most important thing is to avoid CARBS and other sugars and to eat a diet rich in fermented foods and fibre.

How important is the state of our microbiome? In truth, we don't fully know yet. After all, with 100 trillion microscopic creatures in our body across 10,000 different species, it is an area of science that we will probably never fully understand. But logic suggests that, as the bacteria in our gut is ultimately responsible for our immune system, then we should do everything we can to nurture them and keep them on our side. And talking of our immune system, did you know that 80% of it is located in our gut? What's your gut reaction to that fact? Hopefully it is to start taking better care of it!

With such a diverse range of tasks and skills, many scientists regard the gut as the second most complex engine in our body, only surpassed by the brain. It is now believed that a lot of the feelings that we can't always easily explain, such as depression, anxiety and stress, are driven from the gut and not from the brain. It is becoming increasingly evident that there is a connection between gut health and mental illness.

Many medical journals go as far as claiming that the gut is, in fact, our second brain. Think back to the small intestine, with its sensors the size of a tennis court. Compare it to all of our other sensors, such as our eyes, nose, ears and touch. It is vastly larger. It monitors way more than all of our other sensors put together, but we never give it credit or apportion blame for our feelings. Science is now discovering that we absolutely should. The 'gut feeling' is something we should not ignore any longer. In her book *Gut*, with the apt subtitle, 'The inside story of our body's most under-rated organ' author Giulia Enders says, "Cooperation between the gut and the brain begins very early in life. Together, they are responsible for a large proportion of our emotional world when we are babies".

Dr Patrick Holford

The undesirable organisms that reside in the guts of many people are called pathogens. We all have approximately 1.3kg (3lb) of about 300 different strains of bacteria living within our gut. Some can be classified as good and others as bad. However, the potentially 'bad' guys are not a hindrance as long as there are enough of the good guys around. These bacteria help us to digest food and fight off bad bacteria that enter the body, and they even make some vitamins. But the presence of the wrong kind of bacteria can cause ill health – especially if the gut wall is permeable and they enter the bloodstream.

Where Did Our Bacteria Originate?

First things first, this planet that we inhabit is really their domain and not ours. Earth formed some 4.5 billion years ago and, while us humans have only inhabited it for less than one thousandth of that time, it's been the home to single-celled bacteria for some 3.8 billion years! As you will read over the next few pages, we would be wise to view Earth as their planet and not ours.

Bacteria, plankton and single-celled organisms are far more shatterproof than us fragile humans. They can withstand temperatures so low that we would freeze to death in seconds. They can thrive, and indeed multiply, in temperatures so high that our skin would melt instantly. They have survived our planet's hostile environment through toxic periods, caused by mass volcanic activities and colliding tectonic plates, that would wipe us out in a heartbeat. Compared to us Homo Sapiens, some species of bacteria are virtually indestructible. They were the first living life form on planet Earth and, in my mind, will ultimately be the last. To picture how long they have been on Earth, if you imagine a 24-hour clock, bacteria have thrived on our planet for the whole 24 hours - and us humans have only cohabited with them for the last two seconds!

In *The Diet Myth*, author Tim Spector writes, "These microbes are the true and permanent inhabitants on Earth; we humans are just passing through". I love this quote because it really makes me think hard about how important it is that we create harmony between our body and our microbiome.

Dr Martin J. Blaser says in *Missing Microbes*, "If you were to gather them all up, not only would they outnumber all the mice, whales, humans, birds, insects, worms and trees combined – indeed all of the visible life forms we are familiar with on Earth – they would outweigh them as well … Without microbes, we could not eat or breathe. Without us, nearly all microbes would be just fine". Whether we realise it or not, the bacteria in and on our body has played a huge part in the evolution of our species, and how we look after them and treat them today is very different to the way we have partnered with them since our evolution as a species. For more than 2 million years, we did nothing out of the norm to upset our bacteria. Every aspect of human life, until the agricultural revolution some 12,000 years ago, saw us living in harmony with our microscopic inhabitants. Our bacteria felt safe and unchallenged. After all, they greatly outnumbered the cells in the humans they became attached to. But fast-forward to today, and they are at constant war with a barrage of unhealthy, highly engineered and chemically enhanced foods that they are as estranged to, as we humans are.

Here is another fantastic quote from *The Diet Myth*, "Over millions of years we have evolved together with microbes for mutual survival, yet recently this fine-tuning and selection has gone wrong".

What Role Do Bacteria Play In Our Body?

It's important to point out that not everyone will agree with what comes next, but what you will read is both highly researched and backed by lots of up-to-date independent data. Whenever you participate in an activity, say a game of football, golf, tennis or a netball match, there is always a result. Put simply, the activity leads to a conclusion. Similarly, the bacteria in our microbiome participates in a whole host of activities, which in turn eventually lead to a whole host of different results.

Let's look at just some of the activities the bacteria in our body's microbiome play a part in; detoxification, inflammation, the functions of our immune system, neurotransmitter production, nutrient absorption, the control of many hormones and how we utilise or store our macronutrients. Those activities in which our bacteria play an attacking role may lead to the following conditions (to name but a few); ADHD, Alzheimer's, asthma, autism, cancer, depression, diabetes, gum disease, high blood pressure, multiple sclerosis, obesity and Parkinson's disease.

To highlight how important our microbiome is to our health and wellbeing, let me start by asking you another question. The bacteria inhabiting our body are microscopic little things, containing just one cell each. If you could remove them all in one go and place them on your bathroom scales, what weight would you predict they would be? How about if I told you the bacteria inside our body weighs about the same as our brain? I hope that shocked you, because it certainly caused me a mild panic.

Why Do Microbiomes Collapse?

Before I scare you half to death with what I am about to say, even if our microbiome is currently completely shot, broken beyond what you might believe repairable, I am pleased to announce that it is a graceful ecosystem, and with the right nurturing and conditioning we can return our intestines back to the positive working bacterial environment that nature designed. As Dr David Perlmutter reminds us, "Thankfully, the gut's microbiotic community is wonderfully receptive to rehabilitation".

It is now believed that, while in the womb, we don't have any bacteria in our body. But as we travel through the birth canal, a female organ rich with friendly bacteria, our skin acts like a magnet attracting billions of wonderful bacteria to climb on board. Those born by C-section never benefit from this microbiotic kick-start. What's more, most caesarean births (and according to recent research over a third of births now include major surgery) are conducted simultaneously with a course of antibiotics. As their name suggests, antibiotics are 'anti' our body's 'biotics', a.k.a. our bacteria. Sadly, they are not all that good at isolating and attacking just the bad bacteria, but often cause complete genocide, mass-murdering the good bacteria too. If you were born by C-section with antibiotics, and then didn't benefit from bacterial-rich breast milk, then your microbiome really did get off to a poor start (even though, of course, this was neither you nor your mother's fault).

There is also mounting evidence that people in built-up cities experience more immune diseases than those living rurally. Why is that? Because those of us living in built-up environments are living in a clinical, overly sterilised bubble. Our kids no longer bring muddy boots into the house, and at the first sight of a bit of muck, antibacterial wipes are whipped out! My daughter Lili screams at me every time I leave the toilet, "Wash your hands daddy!" The whole world seems obsessed with cleanliness, when the reality is that we are mass-murdering our friendly bacteria. As I am writing this sentence, Lili is sitting next to me on the sofa, still insisting that I need to wash my hands - and while she might be right when it comes to toilet visits, there are many other instances where we would be better off just being a little bit grubby!

Many scientists now believe that our obsession with hand sanitisers and bacterial wipes is not only killing off the bad bacteria, but the good bacteria too. Dr David Perlmutter in *Brain Maker* says, "There's immense value in being unhygienic. Astonishingly new studies show a relationship between our increasingly sterile living environments and incidence of chronic illness, from heart disease and autoimmune disorders to cancer and dementia".

Sadly, as of yet there is little publicity about how protecting our microbiome is as crucial for our health and longevity as preserving our rainforests, oceans and corals are to the survival of our planet.

Dr Patrick Holford

Fifty thousand tons of antibiotics are used each year throughout the world on humans, animals or plants. In the UK alone, doctors write over 50 million prescriptions for antibiotics annually – roughly one per person per year. Not only are antibiotics intestinal irritants, wiping out healthy intestinal bacteria that can take over six months to be restored, but their widespread use is leading to the development of drug-resistant strains of life-threatening bacteria, from staphylococci to mycobacterium tuberculosis and streptococci; which are responsible for most sore throats.

How To Recolonise Our Microbiome

Later, we will discuss fermented foods and discover which are rich in positive bacteria. After being missing in action from supermarket shelves for decades, these probiotics foods - which were the norm - are mounting a resurgence. Regularly eating fermented foods (probiotics) such as yoghurts, kefir, sauerkraut and certain pickles will undoubtedly help rebuild most lacklustre immune systems.

Getting the gut back in good working order is actually a two-step process. We need to eat foods that are rich in healthy bacteria, as well as foods that the bacteria themselves like to feed on. These are known as prebiotics, and they are insoluble fibrous foods that cannot be absorbed or broken down by the gut, and as a result they remain there long enough to feed and fertilise our legions of healthy bacteria. While we can take prebiotics as a supplement, artichokes, raw garlic, chicory, onions (raw or cooked), raw asparagus and raw leeks are all natural sources.

Another way to take care of our microbiome is to regularly put our body into a ketogenic metabolic state. Research has shown that this increases the healthy variety of bacteria known as bacteroidetes and decreases the undesirable firmicutes. Let's remind ourselves what this means. Among other things, firmicutes are able to extract the most energy out of food, effectively stripping out maximum calories and leading to us putting on weight, getting fatter and eventually obese. Being ketogenic is effectively a spiral of upward health benefits. Our body not only consumes its own fat for fuel, but also removes the bacteria that over-extracts calories from food too.

A ketogenic diet is a positively healthy double dose of goodness, where in collaboration we burn our own body fat as our primary fuel source and the good bacteria redirect any excessive incoming energy straight to the exit!

The Bacteria That Makes Us Fat and That Which Keeps Us Lean

I mentioned earlier that it's all too easy to criticise fat and obese people for overindulgence and being too lazy to exercise. It's a natural conclusion for those unaware of the effects of our bacteria. But knowledge is power, and I am hopeful that these next few sentences will help you understand one of the hidden secrets of why some people eat rubbish food and almost instantly get fat, while others seem to be naturally fat-defiant without any real effort. You see, even though there are thousands of different bacteria in our gut, much of it is killed off in the Western human, leaving just two to dominate the entire digestive system. I have mentioned them a few times already, their names are firmicutes and bacteroidetes. It is believed that, together, they might account for more than three-quarters of the bacteria in our body - the combined weight of their armed forces being in excess of 0.9kg (2lbs)! If we want to lose weight, we need to work out how to reduce the volume of firmicutes in our gut. These clever creatures are superefficient at extracting maximum calories from the food that we eat. Bacteroidetes just aren't as qualified at unbundling energy.

Remember the saying 'we are what we eat' or when it comes to meat, 'we are what we eat – eats'? In our gut, our bacteria are forced to eat what we eat. Different bacteria thrive and survive on different foods. This is one of the key reasons why we all have very different ecosystems. Is your diet encouraging the right bacteria? Is it providing a safe harbour for firmicutes? If it is, then you're most likely overweight. But don't take it the wrong way, because getting our weight down might be as simple as working out how to balance our microbiome. Once we have balanced our firmicutes and bacteroidetes, the next thing is to encourage the widest variety of gut bacteria possible.

In *Brain Maker*, Dr David Perlmutter writes, "It's now firmly established that the gut community of lean people resembles a rainforest filled with many species and that of obese people is much less diverse".

At the University of Gothenburg in Sweden, Professor Fredrik Bäckhed, an award-winning expert in cellular microbiology, has performed numerous clinical studies with mice to uncover more about the critical role that microbes play in our gut. In 2004, he took a selection of skinny mice that were all born by C-section, and who had lived in a sterile environment to ensure that they didn't have any bacteria in their guts and began his experiment. He took bacteria from the caecum (the pouch located between the small and large intestine) of normal mice and placed it in the fur of the sterile mice. So, as they licked their fur, the microbes started to arrive in their guts. Within weeks, even without changing their diets, these mice - which had been lean for their entire life - became fat. Seriously fat. Within just weeks, on average they put on 60% more weight.

The professor then reduced the amount of food the mice were eating and they still put on weight. So, without doubt, when it comes to mice, certain varieties of microbes make them put on weight. You might now question if there is any relevance to what goes on in the stomach of a mouse and that of us humans, but let me just remind you that while the vessel might be different, i.e. mouse vs human, the crew is exactly the same! Certain microbes are able to extract more energy out of food than the body can on its own. Whether they reside in mice or humans, a microbe is a microbe. If they are experts at extracting energy from food then they will perform their tasks regardless of their host.

So, if we are fat or obese, the fault might not lie in just our food choices, but the state of our microbiome. In fact, the microbiome can also affect how good our body is at producing the hormone leptin, which informs our brain when our stomachs are full and therefore when we should stop eating. If we have damaged our body's ability to produce sufficient leptin, and we have too many microbes that are experts in extracting energy, then we could lay the blame of every excess pound of body weight at their door!

In *10% Human*, Alanna Collen describes another mice experiment, this time carried out by microbiologist Ruth Ley in America, where she studied the DNA of a variety of supersized mice that are known as ob/ob (their name appropriately derived from their obesity). These mice are almost round in shape, and because they just won't stop eating, they are three times heavier than normal mice. Alanna writes, "Although they appear to be a completely different species of mouse, they actually have just a single mutation in their DNA that makes them eat non-stop and become profoundly fat. That mutation is in the gene that makes leptin, a hormone which dampens the appetite of both men and mice if they have a decent supply of stored fat".

Hang on a minute, if it's as simple as the satiety hormone leptin controlling our hunger, why can't we take leptin tablets or have leptin injections? Sadly, it's not so much a lack of the ability to produce leptin, but also the brain becoming insensitive to it. Just as type 2 diabetes can occur when cells stop accepting insulin (insulin resistance) due a long period of overwhelming abundance, the brain ignores the cries of leptin to stop eating if it has sustained periods where we have over-eaten when we were already full. To the brain, leptin's performance is viewed as a cry wolf scenario.

Dr Dan Maggs

Watch this space! This is such an exciting area of medical research and we're only just starting to learn how important our microbiome is.

More Gut Facts

Serotonin

If you take antidepressant tablets, their role is to simulate the brain's happiness neurotransmitter serotonin. However, some scientists suggest that as much as 90% of serotonin is not, as you might assume, created in the brain, but in our intestines. When we feel depressed, my recommendation would be not just to pop a pill and create temporary relief, but to spend time figuring out how to get our gut in order. Did you know that serotonin is synthesised from tryptophan, and foods rich in tryptophan include eggs, cheese, pineapple, salmon, turkey, pork, nuts and seeds?

Stress

I know I have already covered the negative effect to our health caused by stress, and some of what I am about to say you have already read, but it's so important to our wellbeing that it's worth repeating. Stress plays havoc with our microbiome. It can send our bacteria into a frenzy. Short sharp moments of stress, such as what we experience during sprinting and weightlifting, don't set alarms bells off in our internal bacterial network. But persistent stress – caused by endurance sports and horrible bosses, for example – does. Our microbiome sees prolonged stress as a potential threat to the body and summons the support of both steroids and adrenaline. Together, this mighty taskforce summons the help of a built-in safety device called inflammation. However, nature invented inflammation to protect injured joints, to isolate snakebites and other such dangers. Summoning inflammation when it's not really needed can lead to a whole host of diseases, from cancer to Alzheimer's, from MS to depression. It is therefore important to avoid stress at all costs.

If we don't avoid stress, the Guy Fawkes in our microbiome is going to start setting fire to many of our internal systems, leading to mass-inflammation. If we have a lot of healthy fire-fighting bacteria protecting our corner, then we should be okay at dealing with short exposure to stress. But if they have already left the building due to our diet or sedentary lifestyle, we could be in for big trouble. It's for this reason that many people who suffer from stress also suffer from a myriad of gut-related illnesses. For those that have never got to the root cause of their irritable bowel syndrome, reducing stress levels and rebuilding the health of their microbiome may resolve the issue.

GALT

The immune system has been mentioned several times throughout this book. It is effectively the body's inbuilt self-defence system, which is activated when potential trouble arises. Highlighting the importance of our gut, the Gut Associated Lymphatic Tissue (GALT) represents approximately three-quarters of our entire immune system. Why does the immune system deploy the vast majority of its army in our gut? Because this is where our body needs its defence bolstered in order to stop the enemy breaching the delicate lining of our intestinal wall, which is only one cell thick. Yes, the only thing that stands between all of the nasty stuff that we swallow, that keeps harmful ingredients inside our gut, is just one cell wide. When the bad guys penetrate the immune system's defences, it is referred to as a leaky gut.

Irritable Bowel Syndrome

Irritable Bowel Syndrome (IBS) is rife, with around 10% of the adult population suffering from it, and two out of three people affected by it are female. This common disorder affects the large intestine and causes, among other things; cramping, abdominal pain, gas, bloating, diarrhoea and constipation. While it tends to be used as a catch-all diagnosis when doctors can't pinpoint the exact cause of a patient's discomfort, I believe that, for many sufferers, the cause is an imbalanced microbiome. However, with thousands of varieties of microbes in our gut, where should sufferers turn for a solution? I am a big believer in the Pareto Principle, named after the Italian engineer, sociologist and economist Vilfredo Pareto (1848 - 1923), where 80% of an effect comes from 20% of the causes (also known as the 'law of the vital few'). Therefore, with firmicutes and bacteroidetes occupying around three-quarters of our gut bacteria by volume, weighing in at about 0.9kg (2lbs), more than three times heavier than the human heart, I am confident to recommend to IBS sufferers that they try two things – firstly commit to a diet that creates an environment that firmicutes do not like, and secondly, do everything possible to reduce stress in their life.

Dr Dan Maggs

We must ensure that the good bacteria in our guts outnumbers the bad (collectively known as pathogenic bacteria).

Obesity

Like I previously stated, I have to be careful not to oversimplify something that is regarded as a complex matter. In all walks of life, I often feel sorry for professionals where too much knowledge can cloud their vision and make it difficult to accept a simple solution. In business, I always ask my team to stand back from the coalface and search for a simple solution. But, could obesity in the main be caused by a negative microbiome?

I have already mentioned the brilliant research carried out by Professor Ruth Ley. In another experiment she evaluated the balance of firmicutes and bacteroidetes in both lean and obese mice, and then repeated the experiment across lean and obese humans. The result: obese mice and obese humans have a higher number of firmicutes than bacteroidetes. Lean mice and humans have higher number of bacteroidetes than firmicutes.

Professor Tim Noakes

The dramatic change in the nature of the foods eaten on low CARB high fat diets, may beneficially alter the gut microbiome in such a way that it increases weight loss, for we now know that the bacteria in our gut 'talk' to our brains!

Microbiome Conclusion

Living in Great Britain, where antibiotics and antibacterial wipes are the norm, where packaged food is stripped of nutrients, we are in danger of developing a microbiome depleted of so many species of microbes that the human body was designed upon. To restore the very foundation on which nature created the human body, we all need to take steps to rebuild and then maintain our microbiome.

Chapter 10 Highlights

- It will come as no surprise to you that one of the best ways to get our microbiome under control is to follow the principles in this book.
- With such a diverse range of tasks and skills, many scientists regard the gut as the second most complex engine in our body, only surpassed by the brain.
- Over millions of years we have evolved together with microbes for mutual survival, yet recently this fine-tuning and selection has gone wrong.
- Eat as many organic vegetables and fermented foods as possible, and take a quality probiotic supplement.
- There are 100 trillion microscopic creatures living on and in our body.
- Three-quarters of the weight of our faeces is bacteria.
- There are more than 10,000 different species in the human microbiome.
- Our faeces are made up of more than 4,000 species.
- Individual bacteria cells live from a few days to a few weeks.
- Around 90% of illnesses can be traced back to the gut.
- We are 90% bacteria, fungi and microflora and only 10% human.
- 80% of our immune system is located in our gut.
- Microbes have thrived on our planet for more than 3.8 billion years.
- Firmicutes make us fat.
- As much as 90% of serotonin is created in the gut.

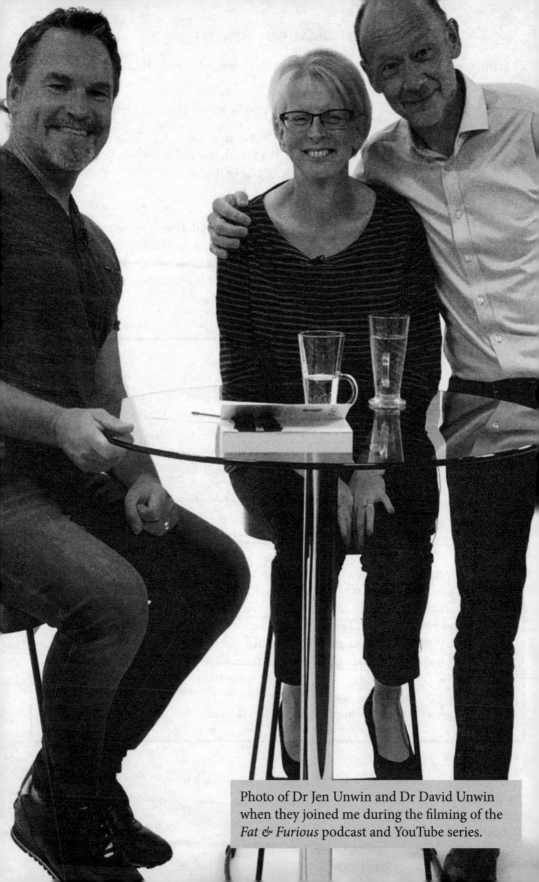

Photo of Dr Jen Unwin and Dr David Unwin when they joined me during the filming of the *Fat & Furious* podcast and YouTube series.

CHAPTER 11

OPTIMAL NUTRIENTS
VS MEDICINE

"Let food be thy medicine and medicine be thy food."
HIPPOCRATES

This chapter explores the essentials nutrients needed for optimal health and how they can be obtained either from our diet or supplements. Plus, we look at the limitations of modern medicine and why we shouldn't always rely on drugs to fix us.

In the 1930s, in order to better understand tooth decay, a pioneering dentist named Dr Price travelled the globe looking at the diets and lifestyles of remote communities. To his surprise, he found communities with none of the Westernised diseases people were suffering from in America. Amongst the places he visited, he spent time with Inuits, Aborigines, the islanders of Thursday Island and the New Zealand Maori. Part of his research involved shipping back the traditional food of these remote communities to his laboratory in America. There he tested them and found that when compared to the average dinner plate in the USA, they were on average:

- Seven times richer in calcium
- Four times richer in magnesium and copper. However, in some cases, the concentration of magnesium was as much as 20 times higher
- Often 50 times richer in iron
- Often 50 times richer in iodine
- A far higher concentration vitamin C and B was repeatedly seen
- Significantly higher concentrations of vitamin A, D and K

Did our primal ancestors take supplements? Of course not. So, ideally, I wouldn't want to recommend them. However, even when we buy everything organic, eat very few processed foods, avoid the deadly CARBS, even when we are completely abstaining from added sugars and as best as we can avoiding toxins, our health is still at a slight disadvantage to our primal ancestors. You see, they ate hundreds of different plants, bugs, insects and animals and, as the seasons changed, so too did their food options. Their diet was far more diverse than what we eat today. Their soils were not full of toxins and chemically produced pesticides and they were not breathing in pollutants.

Ideally, just as our primal ancestors did, we want to get all of our nutrients from our food and not have to worry about the state of our microbiome. However, while our body has yet to evolve to be in sync with the world around us, so much has changed in Great Britain in terms of our food and our environment, that a life without supplements leaves many individuals lacking in various areas.

With so much of the nutritional value in our food being suppressed, we would have to eat copious amounts of some items just to satisfy our basic requirements. Even with some organic foods, the soil has been so badly depleted over the years, they aren't able to soak up as much nutrients through their roots as they have done historically.

Our view on vitamins and minerals is quite straightforward. Eat as much organic and nutritionally loaded, naturally dense food as possible and then supplement to meet any dietary shortfalls.

Dr Patrick Holford

I will often ask my students; do you know why we need to supplement? The normal response is that the soil is no longer good, and we don't choose the right foods, all of which is true. But I actually think there is a much simpler and obvious answer. And that is that we don't eat enough. We eat a fraction of the food that our distant ancestors ate, before there were cars and fridges. We talk a lot about the Mediterranean diet, where the average man in Crete was walking seven miles every day, before cars and fridges. And without fridges, all of our food was fresh and organic, and we had to eat a lot more of it because we had to chop wood and fetch the water. And we moved around so much more. And all of this organic food, in probably three times the quantity, provided a far higher level in vitamins and minerals. A recent study at The Royal Society of Medicine looked at what a mid-Victorian worker diet provided in the way of micronutrients and it concluded that even if you or I wanted to achieve the same level of vitamins, essential fats, minerals, vitamin C for example, as a worker did in the mid-Victorian age, we would have to either supplement or eat two or three times the amount of food we do today.

Introduction to Vitamins and Minerals

Firstly, what are vitamins and minerals? The word 'vitamin' is derived from the Greek word for 'vital for life'. Vitamins are organic compounds made by plants, animals and us humans. In other words, vitamins are derived from living things. Minerals are inorganic, occurring naturally in water and soil.

As we already know, the vast majority of the food we eat is made up of three main macronutrients: CARBS, fats and protein. In terms of weight, the three headline acts make up more than 90%. You will know by now that, when we want to get our weight under control, the balance of these three ingredients is essential, and that after digestion our body converts all CARBS into sugar, most proteins into amino acids and fats into fatty acids.

On top of our fuel, it's also necessary to top up our engine with certain things that are going to make it run smoothly, efficiently and for as long as possible. You might see these as the oils in our engine or the additives they add to premium unleaded fuels. As BP say on their website about their finest fuel, "A formulation designed to bust the dirt in your engine and restore performance". Welcome to vitamins and minerals, the premium fuels for our body.

Vitamins

Let us first get a basic understanding of vitamins. Vitamins form in all living things from cows to humans, from grapes to broccoli. While not every organic compound found in plants and animals are essential in our diet, some are. When our body's health is negatively affected by a deficiency in an organic compound it is then labelled as a vitamin.

All vitamins are considered essential for a healthy life and it's ironic that there are 13 of them. Maybe it's unlucky to miss by just one!

The 13 vitamins that are essential for the human body fall into two categories: either they are fat-soluble or water-soluble. Fat-soluble vitamins are A, D, E and K. I remember these with a mnemonic – 'A Drunken Elephant Kills'. Those that are soluble in water are all the B vitamins and vitamin C. These are easier to remember if you picture a stuttering news reporter struggling to announce their employer – 'BBBBC'. But why is it good to remember which are which? The answer is because, as A, D, E and K aren't soluble in water, the body is very good at storing these vitamins and therefore worrying about our precise daily consumption isn't always necessary. For example, experts once measured sailors in a submarine and found that after 10 weeks below the ocean, their vitamin D level fell by only 50%. However, vitamin C and all of the B vitamins dissolve in water, making them harder for our body to retain, and for this reason we should try to ensure that we consume them in our daily diet or through the use of supplements.

Vitamins, just like minerals, don't just work in isolation, but in partnerships too. Some vitamins need the presence of others to perform certain tasks, while others partner with minerals to get their job done. For example, we all know that calcium is good for our bones, but our body needs sufficient levels of vitamin D in for our skeleton to make full use of it.

Dr Patrick Holford

In the 1980s, we did an experiment with 90 children. We first measured their IQ and then put a third on to a high strength multivitamin and mineral tablet, a third onto a dummy pill which looked identical, and a third took nothing. The study was run by a professor of phycology, David Benson, who actually thought we were nuts. He really didn't believe that by simply taking a multivitamin tablet, it could change your IQ. The BBC Horizon program filmed it. At the end of the seven months, we had an increase of ten points on what is called the non-verbal IQ for those taking the vitamins and three points on those taking the placebo. A seven-point difference. And that would be enough to get half of all children specified as special educational needs, back into the normal category. After the news broke, the very next day, virtually every multivitamin in the UK sold out!

Government Guidelines for Vitamins

Alongside all vitamins and minerals mentioned on the following pages you will find the official daily recommended amount that we should consume. But before you get brainwashed by governmental data, let me start by saying that all these guidelines are founded on the basis of deficiency. Set by a panel of EU nutritional experts, the recommended Nutritional Reference Values (NRVs – or as I call them the Not Really Viable doses) are said to represent the required intake levels of all vitamins and a selection of minerals to help prevent deficiencies in the vast majority of healthy people in Europe. And always remember that the European Union NRVs are assembled around avoiding deficiency, not optimal health. Let me also provide an example of how you have to take them with a pinch of salt; how on earth can the minimum level of vitamin D be the same for someone who works outdoors in the south of Italy as an office worker in Great Britain?

Understanding NRV Amounts:
Mg = 1/1,000th of a gram (one thousandth of a gram)
µg = 1/1,000,000 of a gram (one millionth of a gram)

When it comes to vitamins and minerals, we should always consider the recommended Nutritional Reference Values (NRVs) like we do a minimum wage, it's kind of a safety net, an entry point, not necessarily the optimal amount anyone would really desire. And as I have pointed out several times, we are all very different. We eat different diets, are different ages, experience different stresses and lifestyles. We all have different microbiomes and even everyday our own nutritional requirements will vary a little. The key thing to remember is this; most chronic illnesses are a result of a nutritional deficiency. Whether it be a short-term deficiency or one that has built up overtime, it is crucial for our wellbeing to understand that the key to our own health, happiness and longevity lies in fuelling our body with optimal nutrients, especially vitamins and minerals.

Let me introduce you to a new word and one that if more people knew it, would certainly halt our nation's decline into ill health. 'Orthomolecular' medicine. The phrase was first coined in 1968 by American biochemist Linus Pauling and refers to an approach to health that involves not the use of drugs, but a focus on nutrition. Or as one orthomolecular practitioner, Dr Carl C. Pfeiffer, says, "For every drug that benefits a patient, there is a natural substance that can achieve the same effect". And, whilst 'cure' might have been in the title of my first health book, prevention by ensuring our bodies are optimally fuelled with sufficient vitamins and minerals is what I 100% recommend.

Fat-Soluble Vitamins

Vitamin A (NRV 800 µg)
Plays an important role in maintaining healthy vision (especially improving our sight in low light), neurological functions and our immune system, and helps maintain healthy bones.

Vitamin D (NRV 5 µg)
Plays a vital role in calcium absorption in our bones, helping to fend off osteoporosis. By boosting the immune system, amongst other things, vitamin D helps the body to defend against cancer and Alzheimer's. Getting plenty of sunlight is a great way for the body to synthesise vitamin D.

When it comes to food, we can find rich sources of vitamin D in oily fish such as tuna, mackerel and salmon, plus dairy products and eggs, are all useful secondary sources. Plus, most multi-vitamin tablets also contain a sufficient quantity. When you think about how much vitamin D you personally need, try and compare your lifestyle to that of the caveman. How much time do you spend outdoors compared to the caveman leaving his cave?

Vitamin E (NRV 12 Mg)
A powerful antioxidant and plays a vital role in the body's fight against free radicals. Among many other things, vitamin E helps protect against Alzheimer's and high blood pressure. Our Superfood list is full of natural sources, the best being sunflower seeds, almonds and hazelnuts, and just one portion can surpass our daily needs. If you are not big on nuts and seeds, then a secondary source is greens such as broccoli and spinach and one the biggest superfruits of all – avocado.

Vitamin K (NRV 75 µg)
Plays a leading role in keeping our bones healthy. If we cut ourselves, the blood clotting self-defence mechanism that kicks in is courtesy of vitamin K. It also fights against cancer and maintains a healthy heart. There are actually two types of vitamin K, simply called K1 and K2. K1 is found in vegetables such as kale; it is also one of the best sources with just half a cup providing more than 100% of our recommended daily intake. We also get vitamin K1 from broccoli, cabbage, spring onions and spinach. K2 is found in dairy products, and a healthy microbiome will also synthesise K2.

Water Soluble Vitamins

Vitamin C (NRV 80 Mg)

A powerful antioxidant with numerous health benefits including curtailing high blood pressure, protecting against gallbladder infections, and defending against both strokes and certain cancers. It's also great for keeping wrinkly skin at bay, as well as colds and the flu too. The only problem is that the body can neither create nor store it. Therefore, we must consume plenty of vitamin C on a daily basis.

The best source is the Indian fruit guava, where consuming just one provides six times the daily-recommended amount. The trouble is, in the UK it's hard to get hold of it anything other than a juice. Alternatively, a cup of blackcurrants or raw red peppers will provide three times our daily requirement, with a kiwi or a cup of raw green peppers doubling what we need. An orange, a cup of strawberries, a portion of broccoli, kale or Brussels sprouts will also suffice. Or a cupful of grapefruit or pineapple chunks would do nicely too. All of the following either surpass or come very close to providing us with our daily requirement of vitamin C:

- 1 yellow bell pepper (5 x NRV)
- 1 red bell pepper (3 x NRV)
- 1 green bell pepper (2 x NRV)
- 1 kiwi
- 1 cup of broccoli
- 1 cup Brussels sprouts
- 1 cup of green peas
- 1 cup of cauliflower
- 1 orange
- 1 grapefruit
- 2 large tomatoes
- 2 cups of blackberries
- 2 cups of raspberries
- 5 large strawberries

However, there is a word of warning. I actually believe the daily recommendation for vitamins, especially vitamin C, is way understated for most people. While the recommendation is just 80mg per day, I personally feel that we need closer to 2,000mg (2 grams).

You will find a great speech by Dr Thomas Levy on YouTube, where he claims vitamin C is the very best antioxidant of all. Also, in his bestselling book *Stop America's Number 1 Killer*, he claims that atherosclerosis (the build-up of plaque in the arteries) is preventable and even sometimes reversible through high dose vitamin C and that it is the lack of vitamin C that causes it. Put simply, Dr Thomas Levy believes the number one cause of heart disease is a lack of vitamin C. He is not alone. Linus Pauling, a winner of two Nobel prizes, very vocally promoted vitamin C as he believed that a lack of vitamin C primarily caused CVD, and to prevent it you just need to take a higher daily dose of vitamin C. Tests on guinea pigs (just like humans they can't make their own vitamin C) in the 1960s showed how vitamin C deprivation causes atherosclerosis and heart disease.

Vitamin B

Vitamin Bs can be a little confusing as there are eight of them, but there isn't a B4, B8, B10 or B11. It's all to do with when they were discovered, and how some vitamins that were once thought to be one vitamin later turned out to be several different types. To avoid confusion, many in the scientific and medical community prefer to use names for B vitamins instead of numbers.

Vitamin B1 - Thiamine (NRV 1.1 Mg)

Boosts the immune system, and is believed to be great for cognitive functions, reducing both stress and memory loss. In January 2017, The Independent newspaper ran an article with the headline, "A diet rich in thiamine can reduce your risk of getting Alzheimer's disease, but some groups, such as the elderly, aren't getting enough". Levels of vitamin B1 are often deficient in individuals who consume too much alcohol, as it blocks its absorption. Vegetables, meat, fish, seeds and nuts are all good sources of thiamine.

Vitamin B2 - Riboflavin (NRV 1.4 Mg)

Like several other B vitamins, B2 works alongside other co-enzymes to help us extract nutrients from protein and carbohydrates. It is yet another vitamin that acts as a powerful antioxidant, and as we age it can prevent cracks from appearing around the mouth and nose, as well as counteract depression and sore throats. Food rich in B2 include meats and poultry (especially organs such as chicken liver), seaweed, shellfish, cheese, yogurt, eggs and green vegetables such as broccoli and spinach, as well as nuts and seeds.

Vitamin B3 - Niacin (NRV 16 Mg)

B3 is one of the most powerful vitamins of all and plays a role in over 500 different reactions in the human body. It helps to maintain a healthy cardiovascular system, as well as balancing blood cholesterol levels. As we age, it helps with cognitive functions and joint mobility, as well as preventing the skin from drying out. The best sources are chicken, beef, lamb and fishes such as tuna, sardines and salmon.

There is a great book called *Niacin: The Real Story*, where the authors talk about using large doses of niacin to cure a whole range of children's learning and behavioural disorders. It's a must read for anyone with a family member suffering from ADHD. After all, Dr Lendon H Smith believes that, "ADHD is not a disease; it is a nutritional deficiency".

Niacin was almost worshipped by the founder of Alcoholics Anonymous (AA) Bill Wilson, who used mega doses (orthomolecular medicine) to cure many of his patients of their addiction.

Vitamin B5 - Pantothenic Acid (NRV 6 Mg)
Plays an important role in extracting valuable nutrients from food, and a critical role in maintaining the health of our nervous system. As the vitamin is found in lots of fresh foods, its name is derived from the Greek 'pantos' meaning 'everywhere'. However, it is easily lost during processing, so if we eat only packaged foods, beware. Avocado, sunflower seeds, beef, duck, chicken (especially its organs), salmon, mushrooms, eggs, kale, broccoli and yogurt are all rich sources of pantothenic acid.

Vitamin B6 - Pyridoxine (NRV 1.4 Mg)
Instrumental in producing the happiness neurotransmitter serotonin. It plays an important role in removing excessive homocysteine (a form of amino acid) from our blood after eating meat. Some researchers therefore suggest it is as important to monitor our pyridoxine levels as it is cholesterol. Just like vitamin B1, individuals that consume too much alcohol can often suffer from pyridoxine deficiency. Good sources include vegetables such as carrots, spinach, meat and poultry (especially turkey and organs such as liver), fish, milk, cheese, nuts and seeds, avocado and eggs.

Vitamin B7 - Biotin (NRV 50 µg)
Often referred to as the beauty vitamin, as it thickens hair, nails and beautifies skin. So much so, you are likely to find biotin added to many beauty products in your bathroom cabinet. There are, in fact, eight different types of biotin, but only one is natural with all seven others being synthesised. Don't believe any company who tells you that the synthetics are just as good.

Marketeers who talk of vitamin H (for hair) or vitamin 8 are normally referring to synthetic versions of biotin. Vitamin B7 works as a coenzyme with other vitamin Bs to metabolise all three macronutrients. Sources include liver from both meat and poultry, eggs, salmon, nuts, cheese, avocado and berries.

Vitamin B9 - Folate (NRV 200 µg)
Plays a leading role in producing and repairing damaged cells, as well as supporting nerve and immune functions. It is said to prevent both cancer and cognitive decline. Some experts say that, in sufficient quantities, it delays or even prevents the onset of grey hair… I wish I had known this a few years ago, so I could have avoided my silver highlights! People who consume too much alcohol are often deficient in vitamin B9. Liver, vegetables such as spinach, asparagus, broccoli, Brussels sprouts and fruits (especially mango, avocado and oranges) are rich in folate.

Vitamin B12 - Cobalamin (NRV 2.5 µg)
Plays a major role in creating new red blood cells (preventing anaemia) and maintaining the nervous system. It also helps vitamin B6 in controlling homocysteine and is said to influence many parts of our health including energy levels, mood, digestion and cognitive functions. It's a unique vitamin that contains a mineral, and it's also the only one that's not found in plants. The best source for vitamin B12 is to get our gut in order and have bacteria produce it for us, but food sources include liver

from cows and chickens, fish such as salmon, mackerel, sardines, tuna and trout, plus dairy products such as yogurt and milk. B12 also highlights another flaw in the subject of NRVs, because as we age, our bodies get less efficient at processing this vitamin, resulting in the need for a higher daily intake.

Vitamin Summary

I don't expect you to memorise any of the above, and to be quite frank it would be pretty much a waste of time if you did. But if you scan back through them, you will notice how so many food types appear time after time. This is one of the ways that we compiled our Superfood list. For example, look how many different vitamins olives, green vegetables, offal, avocados, nuts and seeds contain. Compare these to fast foods and packaged foods and the difference is chalk and cheese!

Also, fresh fruits and vegetables are often richer in vitamins than those that are approaching their sell-by dates, and the more raw, uncooked vegetables we can eat the better. When it comes to cooking them, those that are quickly stir-fried or briefly steamed will often retain more vitamins and healthy nutrients than those that are cooked slowly or overheated. And for frozen foods, as they are often packed and frozen very quickly after picking, they can in some instances provide a richer source than those found in the fruit and vegetable aisle in the supermarket.

Dr Dan Maggs

Avoid crap foods void of nutrition and live longer and happier with natural foods full of vitamins and minerals. I also feel that taking a multivitamin tablet is relevant for many people.

Marvellous Minerals

If we were playing the 20-question game, where the first question is animal, vegetable or mineral, virtually everything you will ever eat will fall into the first two categories. Minerals are not naturally found in animals or plants, and only climb on board the food we consume through water and soil. The soil of our primal ancestors' food was rich in minerals, and their water was quite simply mineral water. With the Earth's crust historically providing such a rich layer of diverse minerals, plants absorbed them en masse through their roots, in turn themselves becoming part plant, part mineral. Then, when animals ate the mineral-loaded plants, they too became part mineral.

Being so incredibly clever, nature decided that if plants and animals were constantly consuming minerals, and then in due course so were us humans, it made sense to put them to good use and incorporate them in a multitude of bodily tasks and functions. Over millennia, these minerals have literally become integral to our wellbeing, but sadly, like all good things, they have pretty much come to an end. Over recent generations we have damaged our soil so badly that plants no longer find abundant minerals to absorb, therefore animals lack them in their diet, and as we humans are 'what we eat - eats', we too have become very lacking in minerals.

As the definition of a mineral is 'a solid, naturally occurring inorganic substance', another way we might want to picture them in our diet is as a foundation. In the same way that houses are always built on a solid foundation, so our diet should be too. See minerals as building blocks for the body. They help construct healthy bones and teeth. They participate in producing muscles, skin, hair and blood, and are an essential tool in the metabolic process.

Depending on what definition we apply to nutrients, there are between 40 to 70 of them that are essential to our health and that we must ingest frequently. But, as over the past few generations we have completely ruined our soil with chemicals and pesticides, very little is available to be absorbed by today's plants. This is another reason why more than ever; we need to get a diverse healthy diet. Let's say one vegetable contains ten minerals that the body needs, that leaves some 30 to 60 that are missing. The answer is to eat a wide and varied diet of natural organic food, just as our primal ancestors did and to also take a quality multi-vitamin and mineral tablet.

Just like we separate vitamins into two separate groups – water-soluble or fat-soluble – we are going to do the same with minerals. Some we need in big measures, normally milligrams (Mg), as these are the building blocks on which some bodily functions are cemented, while others we only need tiny trace elements.

Calcium (NRV 800 Mg)

Helps build strong bones and healthy teeth. In fact, our skeleton and teeth contain about 1.5kg (3lbs) of calcium, and for this reason we need to make sure we keep our levels regularly topped up. It is also used by our nerve cells to communicate with one another, and for keeping our muscles nice and flexible. It's believed that calcium helps us to fight off certain cancers, in particular colon cancer. And for those looking to shed a little weight, calcium is a definite fat buster. While there are several cases to be made against milk, it certainly packs a punch when it comes to calcium, with one pint of whole milk containing around 85% of the NHS's recommend daily intake. Our mothers were correct that milk is a rich source of calcium, but so too are other dairy products such as yogurt and cheese. Leafy greens such as broccoli and cabbage also contain it, as well as some nuts and seeds and small fish such as sardines, pilchards and white bait.

Phosphorus (NRV 700 Mg)

Has very similar properties to calcium and is used by the body to build and maintain healthy bones and teeth. Phosphorus is also a messenger between cells, carrying vital information from one to another about our DNA. If we don't have sufficient phosphorus in our system, we might become somebody totally different! Okay, that might be a bit far-fetched, but hopefully you get the message. Phosphorus also prevents our body from becoming too acidic or alkaline (it balances our pH levels). Red meat, dairy produce, fish, poultry, nuts and seeds are rich in phosphorus and therefore it is rare for someone to become deficient.

Magnesium (NRV 375 Mg)

One of the most important minerals, essential for our wellbeing, and is required by more than 300 biochemical reactions in the body. Magnesium plays a leading role in regulating our body temperature, detoxification, formation and maintenance of healthy bones, blood glucose control, regulation of blood pressure and much more.

Researchers in America found that approximately 75% of people tested were deficient in magnesium, and this is a real health issue. Being deficient in a mineral that is critical for us to function properly can lead to an onslaught of illnesses, especially as we age. In her bestselling book *The Magnesium Miracle*, author Dr Carolyn Dean quotes 56 conditions that are associated with magnesium deficiency, including acid reflux, Alzheimer's disease, angina, anxiety attacks, arthritis, asthma, blood clots, bowel disease, depression, diabetes, heart diseases, hypertension, indigestion, inflammation, insomnia, kidney stones, migraines, osteoporosis, Parkinson's disease, tooth decay and more.

I believe so much in the curing powers of magnesium that I am going to dive into a little more detail:

Magnesium May Reverse Osteoporosis - Numerous research studies have concluded that calcium supplemented with magnesium improves bone mineral density. So much so that many women in the USA who are susceptible to the disease take magnesium supplements as a preservative measure.

Magnesium As A Treatment For Diabetes - Magnesium aids in the metabolism of CARBS which helps control blood glucose levels.

Magnesium Treats Headaches and Migraines - For those who suffer from frequent headaches or migraines, increasing your intake of magnesium might prove more effective in the long term than taking painkillers.

Taking Magnesium Before Bedtime - Can help you get a good night's sleep and can even help those suffering from insomnia.

Magnesium Prevents Cardiovascular Diseases - Magnesium has been demonstrated to lower the risk of coronary heart disease.

Magnesium May Boost Exercise Performance - Magnesium helps move glucose into our muscles and helps remove lactate, which often builds up in our muscles during exercise and can often lead to muscle cramping.

Now that you are aware of how beneficial magnesium can be, take a look at the NRV recommendations by the EU. As you can see these are quite high, but in my opinion still very conservative. Let's look at the types of food that we can find magnesium in, and how much we would need to consume.

Magnesium Rich Foods	Milligrams (mg) per serving	Percentage of NRV
Almonds, dry roasted, 28g (1oz)	80	20%
Spinach, boiled, ½ cup	78	20%
Cashews, dry roasted, 28g (1oz)	74	19%
Peanuts, oil roasted, ¼ cup	63	16%
Black beans, cooked, ½ cup	60	15%
Edamame, shelled, cooked, ½ cup	50	13%
Peanut butter, smooth, 2 tbsp	49	12%
Avocado, cubed, 1 cup	44	11%
Potato, baked with skin, 99g (3.5oz)	43	11%
Rice, brown, cooked, ½ cup	42	11%
Yogurt, plain, low fat, 227g (8oz)	42	11%

As you can see, it's pretty difficult to consume enough magnesium through food alone.

Iron (NRV 14 Mg)
Works alongside the two proteins, haemoglobin and myoglobin, which transport oxygen via the blood to our cells. The human body finds it easier to absorb iron from animals than it does from plants. Liver, meat, nuts, seeds, eggs and leafy greens such as watercress and curly kale are all rich in iron.

Zinc (NRV 10 Mg)
Plays a role in creating new cells, hormones and enzymes. It also aids the metabolism of all three macronutrients. It's a vital mineral, and our body is better at absorbing it from meat and shellfish than from plants. That said, leafy greens are a reasonable secondary source.

Fluoride (NRV 3.5 Mg)
Not to be confused with fluorine, which is poisonous. A small amount of fluoride is believed to be good for our teeth, and possibly our bones too. It's commonly found in toothpaste and in drinking water, and you can always top your level up with avocado and strawberries. We don't require much of it, and as a result the NHS don't detail any daily recommendations for our consumption, however in America they do.

Trace Minerals
Let's now turn our attention to some of the trace minerals that we should ensure are in our diet. While the doses we need are minimal, they are just as vital to our wellbeing as they are to making emeralds green and rubies red! Again, in the chart I have listed them from left to right in descending order of the amount we should consume.

Manganese (NRV 2 Mg)

Helps both create and activate several enzymes, and therefore most of it resides in our glands - with a smaller amount located in our bones. Tea is a rich source of manganese, as well as nuts, seeds, offal and some green vegetables such as peas and runner beans.

Copper (NRV 1,000 µg)

Used in the production of both white and red blood cells, and acts as a trigger to release iron to form haemoglobin - the protein that carries oxygen in blood cells. Copper also reduces free radicals and can help defend the body against certain infections. Offal, nuts, tea and coffee, dark chocolate, most green vegetables and shellfish all contain copper. As we only need a small trace amount, primal diets are rich enough not to overly concern ourselves with it.

Iodine (NRV 150 µg)

Contributes to the creation of thyroid hormones. It also helps rebuild and repair bones, as well as supporting a healthy nervous system. Good sources include fish, shellfish and seaweed. Iodine used to also be found in vegetables, but sadly today most soil is depleted.

Dr James DiNicolantonio

One of the important things about real mineral salts, Himalayan salts and rock salt, is that they contain iodine. We lose 50 to 100 micrograms of iodine per hour of exercise. There are now 36 countries where people are iodine deficient. There are some very important functions that sodium plays with iodine. Sodium helps bring iodine into the thyroid hormone. It also helps form thyroid hormones. So T3 is the active thyroid hormone which has three iodine molecules, T4 which is the inactive thyroid hormone has four iodine molecules.

Selenium (NRV 55 µg)

Prevents damage to cells and tissue, and helps the immune system work properly. Researchers have also suggested that it helps prevent cancer and other diseases including heart failure. Sources include nuts (especially Brazil nuts), meat (especially organs), fish and eggs. In some countries, you can get selenium from vegetables, but in the UK our soil is now so poor that this is no longer likely.

Molybdenum (NRV 50 µg)

Pronounced 'molib-dunum', it helps create and then activate some enzymes. Sources include green vegetables like broccoli and spinach, cauliflower, nuts and seeds, beans, legumes and yoghurt.

Chromium (NRV 40 µg)

Influences how insulin behaves in the body, affecting the amount of energy we absorb from food. Good sources include meat, green vegetables (especially broccoli), nuts and seeds and various spices.

The Six Electrolytes

While it might sound like a band name, electrolytes are a group of nutrients that produce an electrically conducting solution when dissolved in our body. In harmony, they perform many vital tasks in our body. Nutritionist and primal living expert Nate Morrow says, "Your body is a complex and carefully-balanced superhighway of cells, tissues and fluids that, almost every second, directs an incomprehensible array of electrical impulses. This is only possible because those cells, tissues and fluids thrive in a homeostatic [a condition of balance or equilibrium] environment where they conduct electricity well enough to carry the signals to their intended destinations. The key to maintaining this conductive superhighway lies with our friend the electrolyte".

The name electrolyte is derived from the fact that they effectively carry an electrical current around our body. They regulate our heartbeat, enabling our muscles to properly contract in order for us to move. Electrolytes are essential for all of our cells and organs, and maintaining a healthy balance of them is critical. The core six electrolytes are sodium, potassium and chloride, plus calcium, phosphorus and magnesium, which we have just discussed.

Balancing our electrolytes can greatly improve our health, but be aware that if they are way out of balance they can actually kill us. What throws our electrolytes off balance? Dehydration, especially as a result of illness or excessive exercise without fluid intake, is the biggest cause. When we have diarrhoea or are sweating profusely, it's crucial that we up our intake of both water and electrolytes. Other causes of electrolyte imbalances include excessive urinating (caused by various infections), drinking too much alcohol or, believe it or not, even drinking too much water, poor diets and over-exercising.

As we age, we become more susceptible to both dehydration and overhydration, and therefore more prone to abnormal electrolyte levels. This is largely because our kidneys do not work as efficiently as when we were younger. Electrolyte imbalances can cause irregular heartbeats, twitching and muscle spasms, changes in blood pressure, confusion, seizures, numbness, headaches, fever, trouble sleeping, anxiety, weakness and fatigue, joint pain and dizziness, plus various nervous system disorders.

So how do we keep our electrolytes in balance? As we have already discussed, we would be wise to ensure we consume appropriate amounts of calcium, phosphorus and magnesium. In addition, we must consider the level of sodium, chloride and potassium that is in our diet.

Sodium Chloride and Potassium

Salt that we sprinkle on our food is made of sodium chloride. Most people who eat packaged food and fast food will likely have too much sodium and chloride in their diet, and therefore their electrolyte balance might be compromised. The NHS report that the average British citizen eats double their daily recommendation. When we live primally, our healthy diet and exercise routine might mean that we occasionally need to add a little to our food to top up our intake. The governmental daily-recommended amount for sodium is 1,600mg (1.6g) and for chloride it is 2,500mg (2.5g). If you add the two together it equates to about 4g of salt.

Potassium is found in various foods, and while it is recommended that we consume 3,500mg per day (3.5g), it's normally quite easy to do when we are eating primally. Fruit (especially bananas), vegetables such as broccoli, parsnips and Brussels sprouts, nuts and seeds, beef, chicken, turkey and fish are all good sources.

Herbs and Spices

Herbs and spices have been used for centuries as medicines in cultures from Asia to the Native Americans, from Southern Europe to the Aztecs. While, for thousands of years, herbal practitioners had no idea why or how herbs worked, through trial and error they became extremely successful at identifying the right herb for the right aliment.

More than 2,000 years ago, to reduce fevers and inflammation in his patients, Hippocrates used to offer bark from the willow tree, and instruct sufferers to chew on it. Then in 1897, the German pharmaceutical company Bayer developed a branded tablet called aspirin from the very same bark. In fact, most pioneering Western pharmaceutical companies created their pills by extracting nutrients from herbs. Even today, more than 100 well-known pills, medicines and tablets still base their remedies on plant extracts. While aspirin no longer comes from willow bark (it's now synthetic), codeine and morphine are still made from opium poppy seeds.

What I love about using herbs and spices in my cooking is that they add flavour to just about anything. And flavour is really important. As we start living primally, there will undoubtedly be the odd occasion when we are going to miss our fast food or sugar-rich snacks. While it is okay now and again to fall off the wagon and have whatever we want (remember we are not promoting a diet but a lifestyle change), ideally the more times we can stay true to what we were designed to eat, the healthier we will ultimately be. I recommend you experiment with as many herbs and spices as you can get your hands on. Even better still, get out in the garden and grow your own. There is no more a satisfying meal than one where we know the flavour was created in our own backyard.

Plus, when we are trying to encourage our family and friends into a primal way of living, tantalising their taste buds with herbs and spices makes it easy in helping them convert to our healthier lifestyle. And for those that you know who pop too many over-the-counter pills, as you read through the following pages you will be able to amass enough knowledge to be able to advise them to close the door on their medical cabinet, and instead plant their way back to good health.

When it comes to herbs and spices, generally the stronger the aroma and the more pungent the taste, the denser are both their nutrients and curing properties. Let's look in detail at three truly supernatural herbs – ginger, turmeric and cacao – and then list other magically healthy herbs and spices.

Ginger

This miracle root vegetable is brilliant for curing sickness and digestive problems. In 2008, when I crossed the Atlantic with my family in a small sailing boat, we didn't know about the natural stomach-calming effect of ginger and instead, relied on a barrage of tablets to prevent seasickness. The effectiveness of those man-made pills was very questionable indeed. But today, when feeling a bit sickly, whether it be travel sickness or anything else, the entire family opens the fridge and pulls out fresh ginger. While my eldest son and I love the strong taste and are happy just to chew on a small chunk, my younger children prefer to put ginger in the blender with a load of berries and yogurt.

A study carried out at the University of Georgia found that taking ginger supplements after exercise greatly reduced muscle soreness. Ginger is also known to reduce pain far more effectively than many pain killers and is especially efficient at reducing discomfort during the menstrual cycle.

Even more beneficial to our health than ginger's rapid action for sickness and pain is its ability to prevent inflammation. It contains a host of anti-inflammatory and antioxidants such as gingerols, capsaicin, caffeic acid, curcumin and salicylate. Ginger is also a rich source of vitamin B6, vitamin C, potassium, magnesium, phosphorus and folate. The BBC's website *www.bbcgoodfood.com* suggests, "The many curative properties of ginger are widely researched. Used on the skin it can stimulate the circulation and soothe burns. As a diaphoretic it encourages perspiration, so it can be used in feverish conditions such as influenza or colds".

Turmeric

Turmeric is one of the most powerful natural medicines we can add to our food. Just as fatty fish offers the finest source of omega 3 and yellow bell peppers are the ultimate provider of vitamin C, turmeric is the richest source of the antioxidant substance curcumin. It's so beneficial for our health that I have written a far bigger article on it under supplements. I personally love to cook lots of dishes with this heaven-sent spice, but at the same time I still take a daily supplement to make sure I am not missing out on the goodness that it packs. After all, the spice is said to reduce the risk of prostate and skin cancer, brain tumours, leukaemia, multiple sclerosis and depression. It's a natural painkiller that, for aches and pains in certain parts of the body, is said to be as effective as ibuprofen. And while I am a big believer that most research is misleading, as correlation rarely proves causation, I do believe turmeric is part of the reason why in India, where it is consumed by millions, Alzheimer's and Parkinson's are extremely uncommon.

Cacao

Keep a jar of raw unroasted cacao (pronounced 'ca-cow') powder in your primal pantry and, whenever you need to make some sweet desserts for friends, you will be able to fool them that your chocolate looking dish is no different to the regular sugar-infused milk chocolate they consume. But of course, there is a difference - a huge difference.

Cacao powder is produced by cold-pressing unroasted cocoa beans from the cacao tree. Unlike regular cocoa powder, which is roasted at high temperatures, by keeping the temperature cool the process preserves living enzymes. The rawest of all chocolates, cacao contains more than 250 different nutritional ingredients, making it possibly the best source of antioxidants from plants on the planet! Rich in polyphenols, it even has more than a dozen times more antioxidants than the superfruit blueberries. No wonder the Aztecs used cocoa beans as a currency. Always check that what you buy is raw and organic. You can normally tell as it has a slightly lighter colour than roasted cocoa.

You may have noticed how most herbs have similar health benefits. That's great news because, unless we are looking for a specific cure or remedy, then all we need to remember is it that the more we can indulge in organic herbs, especially those that are home-grown, the more primal we will be living and therefore the healthier we are likely to become.

Supplements

There are numerous different approaches to supplementing our food intake with vitamins and extracts. Some experts recommend taking loads and loads of pills, while there are others that don't believe in supplements at all. As you might expect, I don't believe that one approach fits all. For example, if you regularly go on holiday and also eat lots of oily fish, nuts and seeds, then there might be no need to take vitamin D tablets. However, if you rarely reveal your body to the sun, and don't receive sufficient amounts of vitamin D in your diet, then you most definitely would be wise to take it in the form of a supplement. And Public Health England have recently recommended us Brits take a vitamin D supplement throughout the autumn and winter months, as we can pretty much guarantee living in this beautiful country unfortunately means we won't be getting enough vitamin D. Another example would be if someone eats chicken and eggs straight after a workout, then there would be little need for an additional protein shake.

When it comes to vitamins, other than water-soluble vitamin C and all of the Bs, as long as say over a ten-day period we ingest roughly ten times the recommended daily amount, then the aggregation will be fine. Sunbathing is a great example. A one-week holiday in the sun with careful exposure can help our body accumulate enough vitamin D for several months.

My view on supplementing is quite simple: Eat foods rich in nutrients and fill any nutritional, vitamin or mineral shortfalls with reputable supplements.

Everyone is different, so when it comes to supplements, without knowing you personally, it's difficult for me to recommend exactly which ones you should make part of your daily life. If you have both the time and the cash, you can go and have your blood and even your poo profiled. But, for most people just making an educated guess about what is right will be enough to help booster your wellbeing and longevity. And remember, what we are talking about here is not drugs, nor medication, but nutrition.

But aren't supplements dangerous, especially if I take too many? Interestingly, the American Association of Poisonous Control Centre, an organisation that monitors the causes of death each year in the USA, state that over the last 35 years of keeping records, there have been just 13 allegations that vitamins were a cause of death, yet not one of them was ever substantiated.

Furthermore, Canadian biochemist Abram Hoffer said flatly, "Nobody dies from vitamins". Compare that with prescribed drugs, which many experts now believe to be the third largest cause of death, after cancer and heart disease. I am not for one minute belittling prescribed medication, because in many instances they prolong life, I am just trying to highlight as powerfully as possible that vitamins and minerals are simply good nutrition, but just in a different form.

In order to achieve optimal nutrition, let me summarise the use of supplements with four thoughts:

1. Dr Carl C Pfeiffer said, "For every drug that benefits a patient, there is a natural substance that can achieve the same effect". While I don't believe this is always the case post-diagnosis, I do believe that nearly all Westernised illnesses are caused in the main by poor nutrition.
2. Nutritional based medicine (orthomolecular medicine – meaning normal) is non-toxic, whereas pharmaceutical medicine, in the main, tends to be toxic (toxi-molecular).
3. Even though natural, herbal, nutritional medicine has been around since antiquity, as you can't patent a vitamin or a mineral, huge corporations don't get behind them. And, if huge corporations don't get behind them, there is nobody to promote their use to doctors.
4. 'Vit' in the word vitamins, is derived from the Latin 'vita', meaning life, as in vital for life. As in if we don't get enough from our diet we could die!

Dr Patrick Holford

I was taught by the late Linus Pauling to always follow the logic. It's the logic that counts. Randomised controlled trials, they come later. And I have realised in life that if you follow the logic of things, you get to the truth. And if you want to know why we are all so messed up and sick, you just follow the money. The logic is the light, and the money is the greed and the dark.

Years back, we had the erroneous belief that once you had the evidence, everything would change. And now we have got the evidence, and it is not changing for the fundamental reason that you can't patent a nutrient. If you can't patent it, you don't get a monopoly, and you can't charge exorbitant amounts of money. If it wasn't for the ability to patent a drug and not patent a nutrient, we wouldn't be consuming all of these vast quantities of pharmaceutical drugs. We would be dealing with the fundamental underlying causes of most of these diseases, which is sub-optimal nutrition.

Supplements That I Take

For all the adults in my family and to all my friends, I always recommend that they take the following five as a base; a multivitamin, omega 3, turmeric, magnesium and a strong probiotic. To me even without analysing their current diet, these are a no-brainer. To provide you with a further example of what supplements you might want to take, I will now explain what I take to help optimise my nutrition, and the logic behind my selection. Some might not be necessary for you and there might be others that you as an individual would benefit from taking. But hopefully it will show you my thought process and act as a catalyst to help you plan your supplementation. These are the current supplements I take daily:

- Omega 3
- Turmeric
- Magnesium
- Probiotics
- Coenzyme Q10
- Combined multi-mineral and multi-vitamin tablet
- Vitamin C
- Glucomannan & Inulin (SlimShotz)
- CBD Oil

Omega 3

Our caveman ancestor had a diet rich in omega 3. He loved eating whole animals, especially omega 3-rich brains! He didn't face the problem of factory manufactured beef, sourced from cornfed antibiotic-injected cattle, with its resulting omega 3:6 balance artificially adjusted from a healthy 1:1 ration to a noxious 1:7 ratio.

If every night you eat oily fish such as salmon, mackerel, anchovies and sardines and then consume a pack of walnuts as your daily snack, then you might be one of the exceptional few who don't need to take omega 3 supplements. If you're not a fishy person, then taking omega 3 will almost definitely improve your health. I personally eat loads of oily fish and love nuts, but still take an organic cold-water sourced omega 3 capsules every morning. For me, omega 3 is a must-have supplement.

In his book *Super Fuel*, Dr James DiNicolantonio writes at length about the benefits of fish-based omega 3 on reducing the chances of having a heart attack. He displays lots of research and statistics to back this up and says, "If a pharmaceutical company could develop a drug with those kinds of benefits, it would be a gold mine that would no doubt cost you a fortune". He goes on to say, "The incidence of sudden cardiac death in the general population of Western countries is almost twenty times higher than in Japan. The average omega 3 index in Japan is ten per cent, compared to just 4.5 per cent in Western countries".

If you don't want to take a supplement derived from fish, then flaxseed oil makes a perfectly good substitute.

Omega Options

There are three different types of omega 3 (which is not related to the fact it is called omega 3). They are alpha-linolenic acid (ALA), eicosapentaenoic acid (EPA) and docosahexaenoic acid (DHA). ALA is primarily sourced from plants, such as seeds and nuts. When animals such as cows, fish and us humans consume ALA, we convert some of it into EPA and DHA. Oily fish like salmon convert it best. EPA and DHA are the two types of omega 3 fatty acids that are the most superior for our health. While the human body can convert a certain amount of ALA into EPA and DHA, it's not super-efficient at doing so. It is for this reason, even though we might consume enough omega 3 by eating plenty of nuts and seeds, that we still need our oily fish or algae supplements to directly deliver EPA and DHA.

But why is it so important for our health? Omega 3, particularly those rich in docosahexaenoic acid (DHA), is quite simply food for the brain. In fact, one of the key components in the brain is docosahexaenoic acid, and for those of us who were breastfed, our mother's milk was loaded with it. It's not just about prevention either, in some instances omega 3 can cure certain brain disorders! But surely this can't be true, because aren't we supposed to be stuck with the same brain cells throughout our entire life? Recent scientific research has turned this belief on its head. It now appears that we can grow new brain cells on a daily basis through a process known as neurogenesis. The area where neurogenesis is most effective is the hippocampus. This is the area of the brain that is responsible for storing long-term memories and learning new things.

I could list dozens and dozens of other amazing health benefits we receive from taking a quality omega 3 supplement daily, but I would just be diluting this one very important advantage: it is an essential fuel for an active brain.

When it comes to selecting the right omega 3 supplement, it's time to become a quality fanatic. While most soft gel omega 3 capsules on the market today are 1,000mg (1 gram), the concentration of the good stuff, EPA and DHA, can sometimes be woefully low. It always pays to check the labels when buying supplements. With omega 3, there is also a danger of the supplement originating from highly toxic fish, full of mercury and other potentially harmful metals.

Dr James DiNicolantonio

Omega 3 is very important for the brain, especially DHA. The brain is highly concentrated in DHA; in fact, our ancient ancestors used to consume the brains of lots of animals. DHA is even more concentrated in the brain than salmon. It's very important for retinal function, for neuron function, growing new neurons and one of the best ways to get it is fresh wild seafood. Canned seafood is okay, but the problem with canned sardines and canned tuna, not to say that eating those are bad for your health, is that the heat used in the canning process can reduce the benefits. You could also take fish oil supplements, make sure it's a highly regulated supplement, where they test for low oxidisation products, is a great way as well.

Turmeric/Curcumin

From the same family as ginger, turmeric is a brilliant anti-inflammatory herb that can either be consumed as a supplement or used to spice up your food. While tablets and supplement manufacturers often claim their products are ten to 100 times more potent than you would put in your homemade curry, if you are not a big fan of taking too many supplements, then heaping it on your chicken or beef is still very beneficial.

Supplements are made up of a compound found in turmeric called curcumin and not turmeric itself. There are more than 5,000 medical articles and pieces of research online, many claiming turmeric to be the most powerful herb on the planet. The benefits of turmeric could fill an entire book (many books actually – Amazon alone has 301 books with turmeric in their title). Let's look at some of the main benefits of this incredible herb:

- Reduces chronic joint pain
- Reduces the pain of arthritis
- Can boost low energy levels
- It can slow and even prevent blood clotting
- For those that suffer side effects from Ibuprofen, curcumin is a godsend
- In 2009, Auburn University of Alabama published a report that explored how taking turmeric supplements can help reverse type 2 diabetes
- It is a powerful anti-inflammatory
- It helps decrease memory loss
- Medical studies have demonstrated that it helps to prevent certain cancers
- It has one of the highest antioxidant scores (see ORAC scale in the colour insert)

Magnesium

I personally love nuts, seeds, spinach, avocado and many other foods that are rich in magnesium and I consume them regularly. That said, I still don't feel that I regularly eat the 500 to 600mg that I believe I need. Why am I saying 500 to 600mg if the recommended daily allowance for my age, as suggested in the earlier chart, indicates 420mg? The more active we are, and the more we exercise, the quicker we deplete our mineral stores. With magnesium's benefits to health being so vast, I take a supplement every day. For those who don't like taking them, you can always buy bath salts rich in magnesium and, in addition to all of the other long-term benefits, your muscles will become relaxed, especially after exercising.

As magnesium helps us get a better night's sleep, it's the one supplement I like to consume just before I go to bed. To ensure I don't forget to take it, I store it in my bathroom next to my toothbrush, and not in the kitchen.

If you are unsure of whether you are getting enough magnesium, calcium and zinc in your diet, consider that, in 2005, *The American Journal of Clinical Nutrition* stated that 73.3% of Americans were not meeting the daily RDA of zinc, 65.1% were deficient in calcium and 61.6% were not consuming enough magnesium.

Patrick Holden CBE

Because we haven't crop rotated properly with livestock since the end of the second world war when nitrogen fertilisers became available, the fertility of our soil has reached a critically low level. Nearly all the vegetables we eat in the UK today are coming from a vegetable monoculture where they grow vegetables year after year, or pretty intensively, at the expense of the soil fertility and the expense of the mineral and trace element composition. And there are studies to show that the mineral and trace element composition of vegetables that we are eating today has gone down by 50% since the second world war.

Probiotics

Once you have started eating fermented foods in your weekly routine, if you feel the need to take a probiotic supplement, then in his book *Brain Maker*, author Dr David Perlmutter suggests that it's advisable to purchase probiotics that contain the following helpful bacteria: Lactobacillus plantarum, Lactobacillus acidophilus, Lactobacillus brevis, Bifidobacterium lactis and Bifidobacterium longum.

Some brands claim their products contain thousands of different bacteria, but my concern with these is that the more they contain, the smaller the dose of each one. Aim for brands that contain ten to 20 different strands, and if they contain all five recommended by Dr David Perlmutter, all the better. Make sure you don't wash these down with unfiltered tap water, or there is every chance that the chlorine in the water will kill off the helpful bacteria before they arrive in the gut!

Coenzyme Q10

This is the preferred food source for our mitochondria and our heart too. Our primal ancestors ingested lots of it when they consumed entire animals, as coenzyme Q10 is found primarily in the heart, kidneys and liver. Smaller doses can be found in sardines, mackerel and peanuts and even smaller amounts in vegetables such as spinach, cauliflower and broccoli.

Our body naturally creates a certain amount of coenzyme, and for this reason it is not considered a vitamin. However, we get less and less efficient at producing it as we age, and therefore can't provide our hearts and cells with the amount they need to stay healthy.

Therefore, if you're not a big organ/offal eater, and you are more than 40 years of age, you might need to consume this in the form of a supplement. There is no NRV for coenzyme Q10, and I guess this is because it's difficult to identify how much of it our body produces naturally. Dr Jonny Bowden, in his book *The Most Effective Natural Cures on Earth*, suggests that once we pass the age of 40, we should consume at least 60 to 100mg daily. And for those with a family history of heart disease, or those with high blood pressure or high cholesterol, he recommends taking between 100 and 300mg daily.

The US National Library of Medicine suggests that coenzyme Q10 supplements may be useful in the treatment of high blood pressure, muscular dystrophy, heart failure, Parkinson's disease, migraines, certain mitochondrial disorders and HIV/AIDS. However, don't take coenzyme Q10 supplements if you are pregnant or less than 18 years old. In a nutshell, coenzyme Q10:

- Reduces blood pressure
- Is good for the heart
- Energises our cells
- Acts as a powerful antioxidant

In Japan, to reduce both heart disease and high blood pressure, approximately 10% of the population are reported to be talking Q10 medication on the advice of their doctors or medical professionals. If you are stressed or take statins, then you almost definitely would benefit from taking coenzyme Q10.

Ivor Cummins

If you are on statins, there is one supplement you must take, and that is coenzyme Q10. And, if you have an established disease and you are not sure of the cause, you should also be taking coenzyme Q10, and all the key vitamins and minerals.

Combined Multi-Mineral and Multivitamin Tablet

A multivitamin tablet is the first step in the direction of optimising nutrition. With a quality multivitamin tablet costing less than 20 pence per day, they really are a no-brainer. While I always try to eat as healthily as possible, I don't want to risk falling short on any of the minerals my body relies on to function.

So, for the past two years, I have started to take a combined multi-mineral and multi-vitamin tablet that has been specifically formulated for men over 50. For females out there, don't worry – there are plenty of different options for you too. Why are age-specific multivitamins a better choice? Because as we age, we absorb and process certain vitamins differently and therefore it is necessary to alter the dosages.

Vitamin C

I take one effervescent vitamin C tablet in the morning and use the drink to help take my other supplements. I then have one in the afternoon. As the EU upper tolerance is set at 2 grams, that's all I should really recommend. That said, the reality is that I take a lot more. How about this as an interesting fact... According to Dr Suzanne Humphries, a cow makes around 12 grams of vitamin C per day. The average-sized goat produces around 13 grams of vitamin C per day and a sick goat, to fight of toxins, produces up to 100 grams per day. That's a lot of vitamin C!

In fact, we are one of just a few species on our planet that can't produce it ourselves. Dr Suzanne therefore claims that the amount we are recommended to take by the authorities, is a gross under estimation.

But isn't it dangerous if I take more? To answer this question, I would recommend you watch a video on YouTube by Dr Andrew Saul, where he is giving a lecture at the Riordan Clinic. In it he says that according to the American Association of Poisonous Control Centre, there has not even been a single reported death from over doing vitamin C, even though many people are taking doses 100s of times greater than that recommended by authorities. He then goes on to say that doctors should insist on high dose vitamin C – while they ponder the right medicine for almost any illness.

But please don't rush out and start taking mega doses of vitamin C as you might experience gastric discomfort and diarrhoea. Start with 1gram per day and then maybe extend to two. Beyond that I can't in print recommend that anyone goes beyond the EU's guidelines!

Dr Patrick Holford

All animals make vitamin C, except for fruit-eating bats, the Red-Vented Bulbul bird, guinea pigs and primates. The animals that do make vitamin C don't get colds, and they don't get cancer. I'm in my 60s and I have never suffered from a cold for more than 12 hours, because the second I get the first signs of an infection I take one gram, or sometimes two grams to kick it off, every single hour, because you need to get your vitamin C level really high, because it is antiviral. But one of the hottest areas in cancer medicine is intravenous vitamin C; it's effectively safe chemotherapy.

Glucomannan and Inulin (SlimShotz)

When I wrote my first health book, it was prior to us developing the Primal SlimShotz product. While SlimShotz is primarily designed to help people lose weight, regardless of what my bathroom scales are telling me, I take it daily because it both stops me from feeling like I am missing out on snacks and also helps up my fibre intake. Its two main ingredients are indeed fibre superstars.

We have already discussed glucomannan under the subject of fibre, but let me expand on it a little bit more. Glucomannan is an almost magical ingredient from nature. It is extracted from the root of the Konjac plant and has been clinically proven to aid weight loss. In fact, it is the only ingredient to be officially recognised by the EU Commission to contribute to helping us lose weight. A natural plant fibre, in our stomach it expands up to 50 times its weight making us feel full.

Taken before a meal, it reduces our appetite and for some people, such as me, it completely removes the desire to eat snacks. When we consume more than 4g per day, the European Food Safety Authority also confirm that it helps us maintain normal blood cholesterol levels.

How does it work? Glucomannan is a soluble viscous fibre, which dissolves in water, forming a gel-like substance. Viscous fibres are found in the walls of plant cells and have the ability to expand like a sponge. When you take a SlimShotz drink, followed by sufficient water, the glucomannan gel continues to expand inside the stomach. Our receptors on sensing this fullness, trigger our satiety hormone known as leptin. If we then eat a meal approximately 30 minutes to an hour later, we consume less food as the brain already has received a signal to say its full. Plus, there is physically less room in the stomach too. It's kind of like a natural gastric band! Glucomannan also acts as a prebiotic, feeding our guts friendly bacteria. Furthermore, once past the stomach, and inside the intestines, the fibre slows the process of breaking down food, which in turn reduces the glycaemic index of the entire meal, in other words slowing down the release of sugar into the bloodstream. As a result, this means that the body doesn't need to release as much of the fat building hormone insulin.

Now, let's discuss inulin (I know it sounds like insulin, but inulin is a very different thing). If glucomannan is king of the prebiotic world, then the god would be inulin. Our friendly gut bacteria are said to have a feeding frenzy when it arrives. They convert it into short chain fatty acids, which nourish colon cells and provide a multitude of other health benefits. Interestingly, the diverse diets of our cavemen ancestors, included far more roots (inulin is from the roots of the chicory plant and glucomannan from the root of the Konjac plant) and therefore far more fibre was consumed than in the modern diet.

But inulin is far more than just a prebiotic. During Angela Rippon's 'How To Stay Young' programme, they mentioned how inulin helps to reduce internal fats (visceral fats). Then during Dr Michael Mosley's 'Trust Me I'm A Doctor' programme, he discusses how inulin helps us get a good night's sleep.

CBD Oil

Over the last few years, you have probably read or heard about CBD. CBD is one of the compounds known as cannabinoids found in the cannabis or marijuana plant. Yes, I mentioned the word marijuana! But don't think that CBD is going to be making you high. Tetrahydrocannabinol or THC is the primary psychoactive cannabinoid found in cannabis and causes the sensation of getting 'high' that is often associated with marijuana. However, unlike THC, CBD is non-psychoactive, making CBD an appealing option for those who are looking for relief from pain and other symptoms without the mind-altering effects of marijuana or certain pharmaceutical drugs.

Is it primal? Actually, yes! You see, it is most likely that our distant ancestors consumed plenty of CBD via the ruminants they ate which often grazed on hemp. But how does CBD help reduce pain? In the early 1990s, scientists discovered that there is an endocannabinoid system within the human body, which as well as helping us maintain homeostasis, is also involved in many processes, such as pain, mood, stress, sleep and our immune system.

I personally take CBD to relieve pain in my right knee, which is the ongoing result of the surgery I had many years ago, and while I am generally laid back anyway, I feel it relaxes me even further.

Supplements and Weight Loss

Could taking vitamins and minerals as part of our daily routine also help us lose weight? I believe so. You see, I believe that when we are hungry, particularly if this is in the morning, it is not always our body crying for energy. I think there are two reasons why our brains tell us to consume food. I believe that hunger is either a cry for energy or more likely for certain nutrients. Many women, when they are pregnant, begin to crave a whole variety of sometimes very strange things. That is normally driven by the unborn child crying out for a specific vitamin or mineral. I think the same often happens when we're hungry, it is not the body crying for energy, but the brain realising that it's lacking a certain nutrient. It is your brain seeking optimal nutrition. If you are hungry when you wake up, before you start scoffing down food, consider taking your multivitamins, omega 3, etc. You might find that it completely removes your hunger and therefore helps you both enter a state of fasting and weight loss.

Can you take too many supplements? Well, it appears not. First, it's important to remember that vitamins are vital for life. Next, it's important to remember that vitamins and minerals are not drugs. According to the American Association of Poison Control Centres, In the US in 2010, not a single person died from taking a vitamin compared to 1.9 million hospital admissions leading to 128,000 deaths from drugs prescribed to them. And in Europe, the European Commission suggests that adverse reactions to prescribed drugs cause over 200,000 deaths per year!

A Recap of the Necessity of Supplements for Optimal Health

Firstly, let me disclose that I am involved with a company that manufactures and retails supplements. However, this involvement only began after I became aware of the vitally important role that quality supplementation plays in optimising our health. There has been a lot of information in both this and previous chapters to comprehend on the matter, so I thought I would bring it to a conclusion by putting all of the pieces of the jigsaw together:

- Because our primal ancestors were burning far more energy, they ate a lot more food. And as their food was entirely natural and organic, the quality was better too. We would have to increase our meal sizes threefold, to receive similar levels of vitamins and minerals.
- In the 1930s, Dr Price demonstrated how remote communities had diets that were amongst other things; seven times richer in calcium, four times richer in magnesium and copper; fifty times richer in iron and iodine and often ten times richer in vitamins; than the equivalent Westernised diet.
- Because a lot of our food is now grown hydroponically (see next chapter), they no longer contain the measurements of nutrients they are supposed to.
- When fruits and vegetables are protected by pesticides, their natural antioxidants aren't necessary and don't fully develop.
- Because farmers no longer build soil fertility through correct crop rotations, vegetables are not as rich in vitamins and minerals as they should be.
- We no longer eat as many organs and offal as we once did, and even when we do eat meat, the animals have often been fed an unnatural diet.

- We don't spend as much time outdoors as our ancestors did, so we don't get as much sunlight and therefore often don't synthesise sufficient vitamin D.
- We need to increase our nutrition because our livers have to deal with an onslaught of toxins that our ancestors were never exposed too.

If we are to get even remotely close to providing our body with the optimal nutrition it so badly needs, there is today - unless we live in a remote area of the planet and spend our days working and walking outdoors - an undeniable need for supplements.

The Pill Nation

Professor Tim Noakes

The current medical model doesn't work. These diseases are all nutritionally based. The majority of the chronic diseases I am aware of are all nutritionally based, and you can't give medications, you've got to change the diet. And the beauty is that you start helping people.

Hippocrates said, "Let food be thy medicine and medicine be thy food". Isn't it such a shame that most people living in our country seem to have forgotten this piece of advice? How about this for a frightening statistic: A recent article in The Telegraph newspaper titled 'Pill Nation', revealed that, "Half of the nation were now taking prescription medication with rising use of antidepressants fuelling a 47 per cent increase in drugs dispensed over the last decade," and that a recent NHS survey showed that, "One quarter of people are on at least three drugs, with millions of pensioners on at least five types of medication".

In her book *Minding My Mitochondria*, author Dr Terry Wahls says, "Universal health care and free medication only treat existing chronic diseases. This is important, but most conventional treatments only control the symptoms of disease. They usually don't reverse damage that has already been done". So, if we combine the wise words of Hippocrates with Dr Wahls, we can draw the conclusion that they are advising that we should use food and nutrition as a prevention, rather than looking to medicine to control and mask symptoms.

Even though living a primal existence can cure several illnesses, we are all still much better off doing everything we can to prevent health issues occurring in the first place. I want you to consider this for a minute: why is it that we will happily send our car in for a service even when there is nothing wrong with it? Why in business today do we invest more money and effort in preventing problems than we do in building huge customer service teams? Because in everything other than the most important thing of all – our health – we have already shifted our attention to prevention rather than cure.

Due to our present predicament, caused, in my opinion, predominantly by food and pharmaceutical corporate greed and governmental lack of genuine concern, we now have more people that need to be cured than need prevention! And while there are many that criticise our doctors for being too quick to reach for their prescription pad rather than to sit and investigate possible lifestyle changes, I personally don't blame them. I think our doctors are in a really difficult, no-win position. Not only are they overloaded with more and more patients to see each and every day, they are then under immense pressure by being measured and monitored in everything they do. It's far safer for our GP to prescribe a course of approved medicine to help alleviate symptoms, drugs that are produced by the huge pharmaceutical companies paying huge taxes to our government, than to risk sticking their neck out suggesting lifestyle changes that don't make anyone any profits.

While I sympathise with our overworked doctors, I feel the need to scream loudly that too many people are being prescribed drugs to mask symptoms, instead of curing the root of their problems. I often speak to people who are on lifetime medication, when a change in lifestyle would cause the underlying problem to disappear. It drives me crazy that I have got friends on statins, who in my opinion just don't need to be, and even worse when I see antibiotics being handed out for conditions that have nothing to do with bacterial infections.

My lovely wife is beautiful, petite, and for some reason prone to picking up infections. Sadly, over the years, it seems all that the doctors want to do is give her another course of antibiotics. Have you ever heard the saying, 'when all you have is a hammer, everything looks like a nail'? Well, in my opinion, that's what seems to be happening with far too many GPs and their prescription pads, but again it's hard to lay the blame at doctors individually – it's the system that's wrong! Luckily for me, my family and closest friends are now living primally, and approach illnesses by first listening to the advice of Hippocrates. I hope that you will be successful in convincing your family and friends to do the same too.

Why are so many pills being prescribed? Well, according to Dr Thomas Levey, author of *Stop America's #1 Killer!*, big pharma spends a whopping $16 billion on direct-to-physician peddling and another $4 billion peddling their wares direct to the consumer. Current beliefs and medical treatments for heart disease, stroke, obesity and diabetes are based on pharmaceutical models. As professor and nutrition activist Tim Noakes says, "They demonstrably do not work, as global epidemics of all these conditions have shown. They have worked only to fill the coffers of the drug-makers."

Let us all pull together to advocate and campaign on behalf of natural preventative medicine as a first step to wellness and try as many natural methods as we can before we accept prescriptions for long-term medication.

Dr Aseem Malhotra

Aseem made the following interesting comments as we were having an in-depth debate about data, numbers needed to treat with a drug for a positive outcome and the difference between absolute and relative risk statistics.

Even the World Health Organisation in 2009 put out a bulletin, written by a gentleman who I have met called Gerd Gigerenzer, who is considered the world's leading researcher expert in health literacy. He basically said that unless you tell patients this when you are prescribing them a drug, it's basically unethical. I have said this in lectures all around the world, that we have unwittingly been practising unethical medicine. Not deliberately, but unwittingly, by not explaining the statistics and likelihood of success to the patient, to help them make an informed decision in a transparent way. Sadly, 70% of healthcare professionals, including doctors, fail basic tests on their understanding of evidence-based medicine. So, there needs to be a cultural shift. This was not something you learn in medical school. We need to change the way we learn, the way we teach, and the way we communicate with our patients, so we become more open and transparent. The interesting thing that once patients are given all of the information about a drug or a medical procedure, about the chances of benefit in general, you find people will choose less of that. Then we start to look at the alternatives. Good health rarely comes out of a medicine bottle.

Don't Rely On Drugs As A Fix

As you will read in various topics throughout this book, our immune system is very dependent on the health of our microbiome, and every course of antibiotics we take indiscriminately kills off many of the helpful bacteria in our guts along with the bad ones. Even in 1945, when Alexander Fleming won the Nobel Prize in Physiology or Medicine for inventing the first antibiotic – penicillin – he warned, "The time might come when penicillin can be bought by anyone in the shops. Then there is the danger that the ignorant man may easily under-dose himself and, by exposing his microbes to non-lethal quantities of the drug, make them resistant".

In 1942, Anne Miller became the first patient ever to have a course of antibiotics. She became seriously ill after giving birth and was suffering from a raging virus. Within hours of receiving the antibiotics, she started to recover, and the new medicine was heralded a success. But it was so scarce, that doctors actually filtered her urine so that they could recycle it! The reason I mention this story is to show the foresight of its inventor who, even when it was still so rare, was warning of its overuse. Don't get me wrong – without antibiotics the world would be a far deadlier place, but the overuse of it should be of concern.

We really have got to the stage where, for almost every ailment, we turn to pills and doctors for a quick fix, rather than trying to eliminate the cause naturally. Over the past few years, whenever I have hurt myself in the gym, pulled a muscle sailing or developed tennis elbow, rather than going to a doctor my personal trainer and his team have solved the problem by identifying the route cause.

Some 10 years ago I hurt my knee playing squash, and the result was hospitalisation and a major operation to reconstruct my anterior cruciate ligament. Sadly, my eldest son Matt had the same operation in recent years, but for him two separate ongoing rugby injuries led to serious operations on both knees. Having now learnt more from a personal trainer and his team, all three knee operations could most likely have been avoided if we had dealt with the root cause of the issue as soon as we started to feel the symptoms.

Nina Teicholz

We have to remember that big pharmaceutical companies are not profiting if you are getting well. They really have no interest in better health.

In December 2003, Dr Allen Rose, who at the time was the International Vice President of GlaxoSmithKline (manufacturers of numerous drugs for the medical pharmaceuticals industry with a turnover in excess of £81 billion per annum), went public with some alarming statistics. In an article featured on the front page of The Independent newspaper he broke the news that, "The vast majority of drugs – more than 90 percent – only work in 30 to 50 percent of the people". That's a huge confession from someone who has been involved with running one of the biggest drug companies on earth.

Then, in February 2016, Mail Online published an article with the title, 'How big pharma greed is killing tens of thousands around the world: Patients are over-medicated and often given profitable drugs with "little proven benefits", leading doctors warned'. It goes on to say, "The Queen's former doctor has called for an urgent public enquiry into drugs firms' 'murky' practices". Later in the same article there is a quote from Dr Aseem Malhotra: "There is no doubt that a 'more medicine is better' culture lies at the heart of healthcare, exacerbated by financial incentives within the system to prescribe more drugs and carry out more procedures". Dr Malhorta makes three more, very relevant, comments:

- He accuses the drugs companies of 'spending twice as much on marketing than on research'
- That 'prescription drugs often do more harm than good, with the elderly particularly at risk'
- 'One in three hospital admissions among the over-75s are a result of an adverse drug reaction'

I have got to thank my own doctor, Renee Kellerman, who on more than one occasion over the past 20 years has resisted putting me on a course of drugs, instead explaining the lifestyle changes I needed to make. She has always instilled in me the need for prevention over cure. Much to the disadvantage of the huge pharmaceutical conglomerates, she wants her patients to avoid at all costs any drugs that merely suppress the symptoms of conditions and diseases.

Rather than trying to address the root cause, understandably sufferers often reach without hesitation for medication. What does medication really do for us? It masks the real underlying problems and slows down our immune system's ability to deal with them. They often tell our immune system to stop working quite so hard and pass the work over to the highly profitable chemical cocktail created by the drug company. This handing over of the responsibility - from the body's natural repair and defence mechanism - to the scientists working for the corporate giants can have numerous harmful side effects for those that rely on certain medicines. Having said this, I fully appreciate there are certain conditions where modern medicines are totally beneficial to the sufferer. My point is more that there are many illnesses where we would be better trying to address the root cause of them first, rather than being sentenced to a life on medication.

Gary Taubes

We have these diabetes and obesity epidemics, and they are overwhelming our healthcare systems. The burdens to the individuals are just terrible, and they are getting the wrong advice. Doctors are giving them the wrong advice, and this just has to get fixed. And the people who buy into what we are saying, are people like ourselves who look at the research and read the books and say, 'this is interesting, let's see what happens'. And they change their diets and get healthier. And they do the complete opposite of what they are told to do, and they are leaner, are lighter, are healthier, have more energy and a lot of other health problems seem to vanish.

Dr Peter Brukner

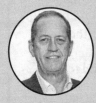

When I began work with the Australian Cricket Team, we were touring in India, and one player in question was having a lot of trouble with regular knee pain to the point where at one stage, he had to stop playing.

He'd been to every doctor and specialist in Sydney, had every imaginable scan, but nobody could figure out what was wrong with him. He was eventually diagnosed with Seronegative Arthritis and prescribed Enbrel, an expensive drug that costs the taxpayer thousands every year.

It made an initial difference. The pain wasn't completely gone, but he was able to play again, so he began injecting himself daily. Each time he felt the pain coming on, he would inject himself, and the pain would temporarily go away.

It helped him recover to the point where he was still in the Australian Squad, but not the first team.

It was reasonably well known by then that I had personally lost a lot of weight by adopting a low carb diet, and he came to me and asked if I could help him do the same. So, we began by taking him off sugar, processed food and put him on a low carb diet. Now, India isn't the easiest place to go low carb. There was plenty of rice and naan bread on offer, and he didn't find it easy but equally he never gave up, was remarkably conscientious and he stuck to it.

Three weeks later, he came to me and said 'Doc, I forgot to take my Enbrel injection because I've had no pain in my knee, should I still take it?'. So, I told him that unless he felt any pain, to hold off, not to take it and to see how he felt.

The pain never returned.

Since he's adopted low carb, he is free from expensive prescription drugs, free from pain, allowing him to train harder than ever and just 12 months later, he was ranked in the Top 10 Batsman in the world.

Chapter 11 Highlights

- Optimising our nutrition is the single biggest step we can take to avoid chronic illness.
- The European Union NRVs are assembled around avoiding deficiency, not ultimate health.
- Vitamin C is the very best antioxidant of all.
- Avoid crap foods void of nutrition and live longer and happier with natural foods full of vitamins and minerals.
- Doctors should insist on high dose vitamin C – while they ponder the right medicine for almost any illness.
- Turmeric is one of the most powerful natural medicines we can add to our food.
- Eat foods rich in nutrients and fill any nutritional or vitamin shortfalls with reputable supplements.
- Omega 3. If you don't want to take a supplement derived from fish, then flaxseed oil makes a good substitute.
- We advocate and campaign on behalf of natural preventative medicine as a first step to wellness and try as many natural methods as we can before we accept prescriptions for long-term medication.
- Professor Peter Gøtzsche at the University of Copenhagen believes that, after heart disease and cancer, prescription drugs are now the third most common cause of death!

CHAPTER 12

THE SUPERFOODS
TO THE UGLY

"One cannot think well, love well, sleep well, if one has not dined well."
VIRGINIA WOOLF

A primal pantry is absolutely stuffed with healthy and delicious things to eat. In this chapter we discover the organic meats, fruit and vegetables we should be consuming, and more importantly the things we need to avoid.

So, now we arrive at the exciting part. Having got this far, you already have a strong understanding of what steps you can take to cure certain illnesses, what food types can kill you, and what nourishment to consume to prevent many diseases from occurring. As you start going through the primal list of foods to eat and those to avoid, you might think that you won't be able to afford to fully take advantage of a primal way of life. However, even though organic foods, quality meats and fish, healthy ingredients and local produce might be more expensive than cheaply prepared and manufactured packaged products, your overall spend might actually go down. Yes, the produce we consume when following a primal lifestyle is definitely in the main more expensive than the cheaper, highly dangerous foodstuffs, but there are loads of areas where we will be saving money.

Top Nine Big Cost Savings When Living Primally

1. As we intermittently fast, regardless of which approach we chose, we will be eating fewer meals and therefore saving money. If, like me, you become an OMAD (One Meal A Day), then your cost of food drops significantly.
2. No more plastic bottled water. We don't want to ruin our oceans and consume leaked chemicals. Instead we are going to drink readily available, filtered tap water.

3. No need to subscribe to health magazines, as my *www.primalliving.com* website, app and blogs are updated frequently, and completely free.
4. Less time off work through illness. Even if you're paid sick leave, trust me it eventually hurts your career prospects if you are known as 'Sick Note Jo'.
5. No more fizzy drinks, which are possibly one of the most profitable and overly priced killers ever invented.
6. No need to sign up for membership of diet clubs. If these things truly worked, then they would have no long-term members at all.
7. By growing some of our own herbs, we won't need to go out and buy expensive, sugar loaded sauces.
8. Our wardrobe gets cheaper too. The yo-yo dieters constantly need new wardrobes to fit their ever-changing size. Once we have gone primal, and bought all our new, slimmer clothing, there is little chance we are going to put a lot of weight back on, therefore our clothes are going to last far longer.
9. No more need to snack. Imagine how much money you will save by not eating crisps, sweets, chocolate and cakes.

Professor Tim Noakes

Anyone that tells you that the diet is expensive, that's wrong. It is nonsense. We are trying to reverse diabetes in South Africa across all demographics. We have come up with a diet that cost the equivalent of about £1.50. And it gives great nutrition and leaves people feeling full up and can help people start to reverse their diabetes.

We begin with eggs, and then canned pilchards and sardines, which in South Africa are cheap (they are also cheap in the UK, supermarket own brands start at as little as just 40 pence). Then we add offal, which is cheap. Then we teach people to work together so they can buy communally. And then to go to the expensive supermarkets and ask for the fat that they have cut off the beef. And what is so exciting is that their health starts to improve dramatically. Just by changing their food intake, they start reversing all these diseases.

Other than the quality food we are consuming, all other LEON (Lifestyle, Environment, Optimal Nutrition) principles for living primally tend to be cheaper than the alternative. We are walking more, exercising more and lifting weights that could be done at home. We are getting more enjoyment out of life, and therefore not indulging in purchases just to make us feel better.

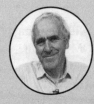

Patrick Holden CBE

In the 1970s, a third of our disposable income was spent on food. Today it is something like 9.9%. So, we are only spending a third as much today! We have shifted away from putting a priority on food, and are spending it in other areas.

The Top 20 Primal Superfoods

In this section, you are going to discover foods that are both genuinely primal and are what I like to call 'nutritionally dense'. Gram for gram, they are going to provide you with more vitamins, minerals and healthy oils than virtually any other food on the planet. If you would like some great delicious Superfood recipes, then please pay a visit to *www.primalliving.com* where we add new recipes every week, or purchase *Primal Gourmet*, which I co-wrote with the incredibly talented Hannah Anderson.

While many of the Superfoods are individual performers, like avocado, spinach and garlic, others are Superfood groups, such as organic meats.

1. Coconut
2. Avocado
3. Eggs
4. Nuts
5. Seeds
6. Berries
7. Cruciferous vegetables
8. Shirataki
9. Spinach
10. Tomatoes
11. Peppers
12. Onions
13. Olives
14. Organic meats
15. Oily fish
16. Garlic
17. Fermented foods
18. Dark chocolate
19. Bone broth
20. Mushrooms

While it is not essential that you read through each of the Superfoods in detail, if you do have the time, you will find some little nuggets of information that will help you better understand how they assist us in optimising our nutrition.

Coconuts

I have already written a lot about coconuts oils, but let's now look at some other ways to consume this incredibly primal Superfood. Before we get going, I want to touch on a few things first. Recently, coconuts have been receiving a little negative press, with some misguided researchers suggesting their fat content leads to high cholesterol and heart disease.

Sadly, these reports are just recycling old news where they linked saturated fats to heart diseases, which as we have already read, has never been established and is just plain wrong! Ignore the ill-informed journalists and instead take note of Hindu mythology, where coconuts are called 'kalpavriksha', which means 'tree that gives all that is necessary for living'.

Coconuts are highly beneficial for our health as they contain vitamins B1, B3, B5, B6, C and E, and come jam-packed with healthy minerals such as calcium, selenium, sodium, magnesium and phosphorous. What's more, they're full of fibre, which today is sadly lacking in most diets.

Interestingly, coconut is a fruit, not a nut as its name implies. Spanish explorers prefixed their nut with 'cocos' – meaning 'grinning face' – because the three little 'eyes' (known as germination spores or stoma) on their base reminded them of a smiling monkey.

Coconut Flour
Simply a gift from heaven, or at least from some very tall trees. If it wasn't for the holy coconut, making bread without grain flour would be kind of difficult. Derived from the dried flesh of the coconut, this is a flour packed with fibre, protein and healthy fats. It's free of both gluten and grain, and it can be used to make tasty breads or cakes, pancakes and desserts. You can also use it to thicken up sauces and curries, and add it to smoothies to ensure you are getting your daily fix of healthy fat.

Coconut Cream and Milk
Unlike cow's milk, coconut milk is completely lactose free! While I am not against organic cow's milk (even though in the true sense it's not really primal), coconut milk is definitely more beneficial to our overall health. Not to be confused with coconut water, coconut milk and cream is produced by grating the coconut flesh and then soaking it in hot water. The thick cream rises to the top, where it is skimmed off, and the remaining juice can be filtered and bottled as milk. Why is it so beneficial? Well, it's no normal fat. As we discussed earlier in the book, it's the richest source of medium-chain fatty acids (MCFAs), which is the closest thing for sale in a can or bottle to human breast milk! As it's very dense, don't drink it like cow's milk.

Even though we don't count calories, if you do want it as a stand-alone drink, just go for half a glass. Even this small amount will provide you with 25g of healthy fat, plus a good dose of manganese, copper, phosphorus, magnesium and iron. Where I find coconut milk comes into its own, is in adding both flavour and thickness to curries. In the summer I have also been known to make a white Russian kahlúa cocktail with it too, but I guess I shouldn't really be mentioning that!

Coconut Water
This is the actual juice extracted from the shell of a young coconut before it develops into flesh. It is naturally sugary, and because of this you often hear people say you

shouldn't drink it if you want to lose weight. Complete rubbish! Well, unless you drink gallons of it. Coconut water contains less than 3g of natural fructose per 100g. Compared to Coke at 11g, it sounds virtually sugar free! And there is less sugar in a glass of coconut water than in an orange! Not only is it an incredibly healthy option when we need to rehydrate our body, in several developing countries, medical centres use it as a treatment for diarrhoea.

As we have already discussed, there are six minerals that together create electrolytes, which rehydrate and recharge our body – which is especially useful after a workout or illness. One of the core six minerals is potassium, of which coconut water is an extremely rich source.

In addition, it also contains smaller concentrations of sodium, calcium and magnesium, all of which are also part of nature's electrolyte-hydration formula. Next time you're about to reach for a sports drink to rehydrate during a workout, do yourself a huge favour and replace it with nature's all-natural sports aid, an electrolyte that has been used for centuries by some of the healthiest nations on our planet.

Nutritionally, coconut water is very different to coconut milk. It has zero fat, around 40 calories per glass and contains 10% of our daily vitamin C requirement, plus it's a great source for vitamin B1 (thiamine), vitamin B2 (riboflavin) and vitamin B6. One glass also contains about 11% of our daily dietary fibre, 6% calcium, 15% magnesium, 17% potassium, 11% sodium and 17% manganese. In short, it is full of natural goodness.

One word of coconut caution. I found nine different coconut water offerings in my local supermarket, but on close inspection only two were completely natural. The others had artificial flavourings, additional sugars and a whole host of other nasties. As with most foods, make sure you always read the label carefully.

Coconut Chunks or Flakes
Both are great to snack on, put into salads or add awesome flavour to curries. I will often sprinkle flakes in with nuts or a bowl of berries topped with probiotic yogurt.

Desiccated Coconut
The definition of desiccated means to remove moisture from something that normally contains moisture. Desiccated coconut is produced from drying the shredded coconut and then heating it. Even though it tastes lovely and sweet, it's totally natural and as none of the fat is removed, all of its amazing health benefits are preserved.

Coconut Aminos
Soy sauce is a popular ingredient especially in Chinese and Japanese cuisine. However, it's not primal and for those looking to avoid gluten, Coconut Aminos makes for a wonderful alternative. It's a dark coloured sauce made from coconut sap and as the name suggests, it's rich in amino acids, as well as vitamin C and several vitamin Bs.

Avocado

The avocado is not just a Superfood, it is one of very few superfruits. While most fruits have numerous health benefits, they are still primarily carbohydrates, so not helpful for us when we are trying to lose a lot of weight, and certainly not good when we consume too many of them. But the superfruit avocado is unique in that it is primarily a fat. There are so many benefits of regularly consuming avocado that, if I had to pick just one food to take on a desert island, it would be a toss-up between avocado and coconuts.

Avocados contain an amazing line-up of vitamins and minerals. First of all, they are 77% heart-healthy monounsaturated fat, 19% carbohydrates and 4% protein. The majority of fat found in avocado is oleic acid (also known as omega 9), which also happens to be the super ingredient found in olives. Oleic acids provide numerous health benefits, including helping to reduce inflammation and warding off cancer. They are full of antioxidants that help, among other things, to protect our sight. There are lots of white papers and studies that suggest that having a high intake of potassium helps to reduce blood pressure (a major factor in heart attacks) and kidney failure. One of the greatest sources of potassium is avocado.

If we eat both halves of an average-sized avocado, then we will be consuming around 150g of delicious healthiness. Avocados are packed full of vitamins B5, B6, C, E, K, folate and potassium. In addition, they contain copper, iron, magnesium, manganese, phosphorus, vitamin B1, vitamin B3 and zinc, and are also a superb source of fibre, and of its huge fibre content, 25% of it is soluble which allows it to feed our friendly gut bacteria.

Eggs

When I was diagnosed with high cholesterol in my early forties, I was told to avoid eating egg yolks as they were high in cholesterol. So, for years, I would spend time delicately removing them before cooking. But now we understand that egg yolks are full of goodness, and even if we are diagnosed with high levels of cholesterol (and don't forget many leading doctors don't actually believe that high cholesterol is a contributing factor in heart disease), the yolk doesn't actually increase it any further.

Eggs are loaded with quality proteins. In fact, they contain all nine essential amino acids, vitamins A, B12, B2 and B5 as well as lots of minerals. They are full of good fats and many traces of helpful nutrients, such as phosphorus and selenium. I guess when you think about it logically, an egg is full of the greatest ingredients nature could create. After all, each shell must contain all of the essential elements to create new life. Nothing added, nothing taken away. Eggs are full of pure, healthy, life-giving goodness, and each one contains a small amount of almost every nutrient we need.

While a little more expensive, it is crucial to try to buy organic eggs. There is a huge difference in the balance of omega 3 to omega 6, with some reports suggesting that the difference can be tenfold!

Egg Box Labelling

According to the Soil Association's website (*www.soilassociation.org*), in the UK we consume 12 billion eggs each year, but sadly only 47% are certified as free range and only 2% are certified organic.

The Soil Association website informs us that standards have been set for organic and 'free range' eggs that stipulate, among other things, flock sizes, stocking densities and how many hens can share a space. Organic standards go further than free-range standards in a number of important aspects:

1. Soil Association organic standards stipulate smaller flock sizes, and lower stocking densities (the number of birds per square metre). Max 2,000 vs 16,000 in free-range systems.
2. Organic farms certified by the Soil Association have to provide more pop holes (exits from the hen house) than free-range farms do, to encourage and promote ranging.
3. No beak trimming – this is a mutilation that can be painful and also prevents the hens from expressing their natural foraging behaviour. The vast majority of UK hens kept in free-range systems are routinely beak trimmed.
4. Organic chickens are fed a GM-free diet. In the UK alone, more than 1 million tonnes of GM crops are used to feed animals, including some free-range chickens.

Also when you find eggs where the label says they are rich in omega 3, they are created by feeding hens a diet of flax seeds, which contain a high level of omega 3.

Nuts

I remember being in Tanzania, when a Maasai approached my Jeep, clutching a bunch of root vegetables he had just plucked out of the soil. As my friend Mark had lived in the country for more than 20 years, I asked them what the vegetable was. It turned out to be peanuts. "But they can't be," I said, "nuts grow in trees". I was surprised that it turns out that the most consumed nut in the world, the peanut, is not really a nut at all but a legume.

When someone has a nut allergy and is only allergic to peanuts, they don't have a nut allergy at all but a legume allergy! And that label you see on some packs of peanuts saying 'may contain nuts' is therefore, of course, factually incorrect!

Botanically speaking, what defines a nut is a dried fruit with one seed (although on a rare occasion it can be two), in which the seed case wall becomes hard at maturity. In reality, there is very little difference between nuts and seeds. The reason why they are so incredibly healthy is that they all are the inauguration of a plant or tree's life. Just as the yolk of an egg is full of nutrients as it carries all the vital ingredients for a chicken to hatch, seeds and nuts are packed full of both energy and nutrients, sufficient enough to sprout huge trees.

Just a thought. Have you ever stopped and pondered why the word 'nutrition' begins with the word 'nut'?

Walnuts, pecans, pistachios, Brazil nuts, hazelnuts, macadamias and chestnuts all have numerous health benefits, and can at the same time add real flavour to our primal lifestyle. "You missed out cashews and almonds", I hear you shout. Well, these are technically seeds and not nuts! That said, as this is a book about how to live primally and not botanical correctness, for simplicity's sake from here on in we will treat these two no differently and not eject them from the nut family.

Why are nuts in our list of Superfoods? All nuts are rich in protein and healthy oils such as omega 3. Most of them also contain healthy levels of magnesium, potassium, iron, copper and various vitamin Bs. But with nuts, we do need to demonstrate a little bit of portion control, while we are trying to keep on top of our weight.

You won't be surprised to hear me say that one thing we should try to do is purchase nuts as unprocessed and as organic as possible. Sadly, many branded nuts are over processed, covered in masses of salt and roasted in hydrogenated oils. All that said, when you are out and about and feel the need to eat something, it's still preferable to buy almost any quality of nuts than reach for sweets or packets of crisps. My view is that any negative or toxic affect from eating processed nuts is still going to be less than the benefits you will receive. Nuts are really good for us. It's that simple. That said, here are some scientific words you might find in articles speaking about nuts and what they really mean:

Phytochemicals
'Phyto' is a Greek word for 'plant'. These chemicals help the plant protect its seeds and nuts from fungi, bugs, germs and other threats. As the word 'chemicals' just sounds too negative, I won't use it in the chart below, but instead replace it with 'phytonutrients'.

Phytosterols
A type of phytonutrient similar in structure to the body's cholesterol. It might sound paradoxical, but when our diet is high in phytosterols, we absorb less cholesterol. In addition, researchers believe that phytosterols may play a role in prevention of Alzheimer's disease.

Polyphenols
A type of phytonutrient with antioxidant capabilities that play an important role in preventing and reducing the progression of cancer, diabetes, cardiovascular and neurodegenerative diseases. They also act as a prebiotic, helping feed our good bacteria.

Flavonoids
A type of phytonutrient that is an extremely potent antioxidant. More than 4,000 different flavonoids have been identified, and they are accountable for many of the vivid colours we see in fruit and veg.

Lignans

These are chemical that activate our bacteria when we digest them. Lignans are considered a form of phytoestrogens, which, as the name implies, are oestrogens found in plants. Research is starting to suggest that lignans may be anti-cancerous, anti-inflammatory and may reduce the risk of cardiovascular disease.

Nuts - The Excellent Eight

These nuts have been designated as Superfoods because they are high in fibre, packed full of antioxidants, and are all a rich source of minerals and vitamins. Those that make up the 'Excellent Eight' are all available in supermarkets in both the UK and the USA. In all forms, they are better consumed than avoided but, if possible, head down the baking isle and look for nuts that have not been salted, roasted in oils or coated in CARBS and flavourings. And while Brazil nuts in dark chocolate are fine, don't try to sell yourself on the health benefits of nuts coated in crispy sugar!

In June 2015, The Independent newspaper in the UK wrote, "Eating just a handful of nuts a day could lower your risk of a heart attack or of dying from cancer and diabetes". They went on to say, "Epidemiologist Professor Piet van den Brandt, who led the study of more than 120,000 Dutch people between the ages of 55 and 69 at Maastricht University, said the findings were 'remarkable', particularly due to the small amount that needed to be eaten daily to make a difference".

- Almond
- Brazil
- Cashews
- Hazelnuts
- Macadamia
- Pecan
- Pistachio
- Walnut

Seeds - The Magnificent Seven

Just like nuts, seeds are in our Superfoods category as they are high in fibre, packed full of antioxidants and offer rich sources of minerals and vitamins. Those that make up the 'Magnificent Seven' are all available in leading supermarkets. As I mentioned with nuts, in most forms they are better consumed than avoided, but if possible, head down to the baking isle and look for seeds that have not been soaked in oils and flavourings.

- Chia
- Flaxseed
- Hemp
- Poppy
- Pumpkin
- Sesame
- Sunflower

Berries - The Fab Four

While there are several other berries that are undoubtedly beneficial for our health, including the currently highly trendy acai and goji berries, plus cherries, cranberries and redcurrants, there are four that, for me, stand above all in terms of nutritional value. You will also notice how they appear high up in the ORAC scale (see the colour insert).

Blueberries

Possibly the most highly antioxidant substance you can swallow is the highly praised and delicious blueberry. In a recent study carried out in America, senior citizens were given two and a half cups of blueberries every day for 12 weeks. Dr Robert Krikorian, who led the research said, "Our new findings corroborate those of previous animal studies and preliminary human studies, adding further support to the notion that blueberries can have a real benefit in improving memory and cognitive function in some older adults".

Blueberries are rich in the flavonoid anthocyanin, which is responsible for their vivid colour. The great news is that we can eat them all year round, as it appears that freezing blueberries has no negative effect on their antioxidants.

Strawberries

Very British, and very good for our health. Full of flavour and fibre, it surprises many people when I tell them how healthy strawberries are. For some reason, many believe they are full of sugar, maybe in a can they can be, but when fresh they are very low in fructose. They are packed with vitamins (especially vitamin C) and minerals, and they're one of the best sources of fruit antioxidants we can consume.

Raspberries

How about this for a key reason to consume raspberries on a regular basis: they are full to capacity with cancer-fighting antioxidants. To put their power in perspective, they are said to be 10 times more concentrated in antioxidants than tomatoes, which in themselves are miracle workers. They boost our mood and help us retain our memory as we age.

Blackberries

I remember as a child picking blackberries from thorny bushes at the end of summer. Just like strawberries, they are naturally very sweet but don't contain many calories. In fact, their nutritional value is tremendously high, with one cupful containing 30% of our daily fibre, and 50% of our vitamin C requirements. Blackberries are also chocka-block with lots of other vitamins and minerals too.

Dr Patrick Holford

The berries have a different type of sugar called xylose. I was talking to a top dentist and asked what are the best things you can do to prevent cavities, and he said xylitol. And in Finland, they give every child a sweet as they arrive at school containing xylitol because what they have learnt is that this sugar, when bacteria in the mouth feed on it, they can't stick to your teeth and it prevents cavities. So, they have the healthiest teeth because of xylose, which is the sugar in berries.

The Cruciferous Family of Vegetables

Pronounced 'crew-sif-er-us', this family of vegetables are descendants of the Brassica genus of plants, famed for their disease-fighting compounds. For more than 30 years, consuming high amounts of cruciferous vegetables has been associated with a lower risk of cancer. Researchers have discovered that it is the sulphur containing compounds (particularly sulforaphane) that, while giving cruciferous vegetables their slightly bitter taste, are primarily what provide them with their cancer-fighting benefits.

An increase of cruciferous vegetables in diets has been indisputably linked to a decreased risk in obesity, diabetes, heart attacks and overall mortality. If that's not enough to motivate us to add them to our daily diet, they also make our hair shine and our skin glow, promote strong bones and nails and, above all, pack more nutrients per calorie than virtually any other food. Plus, as I have already mentioned, cruciferous vegetables contain glucosinolates that help to detox the body:

- Broccoli
- Brussels sprouts
- Kale
- Swiss Chard
- Cabbage
- Cauliflower
- Bok Choy
- Watercress
- Turnips

Here is something that might make you both *Fat & Furious*. We have already learned that rice is not good for us if we are either diabetic or overweight. You may have also heard that cauliflower can be chopped up in to rice sized pieces and cooked to replace the CARB loaded normal rice. But in certain states in America, to protect the rice farmers and I guess the huge taxes they provide the state, they have banned cauliflower rice from being called rice!

Gary Taubes

I asked Gary how is it that green vegetables are good for us, even though they contain CARBS? The names of these diets since I started researching them 20 years ago keep changing. Low carb diets, Atkins, keto diets and lots more. Effectively they are all ketogenic diets. The names keep changing, but the gist of it is that you don't eat carbs because they are fattening, so you avoid the bread, pasta, potatoes and rice, the grain, the legumes, they are all fattening. And instead, you eat a lot of fat and green vegetables. Green vegetables, while they have carbs in them, the fibre and water content dilute all of that, to the point that they are harmless.

Shirataki

For someone who believes that CARBS and other sugars are evil, shirataki appears
to me as nature's culinary magic trick. The word itself is Japanese for 'white waterfall',
which in itself creates an image of health and vitality. Shirataki comes from the konjac
plant (also known as elephant yam) and is largely composed of glucomannan, which
is a water-soluble fibre. It holds water so well, that when cooked it looks like pasta or
noodles, but contains virtually zero CARBS and calories.

There are several shirataki brands starting to appear on the shelves of UK
supermarkets. They come in a pouch of water, which you simply drain off, rinse and
then cook as normal. While they don't contain any flavour themselves, their fibrous
nature means that they easily absorb the taste of the spices or oils we cook them with. I
personally love throwing in lots of herbs and seasonings and serving with a Thai curry.

Here is the magical thing – shirataki can take on the appearance of pasta, noodles or
tagliatelle, yet a serving contains approximately 10 calories, practically zero CARBS
and is gluten free, wheat free, sugar free and normally totally organic!

Whether you consume glucomannan as noodles or as a weight-loss supplement, it
works brilliantly for those that want to lose weight naturally, as it absorbs water like a
sponge, and therefore quickly fills up the stomach and suppresses appetite.

Spinach

This Superfood is a terrific source of antioxidants, full of minerals such as iron,
potassium, zinc, calcium and selenium, as well as vitamin E, K and vitamin B9 (folate).
When you next make a salad, chuck in two cups of spinach and you will add just
15 calories. But in return you will receive two wonderful antioxidants by the names
of lutein and zeaxanthin, which helps maintain healthy eyesight and promotes a
strong healthy heart. As you might expect, with their big green leaves, they are full of
phytonutrients that possess anti-cancer properties. In addition, the vitamins in spinach
strengthen our bones, prevent anaemia, boost our energy and help us fight infections.

If you would like Popeye-sized biceps, researchers at the Karolinska Institute in Sweden
have discovered that nitrate trapped within spinach leaves is the secret behind its
muscle-building properties. The nitrate reduces the need for oxygen when exercising,
which increases the efficiency of the mitochondria that power our cells. Spinach also
contains many flavonoids that help protect our body from free radicals.

As with all big leafy green vegetables, it's absolutely crucial to go organic. With non-
organic spinach, just imagine how much pesticide has landed on their huge surface
areas. And remember, washing vegetables rarely removes the pesticides. If it were as
easy as just rinsing them under the tap, the chemicals wouldn't be able to withstand
rain. If you have to purchase non-organic, the only way to remove man-made
chemicals is to soak the spinach in a bowl with a few drops of vinegar or purchase
FAVwash, which is a specific cleaner for non-organic fruit and veg.

Tomatoes

Tomatoes are believed to contain thousands of different phytonutrients. With more and more research being carried out into how powerful phytonutrients are in the prevention and cure of many diseases, especially in the prevention of cancer, ensuring tomatoes are part of our regular diet makes primal common sense.

Tomatoes are another excellent source of the double act lutein and zeaxanthin, which have multiple health benefits. They have possibly the highest concentration of a super-phytonutrient, known as lycopene. Not only is it the source of their colour, but it's also a powerful antioxidant that has a number of reported health benefits, longer than your average shopping list!

Firstly, lycopene is possibly the most powerful antioxidant of all. In the Westernised polluted world, even when living primally, we simply aren't able to avoid all toxins and pesticides. However, a regular portion of tomatoes, naturally loaded with lycopene, helps detoxify the body. Researchers at the University of Portsmouth suggest that lycopene has the ability to slow the growth of both breast and prostate cancers. It's also great for keeping our brain cells connected with one another, and our bones strong too. In many health shops you can now purchase it as a supplement if you don't like the taste but still want to benefit from the miracle cures offered by lycopene.

Peppers

There are so many different types of pepper that, at first, it can be a little daunting. If you say the word 'pepper', some people immediately conjure up a hot curry and mad dashes for the toilet, while others think of the big, vividly coloured but mild-mannered bell peppers. In fact, let's separate them into two groups – fiery peppers and mild to sweet peppers. With all peppers; as it is with all salad vegetables, it is very important to buy organic. What you will read shortly from Patrick Holden about hydroponics will very likely shock you to your core.

Mild to Sweet Peppers

It is the fabulously talented bell pepper (also known as capsicum) that led me to adding the pepper family to the Top 20 Superfoods. In the main, I wanted to recognise it as a high source of vitamin C, as a big yellow bell pepper has 341mg of it – that's roughly the same as five whole oranges! One red bell pepper equates to three oranges and the green bell pepper, which is a little less sweet, still contains twice the vitamin C found in an orange.

Green peppers are in fact red bell peppers that have not yet ripened. As they ripen, they become sweeter and the vitamin C content increases. Orange and yellow varieties are specially bred to offer colour variety and are also sweeter in taste.

Bell peppers aren't just about vitamin C, as just one pepper provides approximately 10% of our daily fibre requirements, plus they also contain vitamin B6, magnesium and potassium.

Pepper Roulette

There is a small green pepper originating from Spain called the Pimientos de Padrón, where approximately nine out of ten are as mild as green bell peppers, but one out of 10 (and you'll never know which as they all look identical) is as hot as cayenne chilli pepper. They are now starting to become available from a few farms in the UK, and they can make a meal out with a group of friends a lot of fun.

Hot Peppers

Whether you call it sport or a punishment, there are various competitions around the world where slightly insane individuals try to eat the world's hottest chilies. The heat of chilies is measured in Scoville heat units (SHU) named after the American pharmacist Wilbur Scoville, who created the scale back in 1912. The heat in all peppers, regardless of their name, shape or colour, is supplied by the phytonutrient capsaicin, which the plant uses to protect itself from animals, bugs and insects.

As well as proving fun in a curry house, capsaicin offers many health benefits. It has been proven to aid weight loss, cure chronic pain and help fight cancer. In 2006, the UCLA School of Medicine in Los Angeles carried out research to find what effect consuming capsaicin had on prostate cancer. They concluded that it had a 'profound antiproliferative effect'. They also discovered that consumption also significantly stopped the spread of prostate cancer cells. Research in South Korea in 2015 found that it might also be beneficial in helping kill certain breast cancer cells, while in other countries capsaicin is used both in preventing and treating diabetes.

"Hot peppers as a magic slimming pill". It's not quite how they worded it in *The American Journal of Clinical Nutrition*, but they demonstrated how fiery peppers speed up metabolism and thereby we lose weight by burning more energy.

Capsaicin is also used to treat various skin conditions. Today, its miracle cure is so widely acknowledged that we can purchase it as a supplement or a topical cream that we apply to our skin. The cream is really powerful, extremely primal and definitely beats toxic deep heat sprays.

Patrick Holden CBE

The problem with artificially stimulating growth with chemical fertilisers, and then suppressing the diseases with pesticides, fungicides, herbicides, which are actually poisons, is that while we produce lots of food, we compromise the health-promoting qualities of food. Today if you go to a supermarket and buy normal salad vegetables, I am talking about lettuces, tomatoes, cucumbers, peppers, all the salad crops, none of them are grown in the soil anymore! They are all grown hydroponically (hydroponics is the science of growing plants without using soil) in this rockwool, or equivalent. It's like a sort of nutrient holding medium, and they are nourished with fertilisers in solution, and this has replaced soil-grown vegetables. You can't buy soil-grown salads in the UK anymore unless you buy organic. It's even worse in America where the conventional growing lobby have just changed the standards and made it possible to grow even organic vegetables hydroponically! There are bound to be long term consequences on our health. Just imagine if we had a law passed that if you were growing hydroponically, you had to put a label on the vegetables. I think that would have quite an impact.

The future of farming should be about biology and not chemistry.

Onions

Onions, just like garlic, are members of the Liliaceae plant family. After broccoli, Brussels sprouts, shallots and celery, onion is one of the richest sources of polyphenols. These are one of the best types of phytonutrients and include both tannins (as found in red wine), and flavonoids, which are great at protecting against many unhealthy strands of bacteria. As well as their natural antibiotic powers, onions are thought to help prevent certain cancers and lower the risk of diabetes and neurodegenerative disorders, such as Alzheimer's and Parkinson's disease. They also help protect the heart, help maintain strong bones, and at the same time lower the risk of arthritis and asthma.

Due to their anti-viral and anti-inflammatory benefits, old wives tales recommended tying a bunch of onions around our neck to clear sinuses. While that might not look very elegant, there is plenty of research to suggest eating them helps fend off colds and flu. Plus, when we get a nosebleed, holding an onion under our nostrils should act as a natural coagulant to stop the flow!

While growing in the soil, onions absorb sulphur that later turns into the amino acid sulfoxide. When we cut through an onion this is released, causing the familiar sore eyes and crying. Remember that antioxidants found in fruit and veg were once the plant's self-defence system. With onions, especially larger ones, most of the healthy stuff is in the outer section, so when peeling try not to lose too many layers. They also contain plenty of other antioxidants, with two in particular – quercetin and anthocyanin – known to be extremely beneficial.

Just as the phytochemicals were designed to keep away pests and insects, if we rub onion on our skin or put it in a bowl of water, it helps keeps away mosquitoes. Now that's much more of a primal solution than spraying toxic chemicals onto our skin while on holiday. Dice up an onion and one cupful will provide 20% of our daily vitamin C requirements, 10% vitamin B6, 10% manganese, 8% folate, 8% potassium and 5% vitamin B1 (thiamine).

Olives

I am not going to say too much about olives here, as we have already discussed them a lot under the heading of olive oils. Olives and their oil are a staple part of the diet of those living in the Mediterranean, where a combination of lifestyle and food choices dramatically reduces the occurrence of heart attacks and leads to a disproportionate number of centenarians. Enough said!

Organic Meat

All organic meats offer a wide variety of health benefits. While bison, venison and goat are available from several supermarkets, I am going to detail the benefits of the most popular three: beef, pork and lamb.

To be primally acceptable, all meat has to be organic - which means, among other things, that the animals were raised on food they were designed to eat. All those reports about meat being unhealthy might have an ounce of correctness if the researchers were analysing the effect on health of just factory-produced meats. However, when we talk of meats that originate from animals that have lived their entire lives only eating their natural diet, and who have roamed freely, then meat is truly magnificent for our wellbeing. And remember, what we have already learnt from both Dr Robert Lustig and Patrick Holden, that organic grass-fed meats, are not part of the global warming problem, but part of the actual solution.

Whether it is meat from cows, lambs or pigs, they are all rich in both protein and healthy fats. And to those who suggest all meat is bad for our health; let me say it one more time - you are talking complete nonsense! If we weren't designed to eat meat, then our forefathers would have just gathered plants and vegetables. But they didn't. They spent most of their days hunting wild animals, and when they caught them, they feasted on every part. Without realising it, they gained immense health and brainpower by eating all of the animal's organs, which are without doubt full of the greatest nutrients of all.

Today, when you go to a supermarket, look how cheap all of the organs are. Why is it that I can make a liver pâté for just nine pence per portion? The answer is simple – our generation has forgotten how to cook organs and thus there is now more supply than demand. Yet enter a high-end restaurant, and we find plenty of organs on the menu.

For a quick overview of the benefits of meat, I am going to assume that you have bought only organic and totally natural produce. In other words, it has not been packaged or altered in any way (apart from butchering).

Health Benefits of Organic Beef

Rich in omega 3 and an excellent – in fact possibly the best – source of protein, grass-fed beef also contains a secret healing component called conjugated linoleic acid (CLA). Early research into the benefits of CLA revealed how it could reduce tumours by more than 50% in cancers of the breast, skin, stomach, lung, bowel and colon. CLA is also said to help sufferers of asthma, lower blood pressure, fight off cardiovascular disease and reduce the risk of osteoporosis. If you don't eat meat, then there are now dozens of CLA supplements on the market, and they seem to becoming hugely popular in both the UK and the USA. Among their many claims is the ability to help control type 2 diabetes, assist in losing body fat and then maintaining a healthy weight by retaining muscle mass.

Pork

When it comes to pork, look for a pack that carries the organic label. If you want to be put off mass-produced pork forever, then simply listen to my podcast with Patrick Holden or watch 'Food, Inc.' by Robert Kenner. This 2008 documentary goes undercover in a huge slaughterhouse in the US which reportedly processes more than 32,000 pigs every day, in what appear to be the most horribly inhumane conditions. It might cost a little more to buy from real farms rather than animal factories, but it's not just better for the pig, it's far better for our health and the planet too. Let's quickly look at the different labels we might find in the supermarket and understand what they all mean. These are very similar to what you will find for beef and chicken too, and I have listed them in order of preference.

Organic Pork

The EU has a group of requirements for pork to carry an organic label, but better still, try and find pork with the Soil Association's (*www.soilassociation.org*) organic label, as this is a stricter standard. All pigs must be fed organic food without antibiotics. To avoid overcrowding and allow access to sustainable food, there is a minimum amount of land that farmers must have per pig.

Free Range Pork - These pigs are born outdoors and stay outdoors their entire life.

Outdoor Bred - These pigs are born outdoors but tend to be moved back inside at around four weeks old or once they are weaned.

Outdoor Reared - Similar to outdoor bred, but here the piglets get to stay out until they are about 10 weeks old.

If pork doesn't carry any of these labels, we shouldn't buy it. But why eat pork anyway? It's an excellent source of vitamins such as vitamin B3 (niacin), vitamin B1 (thiamin), vitamin B2 (riboflavin) and vitamin B6, plus minerals phosphorus, selenium, zinc, iron, potassium and magnesium. Pork offers a great source of protein without CARBS but is very low in fat compared to other meats. Food:

Lamb

Just like beef, lamb is an excellent source of protein and omega 3 fatty acids. It's rich in minerals such as zinc, iron, selenium, phosphorus, potassium, copper and magnesium, plus it's a great source of vitamin B12, vitamin B3 (niacin), vitamin B2 (riboflavin), vitamin B6 and B5 (pantothenic acid). Both lamb and beef are regarded as red meats.

Have you ever wondered what meat is? For example, if you saw a diagram of a lamb, you would not see the word 'meat', but muscle and fat, organs and bone. When the animal dies, it's the muscle that becomes the meat that we eat. Red meat is a great source of iron. If you feel that you are lacking in it, then adding a few lamb dishes to your weekly line-up of meals should prove beneficial.

The accreditation for organic lamb in the UK is normally carried out by the Soil Association. Unlike cattle, sheep are rarely kept indoors, so the only real question to consider is whether they were reared organically or not.

If you see an organic emblem on the packaging, it guarantees that any dips the sheep have been in are organic, and that the soil and therefore the grass they eat is free from pesticides too. The UK government's website states, "Organic sheep must be fed on organically produced feedstuffs. Maximum use should be made of grazing, and all of the feed required should ideally be produced on the farm".

What is the difference between lamb and mutton? Pretty much globally, lamb is called lamb if the animal is less than one year old. But when meat is sold in Britain as lamb, the age of the animal must be between five and six months. Meat from younger sheep, from three to five months old, is normally called spring lamb. Meat from sheep more than one year old is called mutton.

Lamb is rich in zinc, which among other things provides a boost to our immune system. From some farms, depending on the pasture, lamb can actually provide more omega 3 per gram than beef. It also contains conjugated linoleic acid (CLA), which in some research studies has been shown to fight off breast cancer.

Poultry

If it's not both organic and free range don't buy it. Not just for the sake of our own health, but for the sake of the bird and our planet too. Only organic birds offer a clean source of protein and healthy fat. In the UK, it is estimated that 46% of the protein of the average Brit comes from chicken, and our small nation consumes a staggering 17 million chickens a week.

Let's explain a few details that you might find on the label. First of all, it's important to cut through all of the nonsense. 'Natural', 'Farm-Fresh', 'Premium Chicken' and 'Country Style' are completely meaningless and just marketing fowl play! They're prominently placed on packaging just to encourage us to pick up the produce and feel good about it. Just as I mentioned regarding the welfare of pigs, if you watch the film Food, Inc., I am pretty sure you will immediately be converted to the merits of organic and free range.

Organic Poultry

In the UK this is again regulated by the Soil Association, who limit flock size to 1000 chickens. Every bird must have continuous and easy daytime access to outdoor pastures, and each bird should have a minimum of four square metres each to roam freely. The pasture must be covered with suitable vegetation, and the bird must reach a minimum age of 81 days. The chicken must be fed organic foods and antibiotics must not be used at all.

Free Range
Chickens must have outdoor access for at least half of their life, and there must be the equivalent of one square metre of land for each and every chicken. Minimum slaughter age is 56 days.

Freedom Food
This is a welfare scheme run by the RSPCA that can apply to indoor, organic or free-range chickens. It limits how many can be raised in each space and also details such things as how much straw they get, the size of their perch, etc.

Red Tractor
Seems to be nothing more than a paid-up membership for farmers to use the logo, and their website has very few rules and guidelines beyond what the EU require. That said, it does mean that the food can be traced back to the original British farm ('The Union Jack flag in the Red Tractor logo confirms your food has been born, grown, prepared and packed in the UK').

If you want to see the most detailed report on chicken produce ever, which breaks down the nutritional value between breasts, skin, wings, thighs, whole chickens, drumsticks, drumsticks with skin and many more varieties, then please pay a visit to *www.nationalchickencouncil.org.*

Why is it important to buy organic chickens and only eggs from organic hens? Because those that live indoors are often genetically modified to gain weight more quickly, meaning they take less time to mature and therefore are both cheaper to rear and cheaper to sell. By overcrowding indoor sheds, the cost per chicken becomes lower. With such cramped conditions, many companies rely on the heavy use of antibiotics to fight off diseases. It is said that of the 50 billion chickens farmed around our small planet each year, 70% of them are no longer organic. For the sake of our health, the chicken's health and the health of our planet, always buy organic and local if possible, then be sure to eat the organs too.

Patrick Holden CBE
We need to align our future diets to the output of sustainable farming systems, in the region or country where we live. We need to say right, what would Britain produce if it was all farmed sustainably, what portions of grass-fed red meat, chicken pastured and organic; we shouldn't eat the industrialised chicken at all, it's not even good for us. No more intensive pork because that's all feeding on grain that's produced in environmentally disastrous ways, and then what vegetables can we grow in these crop rotations? Let's look at the proportions and align our diets accordingly and actually we would eat very healthily if we did that, but we all need to become a little bit more expert on these issues.

Only buy chickens that come from a truly sustainable farming system, such as organic. Preferably, those chickens should again drive a lot of their nutrition from grass (about a third), and the grains that they do eat are sustainably produced, which does mean that the chicken that meets all of those criteria, will be four times more expensive. The truth about the cost of the apparently cheap chicken is that the price ticket does not reflect the damage to the environment, the welfare implications or the damage to human health, that the production of that chicken causes. Antibiotic resistance, and also if you look at the analysis of the fats in the industrialised chicken compared to that of the pastured chicken, they are very different. So people think, erroneously in my view that if you want to eat meat, then the least worse meat to eat is chicken, but if it's not pasteurised then chicken is part of the problem and not the solution.

We are probably only ten years away from irreversible climate change, and the single biggest influence on avoiding it is to change the way we farm. Farmers can't change the way they farm without having correspondingly loyal consumer support in the marketplace. It's our buying habits that will force change. Even the politicians won't act, the market is always ahead of policymakers. We need to encourage governments to do more to make sustainable farming the more profitable option for farmers and a more affordable option for consumers.

As a nation, we need to apply the 'polluter pays principle' to the damaging practices and inputs which are causing climate change and causing destruction of soil and which are compromising the health and wellbeing of animals. And if we did that, the difference between the price of the cheap and the expensive chicken would shrink.

How weird it is, that if you farm in a way that causes damage to public health and the environment, it pays better than if you farm in an ecological way. It has to change. Please take a look at the short film we made, A Tale of Two Chickens. You can find it on YouTube.

The Slippery Six - Oily Fish

There are thousands of different edible fish in our oceans and rivers, and the vast majority are healthy to eat. As with all food, there are a few questions we need answering before eating them. After concerns about the environment or sustainability have been met, it's important to check how the fish were caught or raised. One key concern we have with farmed fish is the conditions in which they are kept.

The Food and Agricultural Organisation of the United Nations recently issued a report that stated farmed salmon production had risen 4,000% over the past 20 years, and today most of the produce we are offered in shops appears to be farmed rather than caught. One of the problems with farmed fish, especially those from inland waters, is that the food they are fed is not all natural.

Let's remind ourselves of a primal mantra, 'we are what we eat – eats' and if that is pellets full of synthetic foodstuff, it's not really something we want to be putting in our body. I could go on and on about toxins and the huge difference in nutritional value between wild and farmed fish, but let's get on with the positives of eating fish with just one caveat – all comments about the health benefits of the top six slippery fish relate to those that have been caught in the wild. And by the way, I named them the 'slippery six' because the health benefit linking them together is their richness in omega 3 oil.

The omega 3 found in most seafood is derived from small plant life, known as phytoplankton, that the fish feed on. Virtually all fish and shellfish are sources of omega 3 fatty acids, but their concentrations vary based on the diet of each species, and both the season and location they were caught.

Fresh Fish vs Farmed Fish

One of the reasons most people eat fish is because of the health benefits associated with their high concentration of omega 3. But did you know that fish only contains omega 3 because of what they eat? One of the highest concentrations of omega 3 on the planet is algae. And it is only from fish consuming algae that they too become a rich source of omega 3 for us humans. But if we are consuming fish that have been factory farmed, what happens if the pellets they are being fed don't contain omega 3? Then you aren't going to be receiving any. If you have been eating farmed fish for years, simply in the belief that because they are rich in omega 3 you have been reducing your risk of heart disease and Alzheimer's, then you have every right to be furious!

Salmon

Have you ever noticed how some fish becomes dry even if we just slightly overcook it, yet salmon always appears to remain moist? Guess what – that's the omega 3 holding the fish nicely together in our frying pan. Salmon is one of the richest sources of omega 3 in both our oceans and rivers.

'Beauty is only skin deep, but ugly goes clean to the bone' might be a phrase that relates to some farmed salmon, but when it's caught in the wild, both the skin and the fleshy meat are full of nutrients. Yes, the skin too. In fact, the skin is full of nutritional goodness and I personally love to fry it (in healthy oil of course) until it's really crispy and then serve it separately on a salad.

A typical salmon fillet weighs in at about 150g (5.2oz) and provides us with around 20g of healthy natural fat (approximately 70% of our daily requirement of omega 3), three times our RDA of vitamin B12, one and a half times the vitamin D we need, plus it provides 100% of our selenium requirements and 70% of our daily protein! Wow, all in one small fillet! It also packs in 70% vitamin B3, 67% phosphorus and really big doses of vitamin B6, iodine, choline, vitamin B5, potassium and biotin.

What does all this mean for our health? Pretty much everything! It's simply a miracle food. It's good for our cardiovascular system, our bones and joints, our blood and our immune system, and it participates in the prevention of many diseases such as cancer, Alzheimer's and Parkinson's.

Trout

If you are not a big fan of the taste of salmon, then a close relative that's a lot milder in flavour is trout. Being of the same family, trout are also rich in omega 3 and share many of the other wonderful nutritional benefits that are enjoyed when eating wild salmon.

For a different prospective on the health benefits of oily fish, I thought I would give you the opinion from the people at *www.britishtrout.co.uk*: "There is good evidence for reduction in risk of cardiac death if you eat fish. Evidence also suggests that eating fish is probably associated with a lower risk of stroke and is possibly beneficial for mental health, for example to improve mood and help treat depression. The health attributes of fish are most likely to be long chain PUFAs, although other nutrients in fish (e.g. protein, selenium, vitamin D) may also contribute to the health benefits".

Mackerel

They might taste different, but did you know that mackerel and tuna both belong to the same fish family? Known as Scombridae, they offer a full menu of nutrients for the healthy primal eater.

The Technical Lowdown on Mackerel

I have used a weight of 80g (2.8oz), as that's the typical size of a fillet in UK supermarkets. Each piece will provide us with the following amount of the daily recommendations: Vitamin D 201%, sodium 148%, vitamin B12 160%, vitamin B6 15%, magnesium 12%, potassium 11%, iron 6% and calcium 5%. And of course, let's not forget why we eat slippery fish, as just one small fillet provides us with around 2,900mg of healthy omega 3 fatty acids. That's the equivalent of three of the large omega 3 capsules I take as supplements every day. And for building muscles, there's 20g of protein in each piece of mackerel too.

Tuna

In 2014, off the coast of New Zealand, Donna Pascoe caught a bluefin tuna on her line and wrestled with it for more than four hours. She eventually hauled it onto her boat, and it weighed in at twice the weight of a baby elephant at 411kg (906lbs, or 64 stone). It was said to be so large that it could fill more than 1,700 tins of tuna! However, you can also find tuna that weigh one or two kilos. While historically we haven't seen many big examples in UK waters, over recent years the huge bluefin have started to appear off the coast of Cornwall.

Whether it is in a can or a fresh slice of raw tuna, this fish is full to the brim with goodness. In fact, let's start with the can. We shouldn't buy it with added oil, as when we drain it we also drain away a lot of the omega 3. If the tuna is canned in water, as water and oil don't mix, when we drain off the water, we retain all of the fish's natural oil. A typical small can, where the chunks are stored in water, will depending on the variety of tuna – provide around 300 to 1,000mg of omega 3. While not as potent as salmon or mackerel, it's more easily consumed when we are out and about and don't have time to prepare a full meal.

Technical Tuna

As there are various types of tuna, I won't give percentages for its various nutritional values, but just announce some of its amazing line-up. Tuna is an excellent source of vitamin B3 (niacin), selenium (an unusual and hugely beneficial type called selenoneine, which is an extremely strong antioxidant), vitamin B12, vitamin B6, phosphorus, vitamin B1 (thiamine), vitamin B2 (riboflavin), choline, magnesium and vitamin D.

Sardines (a.k.a. Pilchards)

The word 'sardines' was first used in England to describe small fish towards the end of the 14th century. Its origin probably relates to the warm waters off the Mediterranean island of Sardinia, where small fish were abundant. There are 21 different species of fish that the World Health Organisation (WHO) allows to be classed as a sardine.

While the description sardines and pilchards are often interchangeable, technically speaking sardines are normally under 15cm (6in) in length and pilchards are longer. Small herring, sprats, shad and brisling are all varieties of sardines. One of the great things about sardines is that we don't have to spend time worrying about whether they are farmed or not. All sardines and the bigger pilchards are caught in the wild. They are full of oily goodness and wonderful to eat.

Sardine Specifications

With sardines varying a lot in size and shape it's hard to work out what measurement to use, so I have opted for 100g (3.5oz) as that's roughly what a Cornish sardine weighs. So, of the Nutritional Reference Value (NRV), just one sardine offers 400% vitamin B12, 101% selenium, 75% phosphorous, 71% omega 3, 51% vitamin D, 41% calcium and 35% vitamin B3, plus significant portions of iodine, copper, zinc, vitamin B6, potassium, magnesium and choline. How does this translate for our health? Well, you name it, and sardines will pretty much do it for you! They defend against depression, fight against cancers and infertility, improve our moods and memory, protect our heart, stave off Alzheimer's and Parkinson's disease and so much more.

Anchovies

I won't write a lot on anchovies, as I appreciate they are often an acquired taste. I personally love them and confess that when dishing up a salad at home, my plate always contains the most! There are more than 100 different species of anchovies and some of the very best tasting are from the Mediterranean.

They are full of mineral goodness including calcium, selenium, iron and magnesium, plus they're loaded with vitamins such as riboflavin, niacin, folate, vitamin E, vitamin B6, vitamin B12 and vitamin K. And of course, they provide a rich source of omega 3, where in just 100g (3.5oz) of canned anchovies you will find more than 2,000mg of oily righteousness.

Garlic

I struggled pushing some other foods out of the Top 20 so that I could include garlic. Several friends suggested I should put it under the herb section, alongside ginger and turmeric. Others suggested that, as there are dozens of brands of garlic supplements, it should make its way into those pages. But as garlic is so powerful and so amazing for our health, I felt it needed to take pride of place in the Top 20.

Hippocrates famously said, "Let food be thy medicine, and medicine be thy food", (I love this quote) and he used to prescribe garlic for various ailments. Its use as a medicine has been well documented across many civilisations including the Egyptians, Babylonians, Romans and Chinese. Its main claim to fame lies in its use as an all-natural antibiotic. For thousands of years, people have known about its ability to kill off various unhealthy strands of bacteria and fungi. Its strong aroma comes from a compound called allicin, which provides both its antifungal and antibacterial properties. Garlic is also rich in selenium, vitamins C, B1, B2, B3, and B6, folate, calcium, iron, manganese, phosphorous, potassium, magnesium, sodium and zinc.

Garlic is famed for its ability to lower blood pressure. There is also mounting research that suggests its antioxidant power is one of the best at helping to prevent cancer. For those suffering with spots, eating a few cloves of garlic every day will tackle the root cause of acne and cleanse the skin, from the inside out. For those of us who are a little older, garlic is great for both our hair and skin and slows down our loss of collagen, which is what we need to keep the skin supple and prevent the dreaded wrinkles.

Fermented Foods

In chapter 10 we discussed how important it is to get our gut in good working order. While there are a whole host of supplements we can take in order to create the right balance in our intestines, one of the more natural processes is to eat fermented produce. While it is true that the fermentation of yeasts is used to convert sugar in grapes into wine, unfortunately I am not suggesting that consuming plenty of alcohol is the right approach for the rehabilitation of our gut's friendly bacteria!

Fermented foods go through a process of lacto-fermentation whereby, in the absence of oxygen, natural bacteria feed on the sugar and starch in the food, creating lactic acid. It gets its name from a specific species of bacteria, Lactobacillus, which was first discovered when studying the fermentation of milk. When it comes to fermenting vegetables, they are normally soaked in saltwater or sometimes just their own juice, and given sufficient time the bacteria eats the sugar in the vegetable, turning it into a sour/tart tasting and incredibly healthy lactic acid. But why would we want lactic acid in our gut? It helps our immune system fight off harmful bacteria, acts as a natural antibiotic, defends the lining of our gut and helps control and regulate inflammation, all while protecting our essential levels of vitamins and enzymes. Did you know that the word 'probiotic' to describe food with beneficial bacteria was coined more than 100 years ago by Russian zoologist Élie Mechnikov, the father of immunology and the 1908 winner of the Nobel prize in medicine?

Fermented foods aren't a new concept, in fact before tinned goods became the norm it was the way that most foods were preserved in jars. Sally Fallon, in her book *Nourishing Traditions*, says, "The proliferation of lactobacilli in fermented vegetables enhances their digestibility and increases vitamin levels. These beneficial organisms produce numerous helpful enzymes as well as antibiotic and anticarcinogenic substances. Their main by-product, lactic acid, not only keeps vegetables and fruits in a state of perfect preservation but also promotes the growth of healthy flora throughout the intestine". The US publisher Doctors Health Press ran an article in September 2015 stating, "Aside from the high calcium, potassium and B-vitamins, the major benefit to yogurt and kefir is the probiotic content". This is really why we urge everyone to include them in their primal lifestyle. Probiotics are good bacteria for our gut that provide a number of benefits – many of which are still likely to be unknown. The impact of a healthy and diverse gut bacteria has been tied to many things, including:

- Lower LDL cholesterol levels
- Reduced Alzheimer's risk
- Reduced blood pressure
- Allergy and eczema prevention
- Improved digestion
- Alleviation of bloating and constipation
- Improved mood
- Treating IBS and Crohn's disease
- Treating depression
- Potential treatment and preventative measure for colon cancer

The following are my top 5 fermented food recommendations:

Yoghurt

Just as wine is made from fermenting sugar in grapes, yoghurt is made by fermenting the sugar in milk (lactose). The fermentation process requires the presence of two friendly bacteria, Lactobacillus bulgaricus and Streptococcus thermophilus. Of course, we should only consume yoghurt from grass-fed cows, yoghurt that's totally organic and contains zero added flavourings. Try to choose a natural plain Greek yoghurt, or for that matter any unsweetened natural live yoghurt (these should contain nothing other than milk and added bacteria).

In 2013, there was a study carried out at the Aristotle University of Thessaloniki in Greece to measure the effects of eating probiotic yoghurt. The scientists split a number of lean mice into two groups. The first group ate nothing but fast food and the other ate fast food and probiotic yoghurt. Those eating just fast food became obese, but the group who ate the same volume of fast food but also probiotic yoghurt remained lean. Their conclusion was that supplementing the diet with probiotic yoghurt inhibits obesity. Without doubt, a totally natural fermented yoghurt is full of millions of nature's tiny miracles, and adding just a small daily portion to our diet can do wonderful things for our gut flora. But there is just one slight word of warning. A whole cup of yoghurt can contain 10 to 15g of CARBS, and remember we ideally want to stay below 50g a day, especially when we want to remain in ketosis, so don't go mad on it!

Kefir
The fermented milk of cows, sheep or goats. Its texture is like a cross between milk and yogurt and it is a great source of vitamin B12, calcium, magnesium, vitamin K2 and a whole host of healthy bacteria. If we ever get diagnosed with IBS, then consuming half a cup of kefir each day might just provide a natural primal cure.

Many experts claim that kefir is actually superior to probiotic yogurt in that it is home to a wider array of helpful bacteria. My advice is that we should use both in our weekly routine and benefit from a dietary double dose!

Non-Pasteurised Cheese
When people ask me what the difference is between the Paleo diet and a primal way of living, I always start by saying that we love cheese! Cheeses that are made from raw milk and haven't been pasteurised are a brilliant source of naturally fermented goodness. Soft cheeses are especially rich in helpful bacteria and can cure many smaller digestive issues, while at the same time help boost the immune system. But don't rely on cheese at the exclusion of yogurt or kefir, because many of the helpful strands of bacteria can be lost in the production process.

Pickles
Full of vitamins, minerals, antioxidants and friendly bacteria, pickles work wonders for the gut. As always, it is really important to look for an organic jar and don't buy any pickled in vinegar as this kills off the helpful bacteria. It's okay to purchase them in brine, as not only are they great for the gut, they also often provide a rich source of vitamin K that among other things supports both healthy bones and a healthy heart.

Sauerkraut
Dating back more than 2000 years ago, the Romans fermented vegetables to take on long sea voyages. Made from cabbage, sauerkraut is one of the oldest traditional foods available, and is not only a great source of probiotics, but is also rich in vitamin C, vitamin K and vitamin B. In addition, sauerkraut also contains iron, copper, calcium, sodium and magnesium. As well as helping cultivate a healthy gut, it is believed to boost our digestive system, aid blood circulation, give us stronger bones and fight inflammation.

Another popular form of sauerkraut is the traditional Korean dish kimchi. Just like sauerkraut, its main ingredient is fermented cabbage, but it's more flavoursome, with a host of extra spices and seasonings.

Ten Reasons To Eat Dark Chocolate
Before we get carried away with any old chocolate bar, let me set out the rules from the start. What we are after is real chocolate, not highly manufactured, sugar-stuffed

chocolate bars. Chocolate is made from ground cocoa beans, which grow on cocoa trees in Central and South America. Around 3,000 years ago, Maya Indians discovered cacao and named it 'theobroma cacao', meaning 'food of the gods'. They didn't start by making chocolate, but a spicy drink called 'chocolatl'. As we have already read in the herbs and spices section, I am going to recommend that you put cocoa powder in your primal pantry and make your own chocolate bars and desserts. If you are not a big cook, then purchase bars of dark chocolate where the cacao content is higher than 70%. Most supermarkets have a variety of brands and strengths. Ideally, the closer we can get to 100%, the more beneficial the chocolate will be, but many people find them a little too bitter at first. What you will probably find is that over time your taste buds will change, and you will start to enjoy bars with more than 90% cacao.

The Difference Between Cacao and Cocoa

Raw cacao (pronounced 'ka-cow') powder is made by cold-pressing unroasted cocoa (pronounced 'coe-coe') beans. Because it is unroasted, cacao retains more of its powerful antioxidants. In his book *Tales From the Medicine Trail*, author Chris Kilham says, "If cocoa were a pharmaceutical drug, it would be hailed the greatest medicine of all time, and its discoverer would reap the Nobel Prize in Medicine". While I agree with this, always remember that it is cacao which is richer in antioxidants. Here are 10 health benefits on offer:

1. Increase insulin sensitivity
2. Protect against type 2 diabetes
3. Lower blood pressure
4. Support brain functions such as memory
5. Decrease inflammation
6. Support our cardiovascular system
7. Helps restore flexibility to arteries
8. Prevents white blood cells from sticking to the walls of blood vessels
9. By triggering leptin, the hormone that tells us we are full, it helps us to lose weight. Who would have thought that dark chocolate could actually help us lose weight?
10. Protect against free radicals, thereby guarding against certain cancers. (See the ORAC scale in the colour insert.)

Bone Broth

We have all heard the description of a cavemen hunkered down around a fire, chewing on a bone and extracting the goodness from it - and if you haven't then I'm sure you have seen a dog engaging in a similar act. It's not that the caveman was lazy and couldn't be bothered to track down another animal, but that there was and still is so much hidden goodness to be obtained from the bones.

It doesn't matter whether we are talking chicken or cow bones, they are all excellent sources of nutrients, minerals and vitamins. They are full of gelatin and marrow that are brilliant for curing joint pains and aiding mobility. One of the greatest benefits of boiling up bones into a lovely tasty broth is its ability to break down larger protein molecules of gelatin into a specific amino acid, known as collagen. Its name is derived from the Greek word 'kolla', which translates as 'glue'. In many ways, collagen is in fact the glue that holds the human body together. There is a huge amount of it residing on the inside of bones, in our joints and our tendons, and it also provides the elasticity in our skin (the ability for the skin to bounce back into shape).

As we get older, our body becomes less efficient at creating collagen, and without boosting it through what we eat, we can suffer joint pains, and our skin can become wrinkly. In addition to food, collagen is often found in both skincare and supplements, where it is said to help reduce cellulite and stretch marks.

Without trying to get too technical, for both completeness and to explain some of the supplements we see in health shops, it's good to understand that collagen is made up primarily of an amino acid called glycine. This is not classed as an essential amino acid as our body is able to create it, but according to recent research, we are not that efficient at synthesising it. Therefore, many people in the medical and supplement world are now calling glycine a semi-essential amino acid.

It's the smallest of all the 22 amino acids and plays an important role in the health of our skin, our digestive system, circulatory and nervous system, muscle growth and repair and in managing our hormones. As you can see, glycine gets involved with pretty much everything that goes on in our body. Glycine also helps our body in synthesising, amongst other things, salt - which might be lacking from our primal diet because of the high intake of water and avoidance of salt-loaded packaged and processed foods.

Let's get back to our caveman ancestor for a moment, or man's best friend the dog. By sucking on bones, they are extracting possibly the most important amino acid of all. However, as we would look pretty weird doing the same in a restaurant, instead we should make sure that we put bone broth on our weekly menu. There is plenty of guidance on the web on how to make it at home, but if we don't have time then there are cubes available that you can add to boiling water.

Dr Jason Fung
Bone broth, liver, kidney and blood are all parts of the traditional human diets. Traditional staples like steak-and-kidney pie, blood sausage and liver have disappeared. Ethnic foods such as tripe, pork bung, congealed pig's blood, oxtail and beef tongue still survive. The organ meats tend to be the fattiest parts of the animal. By focusing almost exclusively on the muscles of animals for food, we are preferentially eating protein rather than fat.

Mushrooms
It should come as no surprise that the ultimate superfungi, the mushroom, makes its way into our Superfood list, as we can be pretty certain that our primal ancestors consumed plenty of them. For the past few thousand years, Eastern cultures have

literally worshipped the health benefits of mushrooms. They are rich in protein and fibre and an excellent source of water-soluble vitamins B and C. They also contain calcium, vitamin D, selenium and potassium. They support our immune system and, among other things, are said to help prevent certain cancers. In particular, beta glucans - found in the cell walls of bacteria living on mushrooms - inhibit the growth of cancerous cells, so much so they are available in pill form and often prescribed for people not only with cancer, but also sufferers of diabetes, high cholesterol and HIV/AIDS. Mushrooms also contain linoleic acid that helps prevent the production of excess oestrogen, which is one of the prime causes of breast cancer in women after the menopause.

More recently there has been lots of media attention around the positive effect consuming mushrooms has on our cognitive functions. In January 2017, The Mirror newspaper wrote an article under the headline, 'Mushrooms could be the newest "Superfood", as study shows they can stave off dementia'.

One word of warning about how to buy your mushrooms. Because they are super absorbent, they soak up both good and bad chemicals and minerals from the soil. Therefore, it's crucial that we only purchase organic mushrooms. For our health's sake, if it isn't organic, we should leave it on the shelf and choose something else.

Other Healthy Foods
All the following are excellent sources of micronutrients, and while they just missed out on the Top 20, they made it into the Top 40:

- Shellfish
- Lemon and Lime
- Kiwi
- Celery
- Artichoke
- Peanuts
- Lentils
- Seaweed
- Romaine Lettuce
- Grapefruit
- Pineapple
- Pomegranates
- Asparagus
- Cucumber
- Carrots
- Cheese

Shellfish
Because we eat the entire fish, whether it is an oyster, mussel or clam, shellfish are among the most nutrient dense foods we can possibly eat. With shrimps and prawns,

just like shellfish, we pretty much eat the entire thing and therefore we are getting a
load of bang for our nutritional buck with these small sea creatures. I say small, but let's
also include lobsters and tiger prawns, as they are a rich source of selenium and B12.

Lemon and Lime

If you only put them in gin and tonic, then maybe you're missing the point. Both
lemon and limes are packed full of vitamins and minerals. However, with their very
strong bitter taste, few will enjoy sitting down to a plateful, and therefore we have
added them to the Top 40 for a slightly different reason.

In 1747, Scottish physician James Lind was aboard a navy ship when many of the
sailors became very sick. He conducted what many believe to be the first clinical trial
ever, when he divided the sick into different groups and fed them different foods. The
only group to recover on the voyage exclusively ate oranges and lemons. A century
later, the Royal Navy realised that lime was stronger than lemon, and so in order to
prevent the spread of scurvy they began adding it to sailor's drinks. This amused the
Americans and the derogatory nickname for Brits as 'Limeys' was born. What was
it that prevented scurvy? It was the acid in the lemon and limes, an acid that we call
vitamin C.

These two citrus fruits really do pack an extremely beneficial vitamin C punch. Their
concentration of antioxidants helps prevent free radicals and therefore reduces the
likelihood of many cancers. The short sharp flavour, caused by a phytonutrient called
limonin, literally can halt inflammation and therefore reduce the effect of many
common illnesses. I personally squeeze them into my filtered drinking water, yogurt
smoothies and onto my salads. If I am making a curry, I will often slice up a whole
lemon and put it into the dish while it cooks, removing the slices just before serving.
And the skin of a lime can be grated to produce an authentic tasting Thai curry.

Kiwi

One small kiwi provides our entire recommended daily intake of vitamin C, plus a shot
of potassium, magnesium and iron. Despite their sweet taste, they are surprisingly low
in sugar and their abundant fibres provide a natural counterbalance to the fructose.

With more vitamin C than an orange, the health benefits of a kiwi are huge. Beyond its
high concentration of vitamin C, it's brimming with antioxidants and phytonutrients,
including carotenoids that strengthen our eyesight, polysaccharides that help our skin
to stay youthful by synthesising collagen and it even contains serotonin that helps us
get a good night's sleep.

I could list a dozen more reasons why the kiwi fruit is so healthy, but let me headline
lutein, for which it is one of the richest sources available outside of supplements.
Lutein, also known as a carotenoid vitamin or 'vitamin eye', is said to help prevent
age-related macular degeneration (AMD), cataracts and damage to the retina. It is also
associated with healthy skin and in preventing various types of cancer.

Celery

Used for centuries as a medicine, celery contains an array of phytonutrients that help lower blood pressure and prevent heart disease and inflammation. With their high-water content and array of minerals, they're full of electrolytes that help prevent dehydration.

Dr Josh Axe, who created one of the most informative natural health websites (*www. draxe.com*), says, "It can help prevent or reduce the formation of painful ulcers. A 2010 study published in the *Journal of Pharmaceutical Biology* found that celery contains a special type of ethanol extract that is useful in protecting the lining of the digestive tract from ulcers. Celery extract has the ability to significantly replenish depleted levels of gastric mucus that is needed in the stomach lining to prevent tiny holes and openings from forming".

Artichoke

Not only do they look like the toughest and most sturdy plant we are likely to find on our plate, they are so full of nutrients and goodness that I just had to place them in the Top 40. While most people only eat the heart, the leaves are so full of beneficial antioxidants that we should try to include them in our dishes too. The 'tough guy' image of artichokes is enhanced by their fibrous construction, and their nutritional line-up includes vitamin B12, vitamin K, vitamin C, manganese, magnesium, potassium, copper, iron, vitamin B6 and many other smaller traces of beneficial minerals.

Artichokes are famed for preventing the most serious of Westernised conditions such as diabetes, various cancers and cardiovascular disease. They also help detoxify the liver and help maintain a healthy digestive tract. They contain some pretty powerful phytonutrients including quercetin, rutin, cynarin and gallic acid. These, combined with its high fibre content, have been known to diminish the symptoms of IBS and even cure it.

Peanuts

I didn't include peanuts in the excellent eight nuts, as they are not nuts at all, but legumes. The question still remains: are they good for us? Simply, yes. They are full of monounsaturated fat, which are really good fats, in fact the average peanut is roughly 50% fat and the same healthy type that you find in olives and oleic acid. While legumes as a family didn't make it into the Top 40 and, in the main, should be eaten in moderation, peanuts should be considered differently.

Why are peanuts good for us? A large handful of peanuts is roughly 38 peanuts (28g, or 1oz) and will deliver the following percentages of our recommended daily intake: copper 36%, manganese 28%, vitamin B3 22%, molybdenum 19%, folate 17%, biotin 16%, phosphorus 15%, vitamin E 15% and vitamin B 14%. When it comes to antioxidant content, peanuts are on par with berries and provide a richer array of antioxidant than most fruits. They also have one amazing antioxidant you won't find in other nuts – resveratrol. It's an antioxidant found in red wine and is believed to help prevent both heart disease and certain cancers. So, peanuts are super healthy, but don't eat too many. Even though they are 50% fat, 30% protein and 8.5% fibre, if you consume too many handfuls, especially while socialising at a bar for example, you will undoubtedly not realise how many you have consumed and are likely to create a huge calorie surplus.

While I really don't want you to count calories at any stage (it's really not a primal thing at all), just be aware that each peanut, although healthy, is slightly more than four calories each. So our single handful of 38 nuts is delivering 152 calories! That's more calories than a pack of crisps. Please forgive me for comparing nutritional food to unhealthy processed rubbish – I just need you to appreciate that while peanuts are really healthy, we shouldn't over-consume them.

Lentils

Here's a double-edged sword. Throughout this book, for all of the reasons I have already stated, we have pretty much stayed clear of CARBS. However, I felt it was important to put lentils into the Top 40 for my vegetarian friends, as they offer one of the richest levels of protein we can get from a plant. The CARBS are also very complex, making them fall towards the bottom of GI index. Lentils also contain lots of fibre, folate, iron, manganese, potassium, zinc, phosphorus, magnesium, copper, vitamin B1 (thiamin) and vitamin B5 (pantothenic acid). I don't personally eat them as I get plenty of protein from meat and poultry, but if you are a vegetarian or vegan, then lentils will almost definitely help fill some nutritional gaps in your diet.

Seaweed

If the only time you ever eat seaweed is when it's holding together sticky rice in a sushi roll, then it's probably not going to prove to be a healthy choice. But served in soups or used to roll up avocado and prawns or salad rolls for hors d'oeuvre, then it's simply magical. Seaweed is pretty much the only vegetables we consume from the oceans, and it's full of calcium, folate, iodine, magnesium and a whole host of vitamin Bs. Recent research from the University of Newcastle upon Tyne suggests that seaweed, which is also full of fibre, is great for our guts and helps slow down digestion making us feel fuller for longer.

Romaine Lettuce

I was originally going to give both Romaine and Iceberg lettuce their own Top 40 listings as both leaves are healthy, but the more I researched the more I realised that Romaine lettuce was the hands-down winner in macronutrients. For example, it is more concentrated in vitamin K, so if we are worried about our bones or developing osteoporosis, or have concerns about cancer, then choosing Romaine over Iceberg would again be a wise decision. Romaine also wins hands-down in the two super beneficial carotenoids, lutein and zeaxanthin, so to maintain a healthy eyesight, Romaine is the right choice. That said, if you were to count kale as a lettuce and not a cabbage, then it would be king.

Grapefruit

Oh, how a little knowledge can be a bad thing. One message remains clear to this day as I left hospital after having kidney stones, 'don't eat grapefruit'. Yet medical research in the USA now suggests that it helps to prevent kidney stones. The citric acid in it is believed to bind with calcium in the kidneys, helping the body flush it out. In addition, the citric acid increases the pH in our urine, which is also believed to help in preventing kidney stones.

Grapefruit's somewhat bitter taste is full of antioxidants and fibre, making it one of the healthiest citrus fruits we can eat. It's rich in vitamin C, plus smallish concentrations of various beneficial minerals. Several reports are emerging that suggest that it might help in preventing cells from becoming insulin resistant, therefore preventing type 2 diabetes.

Pineapple

How can something so tasty be so good for us? It's rich in vitamin C and an excellent source of manganese, but most importantly, it's the richest source of bromelain, a mixture of enzymes that are anti-inflammatory and which animal studies suggest protects against tumour growth and cancer. Its ability to reduce swelling makes it an excellent choice for sufferers of arthritis, plus it can cure certain muscle injuries and soreness. Bromelain is also heralded as a natural anticoagulant, therefore can play a role in the prevention of strokes and heart attacks.

The only slight negative is that the pineapple is fairly heavily loaded with sugar, but that said, one portion still contains fewer calories than an apple and way less than a banana. If you are trying to lose a lot of weight quickly, or abstaining from sugar completely, or maybe you're just not a fan of the tropical taste, today there are dozens of brands of bromelain supplements on the market.

Pomegranates

It wasn't until recently that my family added pomegranates to the fruits that fill our fridge. Today, you can buy them in small trays from the supermarket, and they are great to add vital nutrients to a morning yogurt, or to toss into almost any salad. Their health benefits lie in their incredible line-up of antioxidants and other beneficial compounds. When you stop to think about it, they are a cross between a seed and a fruit, and therefore we get a double serving of healthiness.

Rich in vitamin C, vitamin K and potassium, studies have shown that pomegranates may help reduce the risk of cancer and all kinds of inflammation. They are also said to help treat high blood pressure, reduce oxidative stress and hyperglycaemia. They have also long been recognised as an aphrodisiac and a recent study at the Queen Margaret University in Edinburgh suggested pomegranate juice lowered cortisol levels, which can lead to an increase of testosterone not just in men, but in women as well.

Asparagus

I placed asparagus after pomegranates as it is believed to be the finest aphrodisiac wrapped up in a vegetable. The Kama Sutra advised that it should be consumed as a paste, and the Greeks linked it to love in poetry. In history, the French would include it in all meals leading up to a wedding in the belief that it increased libido and therefore prevented embarrassing moments on wedding nights.

However, my own story has nothing to do with sex drive. When I had a kidney stone, my lovely wife did lots of research on how to break the stone up naturally. As I had to check myself out of hospital to attend an important meeting in Hong Kong, and before the doctors who had procrastinated for two days had a chance to zap it, my wife made me eat lots of mushed-up asparagus. Within 48 hours the pain had eased, and when I returned to the UK the doctor was amazed that it had completely vanished. It appears that its high concentration of potassium helps to cleanse both the kidneys and the urinary tract and literally caused my stone to disintegrate.

But back to increased libido, which is frankly far more interesting than kidney stones. Asparagus contains aspartic acid, which can neutralise the excess ammonia in our body which is often a root cause of a drop in libido. On top of busting kidney stones and increasing our sex drive, from its tip to stem asparagus is loaded with other nutrients too.

Cucumber

There are three nutrients in cucumber that aren't mentioned anywhere else in this book, and that are all very beneficial to our health. Lariciresinol, secoisolariciresinol and pinoresinol are antioxidants that support our immune system and are excellent for balancing hormone levels. These three phytonutrients are said to reduce the risk of cardiovascular disease as well as several types of cancer, including prostate, breast and ovarian. Cucumbers also contain another nutrient called fisetin (also found in strawberries), that helps keep the brain in good working order and has slowed down the development of Alzheimer's in laboratory experiments with mice.

Other than its unique phytonutrients, cucumbers have a huge list of beneficial minerals and vitamins, but because they are 95% water their concentration is very slight. That said, the reason why you often see therapists placing them on eyes during a beauty session is that they possess effective anti-wrinkling nutrients known as ascorbic and caffeic acid.

Carrots

They really do help us see in the dark, honestly! They are rich in beta-carotene that the liver converts into vitamin A. When vitamin A reaches the retina, it is further converted to rhodopsin, a pigment that helps enhance night vision. Beta-carotene is also associated with preventing certain cancers, specifically lung, colon and breast. Vitamin A also slows down the ageing of our skin, while boosting the quality of our hair and nails too.

Cheese

While cheese does not feature in a strict Paleo diet, I believe that, as long as you follow a few guidelines, it fits perfectly well in a primal lifestyle. Firstly, I am not talking about mass-produced factory cheeses in brightly coloured wrappings. These are often produced and enhanced in ways that make them not fit for human consumption, or at least primal consumption. Secondly, it's really important to ensure the cheese is organic. The last thing we want to be putting in our mouths is cheese that originated from the milk of a cow that was pumped full of antibiotics.

But isn't cheese full of lactose and isn't lactose essentially sugar? Here is the good news for cheese lovers. The fermentation process that turns milk into cheese significantly reduces its lactose (sugar) content. Indeed, the longer a cheese is aged, the more time it provides the healthy bacteria to ferment even more lactose. Brie, feta, goat's cheese, blue cheese, cheddar, Camembert, Gruyère, Edam, Roquefort, mozzarella and Parmesan all have less than 4% CARBS and in moderation they are healthy additions to a primal lifestyle.

While a lot of people sing the praise of cottage cheese, they tend to have a higher CARB content. As always, avoid any cheeses that say low or reduced fat, as these are most likely pumped with added sugar, sweeteners or other such additives to make up for the lack of natural healthy fat.

Coffee

Coffee is rich in caffeine. The coffee plant produces caffeine in its seeds to defend itself from predators who, if they do have a nibble, go weak, lose their alertness and either fall from the plant, or are easily swallowed up by prey that know better than to consume it. Now it might not send us humans weak at the knees, but it does stimulate our central nervous system. I like to have coffee when I am weight training as it unlocks fat in the bloodstream and turns it into energy.

Some people are more sensitive to the effects of caffeine than others. Personally, I can take a big mug to bed and it has no effect at all on how long it takes me to fall asleep, while others find its stimulation of the nervous system too much and it prevents them from sleeping. As we know already, sleep is really important, so if you find coffee keeps you awake, then as a bedtime drink why not have a herbal tea with ginger, which helps aid sleep. In his book *The IF Diet*, Robert Skinner explains coffee's effect on sleep brilliantly, "Throughout the day, a chemical called adenosine normally builds up, hour by hour. Adenosine dampens down brain activity, eventually allowing us to drift off. Caffeine causes mischief – because it looks like adenosine and jumps into the places where adenosine normally builds up. With the spaces blocked adenosine can't get in to tell your brain 'dim the lights' and we stay… unsleepy".

A slight downside of caffeine is that it's a diuretic, which means it tells our kidneys to pass water. So coffee will dehydrate us a little. As a result, either before or after a coffee I personally try to remember to drink a similar amount of water just to balance it out.

A study in Finland of 1,409 people, aged between 65 and 79, found that those who drank more than three to five cups of coffee a day were a staggering 65% less likely to fall victim to Alzheimer's disease, compared to those that drank either no coffee at all just one or two cups a day. How is this possible? It is to do with the effect coffee has on our microbiome. In the *Journal of Agricultural and Food Chemistry*, researchers reported that gut-friendly bacteria, in particular bacteroidetes and prevotella, receive a 60% growth boost for up to 24 hours after coffee fibres enter the gut. Coffee isn't just great at reducing the risk of mental diseases, its high concentration of polyphenols make it a great antioxidant too. If you don't like coffee you can also get polyphenols in red wine, tea, vegetables and dark chocolate too.

Tea

Tea has for centuries, especially in the East, been regarded as good for health, happiness and wisdom. According to the hugely popular website WebMD, "Studies have found that some teas may help with cancer, heart disease, and diabetes; encourage weight loss; lower cholesterol; and bring about mental alertness. Tea also appears to have antimicrobial qualities". Let's divide tea into two camps – green and other types.

Green Tea

This is possibly the healthiest natural drink you could have, and is created by drying leaves from the tea plant Camellia sinensis. It's full of epigallocatechin gallate (ECGC), which speeds up our metabolism while at the same time suppresses hunger. With every cup we get a double dose of goodness. It increases the hormone adrenaline, which in return produces heat. For the body to produce heat it has to burn energy and of course burning energy causes us to lose weight.

Green tea is not just about ECGC, there are numerous other phytonutrients and antioxidants that boost the immune system, acting as natural antibacterial and antiviral compounds. Its ability to protect us from free radicals and therefore certain cancers is well documented, as too is its ability to prevent symptoms associated with colds and flu. Green tea is so beneficial for our health that, for those who don't like tea, there are plenty of brands that make ECGC supplements.

Other Teas

One day, for a bit of fun, my daughter Jessica and I went to our local supermarket to count how many different flavours of tea were on sale. We found a staggering 97: from ginger with cranberry, rose and sweet vanilla to oat flower with lavender and lime flower. From a tea infused with chamomile that claims to stop us from snoring, lemon balm and lavender to a palate-refreshing triple mint tea containing peppermint, spearmint and field mint. My current favourite is green tea infused with ginger. On the isles of Ikaria and Okinawa, both regions of extraordinary longevity and very good health, drinking organic and local tea is part of their daily ritual.

As someone who has always slightly overindulged in alcohol (although as I write this chapter I am currently on a dry month), I find flavoured teas a great replacement, especially in the evenings. On my fasting days, where I stay alcohol free, if I feel the urge for a gin and tonic or a glass of red wine, I can always put my alcohol monkey (if you have read Chimp Paradox by Steve Peters you will know what I mean) back in its box and satisfy my craving with a flavoured tea. And as a way of keeping tea drinking interesting and varied, I sometimes even put two different bags in the same cup to create different tea cocktails.

According to Dan Buettner in his brilliant book *The Blue Zones*, which features on its cover the subtitle 'Nine lessons for living longer, from the people who have lived the longest', while discussing the incredible number of centenarians on the island of Ikaria he says, "Ikarians drink herbal teas made from wild oregano, sage, and rosemary – all of which lower blood pressure. How they drink them is important too: They drink these daily but rotate the flavours".

Dr James DiNicolantonio

Tea has been used in Asian cultures for thousands of years, where often they have a pot brewing constantly, and they drink the tea throughout the day. Tea contains catechins, plant polyphenols in the tea, which help lower blood pressure, they dilate blood vessels, they increase insulin sensitivity; they can even reduce blood lipids and improve blood glucose. The main catechin in green tea is EGCG.

The 'Okay In Moderation Stuff'

Legumes

Did you know that a mollusc is a sea creature that has a shell that opens and closes on a hinge? Legumes are plants where the fruit is contained in pods, which are casings with two halves that - just like molluscs - often hinge! Legumes are to the land what molluscs are to the oceans. The legume family is normally subdivided into beans, lentils, peas and peanuts.

One of the areas that a primal life differs from the Paleo way of living is in our views on legumes. Firstly, there is growing evidence to suggest that our primal ancestors consumed certain beans and other legumes, such as peanuts, as part of their diverse diet. As a result, I don't think it will be too long before those practitioners of strict Paleo diets begin endorsing them!

Plus, even though I suggested in chapter 2 that CARBS is an acronym for Carbs Are Really Bad Sugars, it was more to highlight the fact that the body eventually turns all CARBS into sugar, rather that we should banish them completely. While it is true that we could survive without ever consuming a single carbohydrate, avoiding them completely would mean missing out on many fruits and vegetables.

Living primally isn't about total CARB abstention, but avoiding those that are devoid of health benefits, such as the white and brown category of CARBS including rice, sugar, bread, pasta and potatoes.

If, like Paleo, we abstained from legumes, we couldn't have dark chocolate and who would want to miss out on dark chocolate? And a chilli con carne would not be a chilli con carne without kidney beans. Plus, I would personally find it too difficult to live life without the occasional handful of peanuts.

While most legumes do contain CARBS, they are rich in protein and fibre and are often very advantageous to the bacteria in our microbiome. Many are full of vitamins and minerals, making them highly nutritious. One of the reasons legumes sometimes receive a bad press is because they often contain the anti-nutrient phytic acid, which binds minerals together in our digestive system resulting in lower quantities being available for the body to absorb.

Legumes, nuts, seeds and grains store the mineral phosphorus in the form of phytic acid. When phytic acid bonds with a mineral it is known as phytate. Even though there are drawbacks of having too much phytate in the body, allowing some useful minerals to be excreted rather than being utilised, some experts suggest that phytate itself may contain protective properties against cancer, diabetes and CVD. With the jury still out, my advice is to consume legumes in sensible quantities. Let's just pick on one legume, the kidney bean, to highlight why I am happy to consume them in moderation.

Kidney Beans

Named because they look similar to our kidneys, kidney beans are a great source of minerals, vitamins, proteins and fibre. Yes, they do contain CARBS, but at least they are of the complex form.

Like other beans, kidney beans are a rich source of flavonols. These are a group of phytonutrients that our body uses as antioxidants to fight against inflammation and also to neutralise free radicals. As a result, researchers believe beans are beneficial in helping to treat and even prevent certain types of cancer. Along with several others, they are said to reduce the bad LDL cholesterol without impacting the good HDL. Research has also demonstrated that kidney beans can reduce insulin levels and therefore help in fighting diabetes.

Kidney beans – in fact pretty much all legumes – help release short chain fatty acids, which strengthen the cells in our intestines, thereby helping us to better absorb micronutrients. Recent research has shown that they also help us to feel full quicker, so are therefore beneficial for those who want to lose weight. One of the few downsides of beans is that they do tend to make us pass wind. The culprit is a certain sugar called oligosaccharide which, unlike other sugars, is not absorbed into the bloodstream. It's oligosaccharide that causes the beans to become musical in our gut, fuelling their embarrassing tunes that we all know tend to announce themselves at the most inappropriate time. Technically this happens as the sugar arrives in the colon, where our bacteria begins to ferment it, a process that unfortunately produces a lot of gas. But, other than the embarrassment of letting one go in public, take pleasure in the knowledge that it's our good bacteria that are getting fed.

Potato and Sweet Potato

Firstly, this is only a brief overview on potatoes. With more than 5,000 different varieties of sweet potatoes and 4,000 varieties of regular potatoes, we could talk about them all day long. With more people on the planet now being overweight than malnourished, it's important to start with a CARBS warning. Both types of potatoes are loaded with them. Personally, I avoid potatoes as they seem to travel straight to my waist. But if you just can't give up on them completely, then try to find a variety of sweet potato that you like and boil or bake them.

Salt

Just like fat, salt has had a bad rap over the past few decades, but it is in fact essential to our health. The best salt of all is coarse sea salt. As we begin to follow the principles of a primal life, we will be drinking more water and eating less processed foods. Therefore, we might need to check whether we are actually consuming enough salt. It is certainly unlikely, when living primally, that we will be taking in too much.

This is especially true if we work out a lot in the gym and build-up a sweat, or on days when we are sprinting or playing a game of tennis or golf, when we might find that we need to deliberately top up our salt intake. If you feel that you are not taking on board enough salt (sodium) and don't like adding it to food for the rest of the family, then add one or two stock cubes (or if you are in America we mean bouillon) to a glass of boiling water and enjoy a quick broth. With your newfound knowledge in nutrition, spend a little time studying the different ingredients from the top brands of stock cubes and you will be surprised at how healthy some of these can be.

Dr James DiNicolantonio

The word 'salary' derives from the Latin word for salt – 'sal'. A common saying is that someone is "worth their salt". The linguistic evidence points to salt being a prized and important commodity rather than something that should be limited and shunned.

The truth is, our most hallowed health institutions cling to outdated, disproven theories about salt – and their resistance to the truth is putting our public health at risk. From an evolutionary standpoint, the evidence does not suggest that we evolved on a low-salt diet. Instead, much of our evolutionary theory seems to support the fact that we evolved on a high-salt diet.

No one truly knows how much salt our Palaeolithic ancestors ate or how much salt our human brain evolved on – but it's probably much more than experts think. Some experts believe that 45 to 60 per cent of our Palaeolithic ancestors' calories came from animal foods that are naturally high in salt.

What everyone needs to understand is the physiology of how our body regulates salt. If you have normal kidney function, you are going to pee out what you don't need. So it is better to get more and pee out what the body does not need, than not get enough of it. Because we can't manufacture or synthesise salt, yet it's an essential mineral, which we have to get through what we eat. To give you an example of how good our kidneys are at filtering salt, they can filter a teaspoon of salt every five minutes. So thinking primally, we used to consume the entire animal, that included the salty blood, the salty organs and all the interstitial and salty fluids. Now you just get a dry piece of chicken breast, and there is no salt there. Even when eating real foods nowadays, we have lost the salt brine that has been encapsulating all of the organs we use to consume. So today, if you are eating real food, you need to add that salt back, or you are not getting it.

Fruit

Berries made it onto our Superfood list because they are simply awesome, so too did the amazing avocado (which is technically a berry as well). Most other fruits are also healthy, but because of their high sugar content just be sure to eat them in moderation.

Does organic fruit make much difference? I want you to answer the question yourself after considering the following; other than those at the very top of the food chain, all animals and plants have predators, and all animals and plants have developed certain tools to defend against these predators. Most fruits and vegetables too are full of a variety of antioxidants to defend against predators such as animals, mould, insects and too much sun.

Our primal ancestors use to eat lots of natural fruits and our body started to use these antioxidants to defend against various illnesses. When we eat organic fruits, our body puts these antioxidants to work. They form a first line of defence against many internal enemies. However, when we consume fruits that are not organic, that have been developed and modified rather than grown exclusively by nature, many of their natural antioxidants are diminished and, in some instances, removed completely.

Think about it like this. An organic fruit or vegetable that manages to survive its harsh environment must be full of powerful antioxidants. Those that aren't wither and die and are therefore never consumed. But when a fruit or vegetable is protected by pesticides, their natural antioxidants aren't necessary and don't develop. What's worse, their artificial life support machine means that they reach their ripening age and can make it all the way to our dinner plate without any antioxidants at all.

Various experts have written articles on the differing quantity of antioxidants found in fruits that are organic compared to semi-manufactured varieties, and I put the median average of all their reports at about 9:1. In other words, on average an organic fruit is nine times more beneficial than an enhanced fruit. In *The Disease Delusion*, author Dr Jeffry S. Bland writes, "Organic fruits and vegetables have a higher phytonutrient index than their non-organic equivalents. Remember that an organic vegetable or fruit has to work harder to defend itself from the stress of its environment. It therefore manufactures more phytonutrient stress-fighters than do foods coddled by pesticides, herbicides and fungicides that do the stress-fighting for them".

Think about this for a minute; isn't it crazy we have had to create a new word, "whole foods" or "real foods" or "organic foods", to define food that is not created in a laboratory or factory. That makes me furious!

Brown Rice

While I have put brown rice in the eat moderately section, if you are overweight or obese, then please cut out this page and Sellotape it into the food to avoid section. And for clarity, although you have probably guessed it by now, never, ever eat the heavily processed and bleached white rice.

Wait a minute I hear you cry. Don't half of Asia rely on rice for their diet and if it is true that it turns to sugar, then surly they should all be obese. I understand your scepticism. This was the first question I asked when I was told about the evil way of CARBS. But before I tell you about Hara Hachi Bu, bear in mind that in Asia, they tend to be far less sedentary than us Brits, intermittent fasting is also common place and in the main they have far less toxins in their homes than we do in Great Britain. In other words, they live far more primally than we do. But what is Hara Hachi Bu? The Huffington Post summarised it best in a recent article, "The Japanese practice something that makes such sense that I can't believe we don't start teaching this to our kids. It's called "hara hachi bu". It means, eat until you are 80% full. You have probably heard about the Okinawan people and how they often live to 100. They are the longest lived, healthiest people on the planet, and they practice hara hachi bu".

The Okinawan people don't eat until they feel full, they eat until they are no longer hungry. Both of these feelings are controlled by hormones, which is the next subject we will take a look at. They also eat a lot more slowly, which also makes them feel like they have consumed more. Eating more slowly has also been attributed to the longer life span of people living in the Mediterranean.

Why do we overeat in Great Britain? Is it simply because we were told by our parents not to leave anything on the plate? Possibly. But more likely it's the supersized portions of sugar loaded takeaways and packaged foods, that have damaged our brains response to a hormone known as leptin.

What To Avoid

As a general rule we should be aiming to eat naturally and not artificially. We should only be looking to consume foods that our body has evolved to eat, and therefore we must avoid anything that has been altered or manufactured by humans since the end of the Stone Age.

Sugar

For the sake of our health, we must avoid sugar wherever possible. Study food labels, where any ingredient ending in '-ose' should in my opinion come with as big a health warning as we now quite rightly slap on a packet of cigarettes. Here we are going to look at just one example: high fructose corn syrup, also known as HFCS, but the same avoidance advice applies to all sugars. I have already mentioned this earlier in the book, but food containing HFCS poses a real problem for those of us looking to live a long and healthy life.

In her exposé of the food industry's biggest secrets, *Swallow This*, Joanna Blythman says of fructose, "While the fructose in whole fruits comes hand-in-hand with fibre which slows and reduces the body's absorption of sugar, this is not the case when fructose is added in a highly refined, 100 per cent purified form, as it is in processed food. When Mother Nature designed fruit, she thought it through properly. The potential poison in it (fructose) comes in the same wrapper as the antidote (fibre), which seems to prevent the former having any negative effects on our metabolism".

HFCS is used in packaged foods because it is cheaper than regular sugar and, as it is a syrup, it's easier to handle. Fructose syrup in packaged food is not only a major contributor to obesity, but also has been linked to type 2 diabetes, hypertension and something I have witnessed my father and father-in-law suffer in great pain with – gout.

Artificial Sweeteners

So, if sucrose, fructose corn syrup and pretty much everything ending in '-ose' are all unhealthy, what about all of the artificial sweeteners such as aspartame, acesulfame and sucralose? Have you seen how tiny these things are? One tiny little pill, less than quarter the size of a Tic Tac, makes our coffee or tea taste like we have put several spoons of sugar in it. In fact, they are all said to be more than 100 times sweeter than corn syrup and the NHS website reports, "Acesulfame potassium, also known as acesulfame K, is a calorie-free sweetener up to 200 times sweeter than sugar and as sweet as aspartame". The fact that these artificial pills are so tiny yet so powerful immediately suggests that something can't be right with these lab-engineered alternatives.

Caveman never ate anything manufactured in a laboratory, so do you really think we are designed to eat anything artificial? The European Food Safety Authority recognises that sweeteners are potentially toxic in larger quantities but has stated that all products it permits for sale are safe for normal consumption.

But, as far as I am concerned, we are back to the magician tossing coins and getting 10 heads in a row! According to Joanna Blythman in *Swallow This*, "Studies have linked artificial sweetener consumption to a variety of negative health effects: migraine, epilepsy, premature birth and brain cancer".

It is also believed that artificial sweeteners cause untold damage to our microbiome, causing good bacteria to run for the hills and leaving the bad guys to flourish. Plus, while the liver is dealing with inbound artificial sweeteners, it has to temporarily suspend producing the satiety hormone leptin.

Processed Food

Caveman didn't have anything processed at all. Everything was fresh, almost fresh or rancid. But even if it was rancid, at least it was 100% natural. I went to a supermarket with four of my children and asked them to spend an hour thinking about what percentage of food in the shop was processed. It's not that my kids are all geniuses, I wanted to see how well they were understanding the primal approach, and to try to figure out how much stuff was truly natural compared to what percentage of food was manufactured. Together, we arrived at a figure of 92% of all the food on sale being processed. So, based on my family's research, more than nine out of 10 items of food in a supermarket are indeed processed.

But is that a problem? Of course, it is, because we are not designed to eat processed food. Let's take bread for example: as t is pure sugar once digested, it doesn't sit well with a primal lifestyle. However, if you bake a loaf at home, while it is still 'one level of evil', it's nothing compared to supermarket bread, which is in fact the devil in disguise. Did you know supermarket bread contains on average seven times more salt than home-baked bread? "A large proportion of the bread we buy is bleached, blanched and nutrient stripped," reported nutritionist Vicki Edgson in an article on The Mirror website in March 2012. "It's made from processed wheat and as well as containing salt and preservatives, some loaves also contain sugar."

Packaged food can last weeks, months, sometimes years before it needs to be consumed. How is that possible? They stuff it full of nasty preservatives. Generally speaking, the longer the shelf life, the more preservatives are in the food. While these preservatives might provide extended shelf life, they tend to kill the helpful bacteria in our gut. Think about it, how do you extend the shelf life of food? You add chemicals that kill off bacteria. However, there is no safety mechanism in these foods to make sure they exclusively kill off bad bacteria. Woefully, once they enter our gut, they kill millions of healthy bacteria that, over thousands of years, nature has ensured we keep alive in our body to fight off both diseases and infections.

Jen Whitington in her brilliant book *Fixing Dad*, explains why, "The dilemma for the food manufacturers or supermarket is a big one: if you make efforts to substantially reduce the levels of sugar, salt or saturated fats in foods you run the risk of altering flavours too much and losing your customers. Sugar, salt and saturated fats make up the holy trinity of palatability in processed foods; if you reduce one you must increase the other to compensate". So what Jen Whitington is warning is that if we purchase a zero fat or low-fat version of a regular product, then it must have extra sugar or salts stuffed into it. Jen, whose husband cured his own father's diabetes by putting him on a low CARB diet and the right exercise program, goes on to say, "These high sugar foods that we have lived on for years and grown accustomed to – even dependent upon in our cravings for them – are massive drivers of insulin. Remember this is a fat-storing hormone".

Genetically Modified Organisms

How un-primal are genetically modified organisms (GMO)? Did our ancestors sit in caves with a chemistry set gluing together different bits of plants in an attempt to produce strawberries in December? Of course not, they were simply too busy hunting and gathering! Don't confuse GMOs with crossbreeding. What is happening in the designer dog world, with a never-ending creation of goldendoodle (golden retriever and poodle) and labradoodle (Labrador retriever and poodle) etc, is very different to artificially messing with the DNA of plants and animals.

How common are GMO foods? Regrettably very! Simply type into Google, 'Top 10 GMOs' and you will find hundreds of different lists. Nearly all websites quote corn, soy and sugar to be the most widely consumed genetically modified foods. The statistics are staggering. In the USA 95% of sugar, 94% of soybeans and 88% of corn is from modified crops. In total it is estimated that more than 80% of packaged food in the USA contains GMOs. In Europe the situation is much healthier, with many GMOs banned from sale and others having to be declared on food labels.

There have been thousands of studies over the past three decades into whether GMOs are safe or not, with much of the recent consensus being that there is no proven difference between GMOs and organically grown crops. But I don't believe this for one minute. While there is no concrete evidence of the ill effect of GMOs compared to non-GMOs, allow me to make three observations:

1. One of the main reasons for their invention was to make crops more robust to pesticides. So, a GMO product is more likely to be sprayed with toxins that we really shouldn't consume.
2. Any toxins sprayed onto food to protect it, reduces the crop's inherent self-defence mechanisms, thereby reducing the amount of beneficial antioxidants we receive when consuming it.
3. The top three GMO crops – sugar, corn and soy – are not recommended to those living primally. So, a GMO label on packaged food might just be alerting us to the fact that we shouldn't be consuming it anyway.

And, even if they were safe for human consumption, which I honestly believe they are not, just remember how Dr Robert Lustig has told us the immeasurable harm they are having on greenhouse gasses.

Fish & Chips

I wasn't going to give this traditional British dish its own heading, but the other evening a good friend of mine began to argue that a primal lifestyle should allow us to eat fish and chips as they have been part of our heritage for over 150 years. He further pushed his case by telling me that Winston Churchill called them 'the good companions'. But as I reminded my friend, even though Churchill was a brilliant leader he was also very overweight! "But Steve, they are just vegetables and fish, both of which you preach we should eat", he continued.

So, I explained that while 'fish like cod is god', the way it's cooked is evil, 'It's the batter that makes you fatter!' and I told him that potatoes, if he were to pay a little more attention to the details, were not a very healthy vegetable as they were loaded full of CARBS. I told him that 'CHIPS' was an acronym for CARBS Hidden In Poisonous Substances, referring to the fact that most chip shops use cheap chemically enhanced oils.

Quinoa – Avoid if Possible

As it's not technically a grain but a seed, there has been much hype and confusion around quinoa over the past decade. Yes, it's not a grain, so yes it doesn't, therefore, contain gluten, but it's still not on the acceptably primal list. While some researchers believe quinoa is exceedingly healthy as it contains omega 3 and all nine essential amino acids, others say it drives the gut crazy! I can understand the reasons behind the claim as quinoa contains saponins, which could potentially damage our microvilli. Saponins got their name because, just like soap, they lather up in water.

However, even one small 150g cup has a GL load of 13 (unlucky for some), which in terms of sugar-loading our bloodstream, puts it in the same ball-park as two slices of pizza or a bag of crisps! Therefore, if you either have diabetes or are looking to lose weight, I would recommend avoiding quinoa if other food choices are available.

Chapter 12 Highlights

- To be primally acceptable, all meat has to be organic which means, among other things, that the animals were raised on food they were designed to eat.
- Always buy organic and local if possible, then be sure to eat the organs too.
- It is said that of the 50 billion chickens farmed around our small planet each year, 70% of them are no longer organic.
- If we don't regularly consume enough Omega 3, then we are more prone to suffer from inflammation, arthritis, joint and muscle pains, allergies, digestive disorders, cognitive dysfunctions and have a higher risk of heart disease.
- Just like fat, salt has had a bad rap over the past few decades, but it is in fact essential to our health.
- As a general rule we should be aiming to eat naturally.
- We should only be looking to consume foods that our body has evolved to eat, and therefore we must avoid anything that has been altered or manufactured by humans since the end of the Stone Age.
- Caveman didn't have anything processed at all. Everything was fresh or almost fresh.

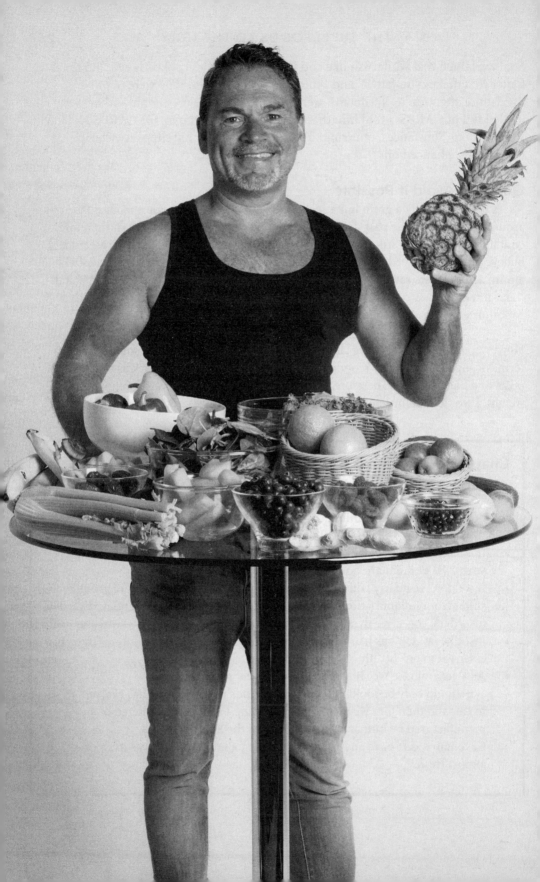

CHAPTER 13

DISEASES THAT PLAGUE BRITAIN
AND HOW TO AVOID THEM

"No disease that can be treated by diet should be treated with any other means."
MOSES MAINONIDES

In this chapter, we will look at some of the main causes of illness, disease and even death in Great Britain and reveal some of the secrets of how to avoid them, and in some cases even put them into remission.

All the illnesses and diseases we discuss in this chapter are Westernised (influenced by the cultural, economic or political systems of Europe and North America) diseases. In other words, they all begin with either the food we eat, the way we eat it, our exposure to pollution and toxic chemicals and our lifestyle in general. Most of the contributors in *Fat & Furious* and I truly believe that the more you apply the LEON principle, the greater your chance is of avoiding them.

Free Radicals - The Ageing Theory

Just like everything else in the universe, our body's cells are made up of atoms and groups of atoms called molecules. Each cell is said to contain more than 100 trillion atoms, which by coincidence is approximately the number of cells in the body!

After we have fully digested our food, the excess energy in our body is stored as adenosine tri-phosphate (for simplicity let's just call it by its abbreviation ATP), and the task of its production is primarily handed over to the mitochondria within our cells. If they are in good condition, and fed plenty of vitamins and nutrients, our mitochondria can remain very good at their job and can convert virtually the entire incoming glucose molecules into ATP. However, if they are not fit and well, they end up creating quite a lot of waste.

When oxygen interacts with this waste, our cells create what is known as free radicals. So, while oxygen is vital to all life, it can have a harmful effect on unhealthy cells (known as oxidative stress). The process goes something like this: the waste becomes oxidised, which creates free radicals – these attack the mitochondria and they are no longer able to turn glucose into ATP. Once the free radicals are done with damaging all the mitochondria (there are normally several hundred in each cell), they turn on the nucleus. As the nucleus holds the blueprint for the cell, the entire cell is damaged.

Free radicals are highly contagious, and often start a chain reaction that turns their neighbouring molecules into free radicals too. Free radicals eventually cause so much damage inside the cell that the mitochondria send a premature message to the nucleus, telling it to kill off the entire cell - and that's what causes premature ageing. Free radicals can also be a direct cause of cancer, strokes and various illnesses of the brain.

One of the fundamental reasons why I don't recommend lots of endurance exercise is that it can massively increase the levels of oxygen utilisation in the cells. This can then lead to the generation of free radicals that damage muscles and other tissues. In his book, *The Low Carb Athlete* (a great read if you are doing lots of sport and are still not convinced that you don't need to CARB load) Ben Greenfield says, "When glucose is used to create energy, a high number of free radicals are produced. Free radicals are dangerous molecules that can damage normal cellular processes. The burning of fat for energy does not create this same cellular damage. In an athlete who is already creating a high number of damaging free radicals from exercise, further damage from high blood glucose levels becomes a nasty one-two combo".

But it's not all bad news. If the right antioxidants are present in our body, they interact with the free radicals and halt the chain reaction before too much damage is done. Fruit, vegetables, nuts and seeds often contain several different types of antioxidants. The strongest antioxidants are vitamin C, vitamin E, carotenoids, beta-carotene and selenium, but as we have already learnt there are hundreds more.

In addition to making sure we eat plenty of colourful fruit and vegetables rich in antioxidants, there is something else we can do to constrain our free radicals. It's to not rely on CARBS and other sugars as our main source of fuel. Remember what was said towards the beginning of the book – sugar is seen as a poison inside the body. One of the reasons for this is that glucose produces more oxygen interaction. If instead of constantly using glucose as our fuel, which free radicals feed off, we burn our own body fat, then it can only be a good thing. But of course, it's a balancing act. To burn our stored fat, we need to intermittently fast, and by doing so we might end up consuming a smaller quantity of helpful antioxidants. This is why when we do intermittently fast, the quality of the small amounts of food that we consume is very important. No matter which type of intermittent fasting we undertake, if we break our fast with a pre-packaged meal or fast food, then we might do more harm than good. But if we end our fast with nuts, eggs, colourful fruit and vegetables and organic meat, we should be able to keep our free radicals under full control.

I mentioned intermittent fasting and its beneficial effects on slowing down the ageing process above. By now, I bet you can guess what goes hand-in-hand with fasting. What can prevent cancer and inflammation and of course radically prolong the onset of ageing? It's moving our body into a state of ketogenic metabolism as often as possible.

Dr James DiNicolantonio

What causes ageing?

Basically, ageing is an accumulation of damage, where our body's repair mechanisms can't keep up with that damage. And we start developing what are called senescent cells, some people call them zombie cells, which are basically cells that our body has a difficult time of getting rid of and can secrete inflammatory substances that damage us. One of the only substances that I know that can break down these senescent cells are called senolytics, you find these in ECGC in green tea and also physiogen in strawberries, those are two comments that are shown to break down those senescent cells. So, again, ageing is this slow accumulation of oxidative stress and damage, and your repair mechanisms aren't able to keep up with that damage.

See also Dr Patrick Holford's contribution on autophagy on page 115.

Inflammation and Autoimmune Disease

If you have ever suffered a sports injury, I'm sure you have experienced swelling or inflammation around the joint or muscle that you hurt. This is the body's self-defence system that protects the damaged area. Inflammation occurs when the body's immune system dispatches white blood cells (plus a few other substances) not only to protect the injured part of the body, but also to create barriers against viruses and bacteria and other stuff it just doesn't understand. Although the science is only just beginning to emerge, it appears that the bacteria in our microbiome play a large role in the creation and control of inflammation. Our good bacteria is acting as the fire brigade and putting out the flames, while our bad bacteria act like Guy Fawkes on a mission to set alight the entire internal infrastructure of our body.

Sometimes Guy Fawkes wins and tricks the immune system into an inflammatory response when there was no need for one. This misinformed inflammatory response is known as autoimmune disease. It is a disease of the protective immune system, causing it to damage its own tissues rather than protect them. For example, arthritis – which affects a staggering 350 million people worldwide is a form of autoimmune disease. But inflammation isn't just restricted to autoimmune conditions. Inflammation can be a silent killer and can progress over years and years without you even realising it. Inflammation is associated with many different modern world diseases. From Alzheimer's to cancer, from heart disease to strokes, from multiple sclerosis to ADHD, inflammation is a root cause of the vast majority of diseases of the Western world.

Think about it logically – if we are living a lifestyle very different to the one we were designed to live, it is going to put a huge amount of stress on our immune system.

The immune system is a complex network of cells, tissues and organs that work as a team to protect our body. But like a modern car with electrical sensors for literally everything, when they go wrong, they can go really wrong. Our body was designed to hunt and gather, to eat healthy foods and to move around more. The immune system was developed to protect against viruses and bacteria. It wasn't created to deal with a daily overdose of sugar, an onslaught of toxins, repetitive over frequent eating patterns and all while sitting on our backsides for 14 hours a day. The immune system has tried to do its best, but it's fighting a battle on multiple fronts that it neither understands or is equipped to deal with!

Giancarlo Caldesi

I had really bad arthritis in my knuckles, and peripheral neuropathy in my feet and my feet are now a good 90 to 95% recovered. To have peripheral neuropathy is really sad because your mobility changes and you become immobile. I made a mistake with my food, but now I have put it right. One of the biggest regrets I could ever have was to not know that the food I was eating was poisoning me. But the most wonderful thing is the food is now making me feel better. I believe in three things; quality, quantity and movement. Good quality food, in the right quantity and then move more. The current lifestyle we have doesn't currently present itself for us to cure ourselves. You have to shut down the manufactured food for yourself and concentrate on the food of nutritional value. And then you will see people get much better, very fast.

Heart Disease

Although it is on the decline, heart disease is still the number one cause of death in the UK, especially in men. Over the past year, I have conducted in-depth face to face interviews with three internationally renowned heart experts; Cardiologist Dr Aseem Malhotra, author Dr Malcolm Kendrick and Ivor Cummins.

From listening to their independent and impartial views, I can honestly say that neither cholesterol (unless you suffer from familial hypercholesterolaemia) nor the consumption of saturated fat, play any significant role in heart disease. Now I know that flies in the face of current thinking, thinking that is very convenient for both the multi-billion statin and sugar industries, but infuriatingly that's just the truth.

Dr Malcolm Kendrick

Throughout history, there have been huge spikes in the rate of death, particularly for men, from heart attacks, linked to social upheaval. There have been many examples where gigantic social upheaval is followed by enormous rates of heart disease. In Scotland, when I was doing medicine, Scotland had the highest rate of heart disease in the world. What happened in the late 1950s and into the 60s, was that half a million people were moved out of Glasgow and deposited in new towns, and the rate of heart disease went through the roof. Then in the 1960s, Finland had the highest rate of heart disease in the world, when in percentage terms it had the largest forced migration of people the world had ever seen. More recently, if you looked around the world and said which countries had the highest rates of heart disease, then many of the top countries are the previous states of the Soviet Union. And then if you say which countries are currently developing a rate of heart disease that is going up and up, it is those countries that are rapidly becoming more modernised such as China and India, where sadly the rate of heart diseases is already exploding. Quite simply, if you take populations and subject them to an enormous degree of stress, heart disease rates go up.

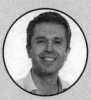

Dr Aseem Malhotra

What are the top five things we can do to avoid having a heart attack? When it comes to food, cut out the ultra-processed food. How do you define ultra-processed? The thing I tell my patients is that if it comes out of a packet and it has five or more ingredients, best avoid it, it's an occasional treat. The reason I mention it is that 50% of our diet in the UK is now ultra-processed, microwaved stuff, stuff out of a packet.

Instead eat whole foods, vegetables, oily fish, olive oil, and a handful of nuts every day. Don't fear fat in the sense of full-fat dairy, cheese, yoghurt and all that kind of stuff. These are the things that should be the base; these are good nutrition. Avoid and cut out refined sugars and refined carbohydrates, and the rest doesn't matter. So, if you get the diet right, you are most of the way there.

Next things, avoid stress. While stress is subjective, if you feel stressed, then you are stressed. Are you getting seven hours of sleep at night? If not, why not? Do something about it! I like meditation, and there is an app I use called Calm. I try and do 20 to 30 minutes every morning. There is good evidence it is anti-inflammatory, it reduces cortisol, stress responses and all of the things that contribute to insulin resistance and inflammation. It is very powerful. I see it with my patients, some of them heart attack patients who transform their lives. They say for them it gives a sense of wellbeing and happiness. So it is also about feeling good.

Get out in the sunshine and then look at your social life. We find when you have a good sense of community, it helps protect against all the other things we have already discussed. I also talk in my book *The Pioppi Diet*, that it helps to have an intimate relationship. For example, we know that middle-aged men who have sex with their partners twice a week, rather than once a month, are 50% less likely to get heart disease. And it isn't about being promiscuous or anything; it's something that reflects a strong relationship with someone who is close to you.

Dr Malcolm Kendrick

Nitric oxide is the single biggest protective substance in heart disease. It sits inside the glycocalyx, which lines the inside of the endothelium (the internal lining our arteries). In Alfred Nobel's (founder of the Nobel Prize) factory, where he invented and manufactured dynamite (which uses nitro-glycerine) they noticed how many of his workers suffering from angina, which is caused by the narrowing of the arteries and reduced blood supply (it's like cramp in your heart), their angina went away. The nitro-glycerine was converted to nitric oxide in the glycocalyx, which relaxes and expands the arteries. And also, nitric oxide is the single most powerful anticoagulant (helps to prevent blood clots) agent known to nature. Anything that boosts nitric oxide is good for cardiovascular health. Interestingly, Viagra does that. In fact, initially, it was developed as a heart drug for angina. Sunshine is one of the very best ways to generate nitric oxide. Exercise increases nitric oxide. L-citrulline and L-arginine increase nitric oxide synthesis, L-arginine is found in meats. Also, beetroot, garlic, dark chocolate, nuts and seeds, spinach, kale, cabbage etc, are packed with nitrates, which are converted into nitric oxide in the body.

Smoking, pollution and lead are three of the worst causes for reducing amounts of nitric oxide in the arteries.

Another thing that can damage the glycocalyx is a raised blood sugar level. People suffering from Diabetes, let's imagine if say the glycocalyx was three feet thick, then if you have high blood sugar levels its now one foot thick. And in fact, spikes of blood sugar really tear it off. Raised insulin levels also damage it too.

My tips to reduce the risk of heart disease:
- Avoid stress (causes narrowing of arteries and increased blood pressure)
- Exercise (creates nitric oxide)
- Sunshine (creates nitric oxide and reduces blood pressure)
- Eat food rich in nitrates (creates nitric oxide)
- Meditation, mindfulness etc
- Reduce sugar and carb intake
- Avoid fake foods
- Avoid pollution
- Don't smoke

Ivor Cummins

Heart disease is an inflammatory problem. Hyperinsulinemia and insulin resistance, high blood glucose and spikes in your blood glucose after a meal, are the top problem in the world driving heart disease. It's not the whole cause. A huge amount of cardiac disease victims, from ages 18 to 80 in recent studies in Europe, across 25 countries, over 70% were essentially diabetic when they looked closely. So, problems with blood glucose, high insulin, high blood glucose and glucose spikes, is the big heavy hitter. There are other things, such as nutrient deficiencies like magnesium, which is a very important nutrient. It's believed that about 70 to 80% of modern western humans, due to depletion in the soil and the foods we are eating, are kind of magnesium insufficient. Magnesium participates in around 300 functions in the body; it regulates blood pressure and countless other things that relate to vascular health. So, I would say low magnesium is another one to really watch out for.

Excessive refined carbs, excessive sugars and I would say excessive seed oils and vegetable oils, poly-unsaturated industrial products, which are in all the processed foods, that triad I would say is the big food problem. And this triad, of course, matches all of the processed and ultra-processed foods, where they use the sugar, refined carbs and seed oils for palatability, extended shelf-life and because they are dirt cheap to produce. And that's where the industry has pushed us over recent decades, into the worst three food types we can eat, because that's where all the profit is.

Eat only natural, wholesome food, eaten in a mixed diet - perfect. But eating processed foods, where the ratios have gone horribly wrong, and all the damage to the molecules and everything else like refined carbs and sugars, you are entering into the synergy which has really driven chronic disease over the past 100 years. You kind of have a fork in the road. Am I going all real food? Whether you do vegetarian with supplements, and that's your choice, or whether you do really heavy meat-eating, either of those are going to separate you from the people who are eating lots of processed food. Choosing real food over processed food is the single big thing that you have got to do. And it's the fact that the three main ingredients of processed foods, refined carbs, sugars and seed oils (which includes vegetable oil) are the three worst things you can eat.

Deborah Colson MSc

What foods are good for a healthy heart? Foods that are important for a healthy heart? I would say the omega 3 fatty acids are very good and as they increase the good HDL cholesterol. Magnesium and taurine are very important for a healthy heart. If you actually look to find where taurine exists in food, it's in the hearts of animals. So it's no surprise that it's also important for the proper function of our own heart. Magnesium is really important for the normal rhythm of the heart. Vitamin E is very important as an antioxidant. Also, you need to look at levels of homocysteine which requires certain B vitamins to keep it under control. Some people have a naturally low homocysteine, but for people who have a higher homocysteine, then they require B vitamins to bring it down. It's probably a more important factor for heart health than the 'cholesterol' story.

Ivor Cummins

You can now have a quick five-minute CT scan to see how much calcium has been used to repair your atherosclerosis (a disease in which plaque builds up inside your arteries). When you are driving the process of atherosclerosis, inflammatory damage to your arteries, it causes little pustules or boils here and there in your arteries. And at some point, the reason you have a heart attack is because one of these becomes big enough to rupture, thus blocking your arteries. But our bodies aren't stupid, and evolution has developed a process. If you are eating all of the wrong things or not getting exercise, or the other bad stuff, calcium will come into these pustules and shore them up and strengthen them up. It's a protective mechanism. But the great news is that if you have a CT scan and your body does not have calcium in your artery walls, your body has had no need to fix any pustules, and you are at very low risk, regardless of your LDL levels.

However, if your calcium scores are high, then you know you need to make lifestyle choices. A person with a high score can have 20 times more risk of a heart attack in the next ten years, compared to someone who scores zero. This scan is a no brainer. It is without question the best technology in the world for non-invasive diagnosis and provides better results and risk prediction than all of the other risk factors put together.

It was invented some years ago, to huge excitement. For the first time in history, we could actually see how much heart disease people had. The professors who invented it said they had patients with no risk factors who actually had huge disease, and they had others with huge risk factors that had no disease. But sadly, it is such a threat to so many industries, and big pharma, that many people don't even know the scan exists. The cholesterol industry does not like it, as it shows there is no link between LDL and heart disease. Every industry is against it. But for the individual its simply amazing.

Type 2 Diabetes

From spending a considerable amount of time with our wonderfully intellectual and talented contributors, plus several days at the office of *www.diabetes.co.uk*, I can tell you for sure, that for many people who have type 2 diabetes it is very possible to put it into remission. Now I know big pharma will say it's not possible and that it is both chronic and progressive, but that is just a convenient myth that they want sufferers to believe. *Diabetes.co.uk*, with their Low Carb Program, has peer-reviewed documentation that they have helped over 50,000 people place their diabetes in remission!

While there are undoubtedly a lot of people suffering from type 1 diabetes, which sadly in the vast majority of cases is not possible to put in remission (there has recently been a report where a handful of people did reverse it immediately after diagnosis), type 2 diabetes is not only avoidable, but for many sufferers, it is possible to put into remission and to deprescribe medication.

As I have already mentioned you could view type 2 diabetes as an equation:

Refined CARBS lead to too much sugar in the blood, which creates too much insulin.

Looking at the above, it's logical to arrive at the conclusion that type 2 diabetes is in fact an intolerance of carbohydrate overloading! Of all the diseases we are about to cover, type 2 diabetes is in some respects one of the more straightforward to suggest a potential cure. Cut out all CARBS and other sugars from anything other than vegetables. If you have diabetes or are close to someone that suffers from this Westernised disease, please buy the book *Fixing Dad*. It's wonderfully written and explains the journey the Whitington family took to rid their father of the condition.

Type 2 diabetes is not a chronic, degenerative, incurable disease. It's caused by insulin resistance which can be lowered by eating foods that don't cause the body to release as much insulin, along with intermittent fasting and exercise. However, the current solution, one that is more palatable to patients, one that generates income for big pharmaceutical companies, is to gradually increase the doses of insulin, which progressively worsens the patient's resistance to it. This makes me furious as it is the advice that my own diabetic father has been repeatedly given by his doctor.

Dr Jason Fung

Most health professionals consider type 2 diabetes to be a chronic and progressive disease. A one-way street, a life sentence with no possibility of parole: the disease continually gets worse until you eventually require insulin injections. But this is actually a great big lie. It is ridiculously easy to prove that type 2 diabetes is almost always reversible.

When the insulin levels can no longer keep pace with rising resistance, blood glucose spikes. That's when the doctor is likely to diagnose type 2 diabetes. Your doctor may prescribe a medication such as insulin injections or perhaps a drug called metformin to lower blood glucose, but these drugs do not rid the body of excess glucose. The blood glucose got better with insulin, but the diabetes got worse. The medication only hid the blood glucose by cramming it into the already engorged cells. The diabetes looks better, but it is actually worse. Here is an analogy. Consider that hiding garbage under your bed, instead of discarding it, allows you to pretend that your house is clean. Once you can't cram anymore in, you put it in your wardrobes and any space you can find. But if you keep hiding your garbage, then eventually it's going to start smelling really, really bad because it is going to start to rot. Instead of hiding your garbage, throw it out.

What happens when excessive glucose piles up in the body over ten or 20 years? Every cell in the body begins to rot, which is precisely why type 2 diabetes, unlike virtually any other disease, affects every single organ. Your eyes rot, and you go blind. Your kidneys rot, and you need dialysis. Your heart rots, and you get heart attacks and heart failure. Your brain rots, and you get Alzheimer's disease. Your liver rots, and you get fatty liver disease and cirrhosis. Your legs rot, and you get diabetic foot ulcers. Your nerves rot, and you get diabetic neuropathy. No part of the body is spared. Standard medications do not prevent the progression of organ failure because they do not help excrete the toxic sugar load.

Dr David Unwin

In the past, I used to say to patients that everything is okay in moderation. But when I think back, that was nonsense. What does moderation mean, is it different for everyone? I used to think moderation in biscuits was six a day but is it? What does moderation mean? Just those six biscuits kept me needing sugar and made it impossible for me to metabolise my own fat. If you have type 2 diabetes, sugar is kind of poison to you, and as you struggle to metabolise it, why would you have more? And as it is a poison for you, why would you want to be moderately poisoned?

Professor Tim Noakes

You can be thin, as I was, and still be profoundly insulin resistant. Being thin does not mean you can eat carbohydrates; it just means your metabolism is slightly different, and you don't store as much fat as other people do.

Dr David Unwin

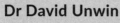

One word of warning on going low carb if you are already on medication for type 2 diabetes. You can't just go low carb without chatting to your doctor about it first, because there are some medications that you may be on, that if you cut the carbs and cut the sugar, and if your medication is also reducing sugar, then you could experience a hypo. A hypo is where you have low blood glucose, and that can also be dangerous. But, if you have just been diagnosed with pre-diabetes or type 2 diabetes, which by the way used to be called 'sugar diabetes', then the best thing to try before being prescribed medicines is to cut out the sugar - it can make all the difference. In my own practice, for most people, they don't actually need drugs at all. Most people, if they go and cut out the sugar and the starchy carbs that turn into sugar when digested, that's the wonderful message of hope. Because instead of it being chronic, progressive and deteriorating, for so many of them they are able to avoid lifelong medication.

What I find if I say to patients: "You have got type 2 diabetes, and we can approach this in one of two ways, we could start the metformin, we could start the drugs today, but that's for the rest of your life, and there are pros and cons, there are possible side-effects. Or are you interested in a lifestyle alternative, where you cut out sugar, and you are able to avoid medication?" And what is so interesting is that I have asked every single patient in this position for six years and not one person has turned down my offer. And we get amazing results. We have actually got to a point now where our practice spends around £40,000 less per year than the average for our area, just on drugs for diabetes alone. And last year, we sent back to the treasury £57,000 of unspent drug budgets.

Giancarlo Caldesi

The big problem when someone comes and tells you that you are diabetic, you have type 2 diabetes, you think – now what? Because 60% of the Eatwell plate is carbs. You think, so I have been having my breakfast as the most important thing, so I have been following this and following that advice, and now I have to take metformin? So really it is seriously wrong advice. In my case, I never took any medicine, I would have if I had carried on, but my levels started falling, by eating no gluten and lower carbs. It worked.

Katie Caldesi

If you have type 2 diabetes, when going to somebody's house or restaurant and they ask if we are allergic to anything, now we must say Giancarlo has a gluten-free diet. But what you should be able to say is 'I am carbohydrate intolerant'. And for people just to say 'I get that'. So, I won't give you potato or rice; I will just give you extra vegetables instead. Just as simple as that. It should just become common parlance that we all know what 'carbohydrate intolerance' means. We all know what gluten-free is now, dairy-free, nut-free, vegan, vegetarian, we all get these; but you should be able to say I am carb intolerant and it should just be part of speech.

Giancarlo Caldesi

It must have been difficult for you as an award-winning Italian chef, who loved his pasta and pizzas, to go low CARB. What first made you decide to change?

I personally managed to turn my diabetes around. If I hadn't by now, I would have lost one leg, that's for sure, maybe both. I had lost the feeling in my foot, and it would soon have been gone. The other thing that sealed it for me was I stopped for petrol one night. It was late after working in the restaurant. I ordered a chocolate bar and a banana. I ate the whole 100g chocolate bar; I was a sugar addict. I was then going down the M40 and all of a sudden I couldn't see anything, it was like a complete fog, it was like driving past a lorry in lots of rain. I managed to get across from the fast lane to the hard shoulder and luckily, I was okay. The short of it was I thought I might have killed someone, so that was it, it had to stop eating carbs and sugar. I lost three stone in about 15 months.

Professor Tim Noakes

My dad tragically died of diabetes. And if you don't die of the disease, you are killed by the treatment. He was told to eat a high carbohydrate diet and snack six times a day. You just have to watch someone die of diabetes, it's a terrible disease. And it's a tragedy because a change in diet could have reversed it. And my dad would have followed that with the greatest of ease because he loved meats, he could have easily cut out the carbs, it would have been no trouble for him at all.

Cancer

In 2010, professor Rosalie David of Manchester University, "There is nothing in the natural environment that can cause cancer. So it has to be a man-made disease, down to pollution and changes to our diet and lifestyle."

I mentioned earlier Dr Price, who travelled around the world visiting remote communities. He once interviewed Josef Romig, an American doctor who had lived with the Inuits and north Indians and found that over 35 years of giving them medical care, there was not a single case of cancer. In every village that Josef visited, as long as they were existing on their traditional diet and had stayed disconnected from Westernisation, that there were no chronic diseases and no tooth decay. But in those villages that had started eating Westernised processed foods, cancer and other chronic illnesses were rife. But it wasn't just the Inuits who were cancer-free. The lead doctor on the islands of the Torres Strait (in particular Thursday Island), told Dr Price that in the 13 years he was posted there, of the 4,000 inhabitants, he did not come across a single person suffering from cancer.

I was going to start this piece by saying something like, "Cancer has only been around for a few hundred years and therefore it is in the main caused by all of the chemicals that are being injected into packaged foods". Then I came across some research where, in a Scythian burial site in Russia, they discovered the 2,700-year-old human remains of a man whose bones were riddled with tumours. But the more articles you read by experts in aetiology and pathogenesis (the study of the history of illnesses), it seems that while cancer may have been around for a very long time, it was extremely rare until the last century. My theory would be that in these rare cases of caveman cancer, they were most likely caused by them being lousy cooks and constantly burning their food (burnt food can be carcinogenic). In *Prescription for Nutritional Healing*, which has sold more than 8 million copies, author Phyllis A. Balch writes, "When burning fat drips onto an open flame, polycyclic aromatic hydrocarbons (PAHs) – dangerous carcinogens – are formed. When amino acids and other chemicals found in muscle are exposed to high temperature, other carcinogens, called heterocyclic aromatic amines (HAAs), are created". Now the worrying thing is not only are these the likely cause of caveman cancer, but these very same chemicals caused by overcooking proteins is, in fact, how they actually induce cancer in animals during laboratory trials!

Back to my main point. The growth rate in cases of cancer is nothing short of a pandemic. According to Cancer Research UK, one in two people will now at some time in their life be diagnosed with cancer. They do go on to say that through advancements in healthcare 50% of people with cancer beat the illness, but the growth in numbers is still concerning. Cancer Research UK state on their website, "More than three-quarters of all people diagnosed in the UK are over the age of 60". So, it seems logical that the older we become, the more precautions we should take to avoid this horrible disease.

In *The Scientific Approach to Intermittent Fasting*, Dr Michael VanDerschelden shares some alarming growth in cancer rates. He says that in the early 1900s only one in 20 people developed cancer. This grew to one in 16 by the 1940s and one in 10 by the 1970s. He finishes by saying that, "Today, a whopping one in three develop cancer!" And of course, we have read above, that with an ageing population there is now a one in two chance that we will develop cancer at some point in our life, most likely after we are 60 years old.

I don't mean to frighten you with the bleak picture painted above, but I do intend to shock you into realising we need to do everything we can to reduce the likelihood of being in the wrong 50%. I lost both grandfathers, my wonderful grandmother and my amazing auntie Avis to cancer. We tragically lost our children's nannie Laura to cancer in her twenties and last year my daughters gifted piano teacher, Carl, sadly died of cancer at just 34 years of age. I am sure you have had similar tragedies. So, let's focus really hard right now on what we can do to increase our odds. Do I really think it's possible? Absolutely. If cancer is growing at an alarming rate, there has to be a cause. If our primal ancestors rarely suffered defeat to cancer, if it affected only one in 20 some 100 years ago, then surely we can change our odds from one in two back to better than one in 20 by adopting a lifestyle and diet from a bygone age.

But what is cancer? While they are all slightly different and can form almost anywhere in the body, in all cases they begin when some of the body's cells start to divide and multiply and spread (metastasise) into surrounding tissues. Under normal conditions, when our old cells die in a natural process known as apoptosis (around 10 billion per day), new cells grow but only when the body requires them. If this orderly process breaks down, cancer may develop. Once cancer starts to develop, old or damaged cells survive when they should die, but at the same time extra new cells that should replace them continue to form. This leads to abnormal growths known as tumours. When tumours are malignant, they can spread into surrounding tissues. Often, they can break off and travel via the blood or the lymph system to other parts of the body. Even after removal, there is a potential that they may return. Benign tumours are contained and do not spread. When benign tumours are removed, they usually don't grow back.

Compiled from the in-depth research I have done and from discussing with our magnificent contributors, here are the top 14 things I believe we can all do to best defend ourselves against the terrible disease that is cancer. And it is not pie in the sky thinking. Even the World Cancer Research Fund believes that 30 to 50% of all cancers are preventable:

1. Don't smoke. Period!
2. Intermittently fast. Frequently put our body into repair mode.
3. Don't consume CARBS and other sugars. This isn't news, 75 years ago Dr Otto Warburg won the Nobel Prize in Physiology for discovering it. He explained, "Cancer, above all other diseases, has countless secondary causes. But, even for cancer, there is only one prime cause. Summarised in a few words, the prime cause of cancer is the replacement of the respiration of oxygen in normal body cells by a fermentation of sugar".
4. Avoid packaged foods, hydrogenated fats and processed meat (trust the cow, not the chemist).
5. Eat organically and avoid poisonous pesticides.
6. Avoid poisons/toxins. We shouldn't put anything onto our skin that we wouldn't be happy to eat.
7. Don't burn food as it can be carcinogenic.
8. Move more, exercise regularly and get active. Adopt the MOMMS principle.
9. Avoid stress.
10. Make it a habit to get between seven and nine hours sleep.
11. Don't consume too much alcohol.
12. Try to tune our body into a ketogenic fat-burning machine (remember that cancer needs sugar to develop and grow). Dr Gary Fettke, both a doctor and a cancer survivor says, "So you think you need sugar? Your cancer needs it more".
13. If you are not feeling well, go and see a GP. While this won't help avoid cancer, most cancers are now treatable if caught early.
14. Avoid obesity. According to Cancer Research UK, obesity is the second biggest preventable cause of cancer in the UK (more on this from Dr Patrick Holford in a moment).

Other than in the listing on the previous page, I haven't yet talked about how a ketogenic diet could help prevent and possibly cure certain cancers. If you have been keeping up with me so far, you might not be surprised by this statement, as going keto means avoiding the very thing that cancer thrives off, sugar. Admittedly, at the moment there isn't heaps of scientific evidence to prove my hypothesis. However, in *Keto Clarity*, author Jimmy Moore quotes scientist John Kiefer, "I've worked with a woman who had stage IV cancer. She was told to go and see her friends right away, because she had less than three months to live. That was six months ago, and now she has a clean bill of health… The power of ketogenic diets is simply astonishing. More accurately, it's astonishing to see how poisonous carbohydrates can be".

Deborah Colson MSc

What role can nutrition play in cancer prevention?
The body is producing cells which could potentially be cancerous all of the time and the immune system is obviously constantly on the lookout. There are about seven different points at which the immune system can intervene to prevent what might be pre-cancerous from becoming full-blown cancer, and those steps, in general, are nutrient dependant. For example, there is one step on the prevention pathway, which cannot happen if you're vitamin D deficient, so we know the size of the role of the importance of vitamin D against prevention. Zinc is another one that's really important along that pathway as well.

Dr Patrick Holford

Patrick, you have written a book called Say No To Cancer. *Please give us some advice on what we can do to decrease our risk of getting it?*
We do know that in most cancers, sugar feeds cancer cell growth. And there is a terribly simple proof of this. If you are suspected of having cancer, you have what is called a PET scan. And with a PET scan, they inject you with fluoridated glucose; sugar, and it finds the cancer cells because the sugar goes to the cancer cell. So, when Cancer Research said that obesity was a big cause of cancer; it's not the obesity that is causing cancer, but the sugar that drives both obesity and many cancers. And for example, recent research in Italy attributes 15% of breast cancer with eating sweets and sweet food; so certainly, sugar is a factor. We also know that the more antioxidants that you can eat in fruit and veg, especially multi-coloured foods etc, reduces the risks. Having a lot of vitamin C definitely reduces risks. And one of the hardest things to get a measure on is all of the chemicals that we are exposed to. For example, pesticides and herbicides are basically substances that are designed to kill, and what happens is that we get a smaller amount of them over a longer period of time. That could be a factor. Stress is also a factor.

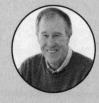

Professor Tim Noakes

I think the next big breakthrough area is going to be cancer. I am not suggesting cancer is purely nutritionally based, but I have read enough now to know that there are many things you can do if you have cancer, you still need some of the traditional treatments but, much reduced.

What happens with cancer is that the treatment is so barbaric, and it's likely to kill more people than it helps. But if you just reduce the dose of those killing treatments, and use a whole bunch of other stuff, and look at nutrition particularly, and the low carb diet is central for almost all cancers. And there is a whole load of other things that you need to do; we can start doing something about cancer in the same way as we are now doing something about diabetes. But unfortunately, just like diabetes, which is controlled by the insulin manufacturers, oncology (the study of cancer) is controlled by the people selling toxic medications. They are not about to suddenly change. But we will relentlessly try and force them to do so.

Dr Patrick Holford

What we have started to realise is that when you go on to a certain kind of ketogenic diet, it triggers a cellular repair process called autophagy, and that is also what happens when you fast. But when you have a lot of carbs, it's growth. And the big problem with humanity is that we are eating non-stop carbs. So, we have over-growth; obesity is widespread. But we also have the growth disease like cancer. Just imagine for a minute. A cell in the body, in order for it to switch to a cancer cell, has to have an environment which is really hostile. So, we have created an environment for ourselves that is so significantly hostile that one in two people are now likely to develop cancer.

Coeliac Disease

More commonly known as gluten intolerance, coeliac disease is, in some ways, the body's self-defence system informing the sufferer that CARBS in the shape of wheat and barley are not what they are dressed up to be and are in fact poisonous. Gluten is the protein found in grain and for some people it triggers an autoimmune reaction in the small intestine.

Several years before we started living primally, at the age of six, my daughter Jessica was described by our doctor as being sensitive to gluten, and we were recommended to cut bread and cereals from her diet. While it is estimated that only one in 100 people suffer from coeliac disease, being sensitive to gluten appears to be far more common. As grains weren't part of our ancestral past and were first farmed just 12,000 years ago, I would argue that, in some sense that all humans are sensitive to gluten, but we don't all demonstrate symptoms.

The website *www.celiac.org* introduces the disease as follows, "Coeliac disease can develop at any age after people start eating foods or medicines that contain gluten. Left untreated, coeliac disease can lead to additional serious health problems. These include the development of other autoimmune disorders like type 1 diabetes and multiple sclerosis (MS), dermatitis herpetiformis (an itchy skin rash), anaemia, osteoporosis, infertility and miscarriage, neurological conditions like epilepsy and migraines, short stature and intestinal cancers". For the sceptics out there still struggling to come to terms with the fact that most neurological conditions start in the gut, hopefully the above description should act as further proof that what we eat affects far more than just our waistline.

When people with coeliac disease eat grains, their body mounts an immune response that attacks the small intestine. These attacks damage the villi inside the gut. When our villi become damaged, whether from gluten or other diseases or intolerances, the gut is unable to properly digest nutrients and therefore we open the door to an onslaught of health problems. In his book, *Brain Maker*, neurologist Dr David Perlmutter says, "My patients often reach me only after they've been to a slew of other doctors and have 'tried everything'. Whether they're suffering from headaches or migraines, anxiety, ADHD, depression, memory problems, MS, ALS, autism or just some odd set of neurological symptoms with no definite label, one of the first things I do is prescribe the total elimination of gluten from their diets. And I continue to be astounded by the results".

One of the simplest ways to avoid gluten is to live primally and eat as our distant ancestors did. As you have already discovered in this book, our gut and brain are inextricably linked. Taking good care of our microbiome is like taking out insurance for the brain.

'Avoid gluten and mass-produced packaged foods stuffed full of high fructose corn syrup' was the first dietary advice I gave my two grown-up children when I started to take my own health and longevity seriously. And, it's a great bit of advice for people who prefer bite-sized chunks of information rather than fully diving in.

Neurological Diseases

My good friend Glenn Lehrer's mother lived to 104 years and Glenn described her as 'bright as a button' until the very end. Why is it that some people can keep their brain in excellent working order for their entire lives while others, including some of the most intelligent people on our planet, have their brains start to fail at a very young age?

Before I jump into the detail, I would like to thank Dr Perlmutter for the vast amount of research he has done connecting so many neurological disorders and diseases with what goes on in our gut. I found his first book, *Wheat Belly*, extremely informative and brilliantly researched, but his subsequent book *Brain Maker* ranks as one of the most insightful and life-changing books I have ever read. The fact you have read this far tells me that you are serious about your health, and therefore let me recommend that you get hold of a copy of these books, in which you will discover exactly what goes on inside our guts.

As a neurologist, on a daily basis Dr Perlmutter is confronted with the outcomes of Westernised brain disorders. He has the devastating task of informing patients about their diagnosis. Through his research and subsequent books, he works relentlessly to try to prevent disorders of the brain from causing more damage. He is very open about what fuels his desire to rid the world of these debilitating diseases as his own father, who himself was a neurologist, is now suffering with advanced Alzheimer's. For me, a highly qualified expert in a field, driven by such personal emotional connection, is the ultimate individual to take advice from.

In *Brain Maker*, Dr Perlmutter writes, "New, leading-edge science coming from the most well-respected institutions around the world is discovering that to an extraordinary degree, brain health and, on the flip side, brain diseases, are dictated by what goes on in the gut". Yes, you read that right. Science is now connecting our gut with the vast majority of disorders and diseases of the brain.

From multiple sclerosis to schizophrenia, from bipolar disorder to migraines, from ADHD to Alzheimer's, from headaches to Parkinson's, from autism to depression, scientists are now starting to look at the gut as the primary root cause and the place to start the fight back against these potentially avoidable conditions. In the USA, more than one in four adults suffer with a diagnosable mental disorder, and globally the number one disability is said to be depression. What's extremely worrying is that the number of people being diagnosed with depression and being put on medication is spiralling out of control. Some go as far as saying it is one of the fastest growing illnesses ever!

We have already discussed that we can remove brain fog by limiting our CARBS, intermittently fasting and by exercising. But here I want to go beyond a foggy brain and look a little deeper. Let's first start by looking at a protein that is synthesised (created) in the brain, called brain-derived neurotrophic factor (BDNF). While it was once believed that we are born with all of our brain cells and we can't make more of them, BDNF is able to make them grow and help them better connect with one another. A better-connected brain makes us more intelligent and helps improve our memory. The best ways to support our brain's production of BDNF is:

- Intermittent fasting
- A good night's sleep
- Exercise
- Sunlight exposure
- Mindfulness
- Move more
- Max out

Why does intermittent fasting synthesise BDNF? It's logical really. Picture the scene: caveman is sitting in his dwelling getting more and more hungry because he hasn't been able to gather any food, and he has also forgotten where he last saw that apple tree. He's been moving around a lot recently and his mental mapping of his surrounding is a little hazy. Now Mother Nature doesn't want him to go hungry, so as he sleeps, he begins to connect more and more cells together, and when he awakes, he experiences a eureka moment and remembers where he last saw the tree. It's not that Mother Nature doesn't want our caveman to starve, but unless he is of older years, she needs him to still create offspring – if he were to starve then the species would soon die out. When he is awake and sitting down chomping on a bone or eating his hoard of apples, nature has no concerns about our caveman fulfilling his procreation duties and switches her attention from brain building to digesting food and extracting nutrients.

If you want to be smarter and remember where you left your car keys, make sure you intermittently fast and get a good night's sleep too.

Nine primal things to keep our brain in good working order:

1. Intermittent fasting – increases neurogenesis.
2. Omega 3 – whether it is from organic oily fish or a quality supplement, omega 3 is simply food for the brain.
3. Use it or lose it – cognitive stimulation increases neurogenesis.
4. Exercise – follow the MOMMS principle to keep the brain healthy.
5. Dark chocolate or a glass of red wine – both are rich in healthy flavonoids.
6. Turmeric – is said to help in the regeneration of damaged brain cells.
7. Coffee – contains polyphenols that are powerful antioxidants that increases neurogenesis.
8. Green tea – the epigallocatechin gallate (EGCG) found in green tea increases neurogenesis.
9. Go out in the sun – vitamin D increases levels of BDNF in our brain.

Dr Emer MacSweeney

One of the really big misconceptions that a lot of people do have is that you reach maybe the age of 65, then you think 'better worry about my brain health'. Actually, we have to be thinking about our brain health from when we're very young, it's actually exactly the same as our heart or anything else and probably more important because the brain is a more complex organ.

The things that we do on a daily basis that positively or negatively impact on brain health are effectively what we call our lifestyle. So, the big things that have been identified as significant factors in terms of brain health are exercise. There are now really big studies which have demonstrated statistically and scientifically that undertaking a certain level of exercise every week does have an impact on risk factors for diseases such as Alzheimer's affecting the brain.

The other thing for the brain particularly is to remember that the brain is a muscle and like any other muscle in the body, it has to be well exercised. So, from the outset learning multiple languages, learning things like musical instruments and just generally keeping the brain active, learning new things, being very sociable - all of this is just very good exercise for the brain.

Diet is really important for the brain. On a macro level, the types of things which are important in the diet are to avoid those things which are bad for us — too much artificial sugar, inappropriate fats and then obviously too much alcohol, smoking etc. But the important thing is to focus on a healthy diet which is really in this context defined as really a Mediterranean diet. So fish oils, nuts, pulses, natural sugars and the right type of fats.

Sleep is very important as well, having an appropriate amount of sleep and an appropriate amount of cognitive stimulation can reduce risk factors for neurodegenerative cognitive diseases in the future by about 33%.

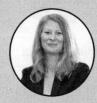

Deborah Colson MSc

There are lots of ways that diet impacts our mental health. There are numerous studies now that show that a diet which is high in refined carbohydrates and sugar really increases things like inflammation and can increase the risks of dementia by 20%.

In a nutshell, food for a healthy mind is good proper fresh, colourful food. There isn't one single food that people should be eating, and there isn't one single diet that people should be on. However, it should not be a lot of beige carbohydrates; it should ideally be fresh vegetables, good quality protein (ideally if possible organic), plus free-range and grass-fed is going to give you a much better-quality protein than intensively reared. Plenty of good fats too, things like olive oil, coconut oil, organic goose fat and butter, which are all good fats. Moderate amounts of fruit too. Fruit has got some health benefits, but it also has sugar so we should look at it as a healthy alternative to sweet treats.

Dr Robert Lustig

Not only is metabolic syndrome related to depression, but it is also related to cognitive decline – and nothing will make you more depressed than losing your intelligence. We've known for a long time that people with type 2 diabetes demonstrate cognitive decline, and that brain insulin resistance correlates with dementia (e.g. Alzheimer's disease).

Alzheimer's

Many professionals are now calling Alzheimer's 'type 3 diabetes'. To visualise what is happening inside the brain over a sustained period of too many sugary drinks, cakes, pasties and in fact all ultra-processed CARBS, imagine the limescale that builds up over time inside a kettle where the water supply is hard. Inside the brain, the Westernised diet leads to a build-up of plaque.

Alzheimer's is a horrible debilitating disease. My good friend Chris' father was a rocket scientist, and not in the hypothetical sense – a real life rocket scientist. Sadly, he was recently diagnosed with Alzheimer's. This disease of the brain can truly affect anyone. Over the past five years, my mother has started to repeat herself many times during the same conversation and often can't remember what we talked about two minutes earlier. As a result, I have spent many hours researching this ruthless degenerative disease of the brain. While we still don't know exactly what triggers Alzheimer's, Dr Shivapour, who is a Professor of Neurology at the University of Iowa, believes that, "Too many physicians do not understand the critical role nutrition plays in brain health". What many scientists are starting to suggest is that regular eating and not allowing the body to self-detox (autophagy) might be a contributing factor. So intermittent fasting might be a way to prevent the disease from occurring, or at the very least delay its onset. Recent research has shown that many people suffering from Alzheimer's and many other brain disorders have a very low level of BDNF (brain-derived neurotrophic factor), and once again diet – in particular ensuring sufficient levels of omega 3, intermittent fasting and exercise – are all recommended to boost BDNF.

Without doubt, of the mass of research papers I have studied, the one recurring belief that seems to now crop up in almost every single white paper on Alzheimer's, is that there is a direct correlation between high blood sugar levels and this awful debilitating disease. In a study of more than 2,000 individuals with an average age of 76, the University of Washington measured the sugar levels of participants over a period of seven years. They found that there is a direct correlation between blood sugar levels and the onset of dementia. Put simply, if we eat too many CARBS and other sugars, our chance of developing dementia, Alzheimer's, Parkinson's disease and many more neurological dysfunctions, not to mention cancer and diabetes, increase dramatically.

On the flip side of the coin, there is now plenty of research that suggests that those of us in our more senior years that consume healthy oils such as coconut, olive and avocado oil, plus those that eat plenty of organic nuts and seeds, are less likely to suffer neurological diseases than those that eat lots of CARBS and other sugars and avoid fat. Let me make this very clear, my mother was a huge believer in low-fat everything since it was heavily promoted as a health benefit some 40 years ago, and now she will remind me five times in as many minutes that the hospital I was born has been pulled down.

Alzheimer's and dementia are caused by inflammation in the brain, which is caused by the brain becoming insensitive to insulin. This is so similar to type 2 diabetes - where the liver becomes insensitive to insulin, leading to many other cells locking the door as well. As mentioned above, many researchers and scientists are now referring to Alzheimer's as type 3 diabetes. But what happens if we change our body from a sugar-burning furnace into a ketone lean machine? Dr Perlmutter, author of *Grain Brain*, tells how research has uncovered that in some patients suffering from mild Alzheimer's, an increase in ketones led to an improvement in cognitive function. When you think about it, this makes complete sense. Just like cancer growths begin to stagnate with the absence of sugar, the development of type 2 diabetes and Alzheimer's must be disturbed if insulin is reduced by the body changing its fuel supply to ketones.

But why does Alzheimer's creep up on people? It turns out that, while the brain is always quick to inform us about problems in all other regions of the body, it doesn't possess any pain receptors in its own backyard. Many researchers are now citing excess sugar and gluten as the most likely root cause of Alzheimer's. Yes, that right – this disease of the brain begins in the gut. Excess sugar molecules in our bloodstream can bind with protein molecules or fatty acids molecules, creating new molecules that can best be described as deformed or irregular. You might have heard of AGE and wondered what they are. AGE stands for Advanced Glycation End products, and this is simply the name given to these proteins or fatty acid molecules that become glued (glycated) as a result of exposure to sugar. The body doesn't recognise AGEs as being normal, so creates inflammation as a response. And as we don't have pain sensors in the brain itself, AGEs can play havoc before we witness any symptoms. Let me say it one more time. Now that scientists have recognised that Alzheimer's relates to an overload of sugar in the bloodstream, many now refer to the disease as type 3 diabetes.

If you are worried about neurological diseases, or know someone who appears to be showing signs of dementia, please purchase a book titled *Alzheimer's Disease: What if There Was a Cure?* It's passionately written by Dr Mary Newport, whose husband was diagnosed with the disease and who through several steps, primarily removing starchy white CARBS from his diet and encouraging ketosis through the use of my beloved coconut oil, managed to reverse her husband's condition. To make it absolutely clear, let me repeat it one more time: elevated blood sugar dramatically increases the risk of developing Alzheimer's, as it does many other diseases.

One final thought. In one of my favourite books ever written on health, *The Orthomolecular Treatment of Chronic Disease*, which carries the subtitle, '65 experts on therapeutic and preventative nutrition', the collective opinion of the authors conclude on Alzheimer's, "It has been known for over a century that aluminium is a neurotoxin. The uncomfortable truth that its widespread use is the major cause of Alzheimer's is now unavoidable. For the sake of your brain, please go and throw out your aluminium foil and cooking pots."

Dr Malcolm Kendrick

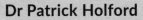

A recent study in Cambridge has shown that B vitamins, including folate, have significant benefits in reducing homocysteine (an amino acid found in the blood that is associated with disease) levels. If you give them in high doses, way above those currently recommended, they may delay or even prevent Alzheimer's disease and reduce or prevent brain shrinkage.

Dr Patrick Holford

Our brains are made of neurons, and they are made up of omega 3; a specific kind called DHA. You get DHA from fish and fish oils; you do not get it from chia or flax seeds. So, if you are vegan, and you think you are getting enough, you are not because the kind you get in vegetables is alpha-linolenic acid. Only 0.05 per cent converts to DHA. DHA is over 90 per cent of the structural fat in the brain.

Now the omega 3 has to attach to things called phospholipids. They are very rich in fish and eggs. The attaching is done by a process called methylation, which is dependent on B vitamins. And you know that you are not good at methylation if you have a raised blood level of something called homocysteine. In America, National Institute of Health researchers have looked at the causes of Alzheimer's, and they attribute 22% of the cause to raised homocysteine, lack of B vitamins and also 22% to a lack of seafood and low omega 3. Now at Oxford University, they took several hundred people with pre-Alzheimer's and originally gave them high dose B vitamins. And by the way, the critical one is B12, because the older we get, we don't absorb it so well. And some of that is to do with medication drugs, antacids. They also had a placebo group. But in the ones taking the B vitamins, they got a 53% reduction in their rate of brain shrinkage in one year. And virtually no further memory loss. But they then went back to the original blood samples and studied how much omega 3 was in the blood and then split the group into a third with the highest and a third with the lowest. Now the third with the lowest omega 3 did not get a benefit from the B vitamins, but the third with the highest omega 3 had 73% less brain shrinkage and no further memory loss.

The point is to build a brain you have got to have both omega 3 and the B vitamins. We are now at a point where we are looking at something close to nine times less shrinkage of the Alzheimer's area of the brain if you get your homocysteine levels down with B vitamins and have enough omega 3. And that is at least one-third of the total risk for Alzheimer's. This is proven in studies and brain scans.

We have a charity website called *www.foodforthebrain.org*, where you can do a cognitive test online; over three hundred thousand people have already done the test, and if your results are not good then you should go and get your homocysteine levels tested by your doctor. If they turn out not to be good, then take B vitamins. And as B vitamins cost only around ten pence per day, if that was done across Europe, we have calculated that would save fifty billion euros in just five years. We could do it tomorrow. It's terrible, and we knew this in 2010. Half a million people in Britain have now got Alzheimer's, simply through ignoring this. The science is impeccable. And the simple reason why I believe it is not happening is because the drug companies can't make any money out of it. In fact, one of the drug companies actually told Professor David Smith (Department of Pharmacology at Oxford University) that if B vitamins were a patentable drug, it would be a 20 billion a year thing!

Here is something that really is amazing. While we have, through our research and trials, got nearly up to 90% less brain shrinkage, the best drug is only 2%. We actually have 30% of people no longer with a clinical dementia rating. Best drug – nothing! The amount of money spent in Britain by the government and all of the research councils on prevention and research of Alzheimer's since 1998 is less than 200 thousand pounds. Yet the amount of money spent by big pharma on Alzheimer's, trying to develop a drug for Alzheimer's, is 200 billion pounds.

Alzheimer's is a preventable disease. Nobody needs to get Alzheimer's. When people say the NHS needs more and more money, it doesn't. What we need to do is to solve the underlying causes of the two disease that are costing the NHS the most, and they are dementia and diabetes, both of which are preventable and both of which can be solvable. Let me put it another way. More people have died in Britain over the past ten years, from diet-related preventable diseases, than died in Britain during world war two.

Migraines and Headaches

Dr David Perlmutter informs us, "Headaches, including migraines are among the most common disorders of the nervous system; nearly half of the adult population wrestles with at least one headache a month". He then goes on talk to about how the pain killers people take in the USA to simply mask the pain and not cure the root cause of the problem leads to about $30 billion a year in sales. Hopefully, you will understand why, in my opinion, none of the big pharmaceutical companies want to tell us the secret of what causes headaches in the first place!

Dr William Davis, in his book *Wheat Belly*, explains how Gliadin (a component of gluten), which is present in wheat and several other cereals, is the cause of many headaches and how cutting back on bread and carbohydrates may totally stop many people from suffering headaches. Personally, since turning primal four years ago, I haven't had a single one! But the big pharmaceutical companies don't want you to know that, because pain relief is a $75 billion market!

As I have previously mentioned, science is just starting to come around to the idea that many diseases and disorders of the brain are related to the gut. While the pain of the headache appears inside our skull, the root cause is most likely to be in the gut.

Osteoporosis

Osteoporosis is a medical condition where bones become brittle and fragile from loss of tissue, typically as a result of vitamin D deficiency, hormonal changes or a lack of calcium. So how do you avoid it? Let's deal with the easy part first: get out in the sun and make sure you are not deficient in vitamin D, or if that's not possible, start topping up your levels with a supplement. One of the main hormonal changes that triggers osteoporosis is an increase in insulin levels. And as you are fully aware by now, to reduce insulin levels you need to eat primally, severely restricting CARBS and substituting them with healthy fats and proteins. The deficiency of calcium is actually linked to insulin too. You see, when insulin levels are too high the body often excretes the stress hormone cortisol. The two hormones then work together to leech calcium from our bones. In addition, women who do a lot of long intense cardio sessions put themselves at higher risk as this also causes cortisol levels to rise significantly.

Many people who suffer with osteoporosis are also at a high risk of cardiovascular disease. The reason for this is that when bones start to leach calcium, while some of it exits the body in urine, a high proportion becomes stuck to the lining of the arteries.

Can living primally and eating the same diet that our ancestors ate in the Stone Age reverse osteoporosis? While most of our bones completely replace themselves every 10 years or so, as we get older the rate of replacement dramatically slows down. So if we are aware of the disease at an early age and if we truly live primally, it is possible to cure the disease, as we will by regenerating our bones through the presence of the right levels of vitamin D and calcium.

Depression

It's really important that we see depression as a disease, and not the fault of the person who is suffering from it. It turns out that one of the biggest causes of depression is an hormone imbalance, and what causes this? Our food. One of the first imbalances to address is the omega 3:6 ratio. Scientists have discovered that those suffering from depression have a low level of docosahexaenoic acid, which is an omega 3 fatty acid. If we ever find ourselves becoming a little moody and are not sure why, we should quickly rush to our local health shop and purchase an organic, cold-water source of omega 3.

In the UK, millions of people now suffer with depression, and in the USA, one in four middle-aged women take antidepressant drugs. The epidemic is spreading so quickly, that the World Health Organisation (WHO) suggests that depression is now the leading cause of disability in the world! If the main cause is diet, why on Earth isn't everyone aware? With the drug companies in the USA raking in more than $12 billion of sales each year from doctors prescribing their antidepressant suppressants (and that is all they are – something to suppress symptoms rather than fix them), we can bet that they will do everything possible to keep the truth a secret. If we start to feel down, we should act quickly by trying to get our gut in good working order.

There seems to be a bigger link between metabolic syndrome and depression, than metabolic syndrome and obesity. And that's saying something. By returning to whole and organic natural foods, you can eat your way out of metabolic syndrome and not only will your waistline drop dramatically, you most likely will become happier too. It's all down to chemistry and biology. For example, people with depression have both lower levels of serotonin and poor serotonin functions, and this can be caused by both processed carbohydrates and processed foods. The very things that cause metabolic syndrome and obesity, also fuel depression. However, in large studies of people eating fish, it was clear that it had an inverse relationship with depression. Eggs, organic meats, nuts and free-range poultry, all can play an active role in beating depression.

Chapter 13 Highlights

I believe the root cause of nearly all illnesses in Great Britain can be traced back to:
- Imbalance of macronutrients (fat, CARBS, protein).
- The poor state of our gut's microbiome.
- Toxins (not just eaten but absorbed through the skin).
- Lack of fasting.
- Lack of certain vitamins and minerals.
- Sedentary or incorrect exercise.
- Stress and lack of sleep.

All seven of these are because we no longer live our lives in the way Homo Sapiens have been programmed. We are no longer staying true to our primal design.

CHAPTER 14

CONCLUSION

*"Your health is what you make of it. Everything you do and think either adds
to the vitality, energy and spirit you possess or takes away from it."*
ANN WIGMORE

Calling this chapter a conclusion goes against the grain a little (if you'll pardon the
pun), as it is in reality just the end of the beginning of a wonderful journey.

I hope now that you have arrived at the end of the book, you appreciate that human
health, above all, depends on sound nutrition. The same nutrition that our primal
bodies are designed to eat. Not unnatural foods. Not manufactured and processed
foods full of sugars, processed carbohydrates and vegetable oils. How crazy is it that
the golden age in our country's health was actually the period between 1850 and 1880,
when due to an abundance of real farm foods, even the working class where eating a
highly nutritious diet and the life expectancy back then, especially for males, was three
years longer than it is today!

At the International Low Carb Summit in February 2015, all of the speakers - including
four of the magnificent contributors to this book; Dr Aseem Malhotra, Dr Jason Fung,
Gary Taubes and Professor Tim Noakes - published a consensus statement, which as
far as I am concerned, is the most concise and important 120 words I think anyone
who wants to live healthier for longer should read. On its own, it could easily have
become the entire conclusion of the book! It states:

*The mainstream dietary advice that we are currently giving to the world has simply
not worked. Instead, it is the opinion of the speakers at this summit that this incorrect
nutritional advice is the immediate cause of the global obesity and diabetes epidemics.*

This advice has failed because it completely ignores the history of why and how human nutrition has developed over the past three million years. More importantly, it refuses to acknowledge the presence of insulin resistance (carbohydrate intolerance) as the single most prevalent biological state in modern humans. Persons with insulin resistance are at an increased risk of developing a wide range of chronic medical conditions if they ingest a high carbohydrate diet for any length of time (decades).

But let's expand on their summary and start by first summarising the principles of living primally, the very roots of my LEON (Lifestyle, Environment, Optimal Nutrition) principle:

1. Eat a diet that is low in CARBS, sugars and processed oils. From now on, before you eat any food simply ask yourself the question, "has this been alive until quite recently"? If the answer is no, then other than frozen meats, berries etc, don't eat it.
2. Intermittently fast
3. Drink plenty of water
4. MOMMS – Max out – Move More - Sprint
5. Sleep – get lots of it
6. Avoid Stress and be happy
7. Sunshine – embrace it sensibly

Then there are four more principle that we have to undertake that are kind of post-primal. In other words, primal man didn't have to concern himself with these, as they relate to protecting our body against the effects of our current environment.

Let's call these our 'Life Beyond the Cave Principles':

1. Toxins and poisons – avoid them
2. Gut – look after it because the soil and environment no longer do
3. Supplement to achieve optimal nutrition
4. First try to fix health problems with nutrition, before evaluating medication

Dr Aseem Malhotra

The good news is most stuff is reversible. And it's reversible quickly. One of the things I discovered during my own research into this is that dietary change impacts on heart disease risks, on the risk of heart attacks, even in just a few weeks to months, just by changing your diet. It's not a long haul. I think it's important for patients to realise this, because if they think it's an uphill battle, if they think 'it's taken years to get here, then it's going to take years to reverse it', it's simply not true. Let me give you one example of how quickly things can improve. In Helena, Montana in America, when they introduced a public smoking ban, just a public smoking ban so the smoke was out of the environment, and within six months, there was a 40% decrease - absolutely decrease - in heart attack rates. The tobacco lobby came in, the law was rescinded, so they got rid of the smoking ban, and within a short space of time heart attack rates went back up. I'll explain that biologically. Just 30 minutes of exposure to passive smoking increases the clot-ability of blood. Remove smoke from the environment, and the clot-ability reduces. Result? Less heart attacks. We should think about diet in the same way. The impacts on diet and health seem to be similar. It is never too late to really make a difference, and you will notice a difference very quickly.

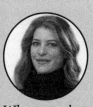

Nina Teicholz

I asked Nina how sure we are that our approach works?
There now over 100 rigorous clinical trials on low carbohydrate diets. And because you are reducing carbs, you must be consuming more fat. And by low carb, I mean below 20 to 25% of your diet is carbs. Whereas, a ketogenic diet is where less than 10% of your diet is carbs. And both of these diets consistently lead to significant weight loss - better than controlled diets and can reverse type 2 diabetes and improve the vast majority of cardiovascular risk markers. So there really is a large body of scientific research and knowledge behind this. And I want to say, compared to the Mediterranean diet, which many believe is the gold standard of diets, there has only been one clinical trial, which only showed a point two per cent improvement in cardiovascular outcomes. So just compare that single Mediterranean diet trial to over 100 low carb trials. What I think it's fair to say is that it is the low carb diet that is truly supported by science.

Helping Others Live Primally

Our health is worth fighting for, right? But with all the brainwashing we have endured over recent decades, with all the advertising by food giants, the ill-funded research and the onslaught of fast food and packaged food with their highly addictive ingredients, going primal is sometimes not easy. What's more, many of your friends and relatives just won't grasp your new approach to health as they will still be suffering from corporate indoctrination. It really is going to require willpower and determination.

As my principles go against much of what we have been brainwashed with over the past six decades, it is unlikely that we are going to convince all of our friends, colleagues and loved ones to join us on our primal journey. Therefore, forget all the copyright stuff, feel free to pass this book around your family. Ensure your family and friends read it cover to cover. Not only will you be helping them prevent certain illnesses and maybe even cure a few, by sharing the principles behind our new lifestyle you will be making your own journey an easier and more rewarding one.

Willpower and Determination

First of all, this primal lifestyle works. Not just a little bit – a lot. I didn't set out to write this book for your benefit, but for my own family. I was fed up of seeing them being held hostage by the big food corporations and had to write down my findings. All of my children are doing well by living more primally, especially my 16-year-old daughter. Jessica has transformed her eating habits to the primal way of living and is reaping the benefits with her body image, ability to concentrate and increased energy levels, simply by cutting out cereal for breakfast and exchanging it for eggs, fermented yoghurts and berries. Going primal really works, we just need determination and willpower to get through the first few weeks, and after that it really becomes both enjoyable and rewarding. As soon as you start seeing results and start feeling healthier, I promise you that you will no longer need determination and willpower – you will simply just love the new you.

But getting through the first few weeks is going to take guts and a thick skin. The new you begins when you, and only you, make the decision to give it a go and make it a habit.

Making the Change

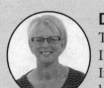

Dr Jen Unwin

To help people make changes in their lifestyle to regain their health, I use an acronym called GRIN. It stands for Goals, Resources, Increments and Noticing. For example, if someone wanted to lose lots of weight, we first need to set goals. Goals really need to draw out the patients hopes and desires. It's important to get patients to really picture a positive image of themselves, where they ultimately want to be. As a colleague of mine says, "It's a long day on the golf course if you don't know where the hole is". Then you need to look at the resources the person has access to. The people around them, access to exercise, do they like to cook, do they read about personal development, would they like details of online support forums etc. Even drawing on their past experiences as a resource. With increments, it's important to remember a journey of a thousand miles starts with the first step. For example, we might take the current position as zero and then look at the small steps they might make to move forward. Ask the patient to describe what one on the improvement scale might look like and how would they feel when they got there. Then as things improve, noticing the positive differences in how they feel. Noticing what's working and feeling the improvements really drives positive psychology. Quite often, looking at graphs and charts of improvement can prove very motivational and help patients stay on the path to wellness.

You're Not Giving Anything Up

Just like I tell my friends who want to stop smoking – not to see it as giving up but escaping – we must feel the same about CARBS, junk food and toxic packaged food.

You're not giving anything up, you're instead escaping the corporate trap of addictive sugar and toxic infused mass-produced rubbish. Once you have kicked the sweet tooth syndrome into touch, your new treats become whole natural foods, flavoured by herbs and spices. You'll see from our recipes and blogs on *www.primalliving.com* that you can still enjoy puddings and snacks, but preferably only those made with 100% primal ingredients. Recipes include raspberry protein brownie bars, coffee banana bread, energy balls and one of my favourite recipes, my CARB-free Primal Spaghetti Bolognese.

Give up the CARBS and other sugars for just seven days and see what happens. Once you have started, I promise you that you just won't want to stop.

Katie Caldesi

It's important to realise that food can still be fantastic. Low carb does not mean horrible food. My challenge with Giancarlo was to make sure I didn't just say 'you can't have pasta', without saying what he could have. You can't have a KitKat, but you can have some walnuts or some dark chocolate. It's important to stress what you can have, not just what you can't. That is why we wrote *The Diabetes Weight Loss Cookbook* and why our cookery school now holds low carb classes.

Nina Teicholz

It's a great joy not to feel guilty about the foods you are eating, and once you know about good nutrition, to just listen to your body. To rediscover truly pleasurable foods that are so delicious that you used to eat with so much guilt and self-loathing, and now they become a source of real joy. For example, the drippings of a roast chicken - they are just divine. I used to fight my father over who got to scrape the pan.

Professor Tim Noakes

Tim, what are your top five tips for living healthier for longer?

1. Attitude. Your goal in life is to die in your sleep at an old age. So, every day when you wake up, you should ask yourself, what am I going to do today, to ensure that I die of old age in my sleep. I get so frustrated with people who just say that they will go to the doctor and get a pill, and everything will be all right. It's just not going to help. You have to take responsibility for yourself. You cannot allow the medication profession to take control of your health; because they will manipulate it, and they will use it to earn income from you, and you can't allow that to happen.
2. Nutrition. If you get your nutrition right, you can pretty much forget everything else. And it has to be low carbs, and the more insulin resistant you are, the more low carb it has to be.
3. Okay, I said it twice. Nutrition.
4. Have good intimate relationships. Be socially active.
5. Exercise. Do weight training, cross fit etc.

Placing People and the Planet Before Profit

As consumers we are starting to become more aware of the issues facing our health and the wellbeing of our small planet. I also believe this is just the start of the consumer revolution and I pray that in the very near future, us consumers become even more demanding and increasingly influential, both in what ingredients go into the food we eat and saving the planet via our purchasing decisions.

I hope that one day stock markets and governments find a way to measure the social impact that businesses have, and that this combined with all of us consumers voting with our wallets, choosing the good over the bad – will help the good companies prevail. I would like to believe that 20 years from now, profits will no longer be the main driving force behind businesses, but viewed equally alongside both the health of people and the planet. Especially here in Great Britain, all corporates need to do their part in restoring the health of our nation.

The Final Word

When Einstein was credited with being a genius, he replied, "The only real genius in the world is Linus Pauling". Pauling was a scientist specialising in the fields of quantum chemistry and molecular biology. He was a peace activist and author, who still to this day, is the only person to have been awarded two unshared Noble Prizes. He wrote a brilliant book in 1986 named *How to Live Longer and Feel Better*, in which he listed 12 things as a regimen for better health. Other than the 23 brilliant contributors in this book, if you are going to listen to anyone handing out advice on how to live longer, then there is probably no more a better person than Linus Pauling, and with whom I would like to finish the conclusion of this book:

1. Take vitamin C every day, 6 grams to 18 grams or more. Don't miss a single day.*
2. Take vitamin E every day, 400IU, 800IU, or 1600IU.*
3. Take one or two super-B tablets every day, to provide a good amount of B vitamins.
4. Take a 25,000IU vitamin A tablet everyday*.
5. Take a daily mineral supplement, which provides 100g of calcium, 18mg of iron, 0.15mg of iodine, 1mg of copper, 25mg of magnesium, 3mg of manganese, 15mg of zinc, 0.015mg of molybdenum, 0.015mg of chromium, and 0.015 mg of selenium.
6. Keep your intake of ordinary sugar (sucrose, raw sugar, brown sugar, honey) to 50 pounds per year, which is half the present US average. Do not eat high sugar foods. Avoid desserts. Do not drink soft drinks.
7. Except for avoiding sugar, eat what you like. But not too much of any one food. Eggs and meat are good foods. Also, you should eat some vegetables and fruit. Do not eat so much food as to become obese.
8. Drink plenty of water every day.
9. Keep active; take some exercise. Do not at any time exert yourself physically to an extent far beyond what you are accustomed to.
10. Drink alcoholic beverages only in moderation.
11. DO NOT SMOKE CIGARETTES.
12. Avoid stress. Work at a job that you like. Be happy with your family.
 One word of caution, please note, unsurprisingly these are higher than those recommended by our government.

Happy Primal Living

When you have got your weight, nutrition and health back on track, please email *steve@primalliving.com* with your story, along with a before and after photo if possible (please take one today, because you are about to change your shape permanently).

FURTHER READING

I am going to list the brilliant books written by our contributors. I am sure that if you follow what you have read in this book that *Fat & Furious* will get you on the right primal path to a healthier life; and for sure the books below will help keep you on it. Many of the contributors have written many more books than those listed here, however, I have only listed those I have read (some in draft form). I have also added one or two additional insightful books that I have read but have yet to conduct formal interviews with the authors. All books are listed alphabetically.

- *The 5 Day Diet* - DR PATRICK HOLFORD – Give your body an MOT by getting into autophagy
- *A Bitter Pill* – DR ASEEM MALHOTRA – A Doctor's Insight into Medical Corruption
- *The Alzheimer's Prevention Plan* – DR PATRICK HOLFORD AND DEBORAH COLSON – 10 proven ways to stop memory decline and reduce the risk of Alzheimer's
- *Alzheimer's Disease* - DR MARY NEWPORT - What if There Was a Cure?
- *Around the World in Salads* - KATIE & GIANCARLO CALDESI – 120 ways to love your leaves
- *The Best Possible You* - HANNAH RICHARDS - A unique nutritional guide to healing your body
- *The Big Fat Surprise* – NINA TEICHOLZ – Why butter, meat and cheese belong in a healthy diet
- *The Big Prescription* – DR SHAN HUSSAIN – Balancing the three principles of enduring health
- *The Case Against Sugar* – GARY TAUBES – Why more than half a billion adults and 40 million children are obese.
- *The Case for Keto* – GARY TAUBES – Rethinking weight control and the science and practice of low-carb/high-fat eating
- *The Complete Guide to Fasting* – DR JASON FUNG & JIMMY MORE – Heal your body through intermittent, alternate day, and extended fasting
- *The Diabetes Code* – DR JASON FUNG – Prevent & reverse type 2 diabetes naturally
- *The Diabetes Weight Loss Cookbook* – KATIE & GIANCARLO CALDESI – A life-changing diet to prevent and reverse type 2 diabetes.
- *The Diet Delusion* – GARY TAUBES – America's most controversial science writer – Sunday Telegraph
- *The Diet Fix* – DR ZOE HARCOMBE – How to lose weight and keep it off – one last time
- *Doctoring Data* – DR MALCOLM KENDRICK –How to sort out medical advice from medical nonsense
- *Eat Rich, Live Long* – IVOR CUMMINS – Use the power of low-carb and keto for weight loss and great health
- *Fat Chance* – DR ROBERT LUSTIG – The hidden truth about sugar, obesity and disease

- *The Fat Chance Cookbook* – DR ROBERT LUSTIG – More than 100 recipes ready in under 30 minutes to help you lose the sugar and the weight
- *Fixing Dad* - JEN WHITINGTON - How to transform the health of someone you love
- *Good Calories, Bad Calories* – GARY TAUBES – Fats, carbs, and the controversial science of diet and health
- *The Great Cholesterol Con* – DR MALCOLM KENDRICK – The truth about what really causes heart disease and how to avoid it.
- *The Hacking of the American Mind* – DR ROBERT LUSTIG – The science behind the corporate takeover of our bodies and brains
- *The Harcombe Diet* - DR ZOE HARCOMBE – Stop counting calories and start losing weight
- *How to Live Longer and Feel Better* – LINUS PAULING – How taking vitamins and minerals prevent diseases
- *The Hybrid Diet* - DR PATRICK HOLFORD & JEROME BURNE – Your body thrives on two fuels. Boost your energy and get leaner and healthier by alternating fat and carbs.
- *The Longevity Solution* – DR JAMES DINICOLANTONIO & DR JASON FUNG – Rediscover centuries-old secrets to a healthy, long life
- *Lore of Nutrition* – PROFESSOR TIM NOAKES – Challenging conventional dietary beliefs
- *The Low-GL Diet Made Easy* – DR PATRICK HOLFORD – The perfect way to lose weight, gain energy and improve your health.
- *The Obesity Code* – DR JASON FUNG - Unlock the secret of weight loss
- *The Obesity Epidemic* – DR ZOE HARCOMBE – What caused it? How can we stop it?
- *Optimum Nutrition for Your Child* - DR PATRICK HOLFORD AND DEBORAH COLSON – How to boost your child's health, behaviour and IQ
- *The Orthomolecular Treatment of Chronic Disease* - DR ANDREW W SAUL - 65 experts on therapeutic and preventative nutrition
- *The Pioppi Diet* – DR ASEEM MALHOTRA - A 21-day lifestyle plan
- *Real Food on Trial* – PROFESSOR TIM NOAKES – How the diet dictators tried to destroy a top scientist
- *The Reverse Your Diabetes Cookbook* - KATIE & GIANCARLO CALDESI – Lose weight and eat to beat type 2 diabetes.
- *The Salt Fix* - DR JAMES DINICOLANTONIO – Why the experts got it all wrong and how eating more might save your life
- *Say No to Cancer* - DR PATRICK HOLFORD – The drug-free guide to preventing and helping fight cancer
- *A Statin Nation* - DR MALCOLM KENDRICK – Damaging millions in a brave new post-health world
- *Super Fuel* - DR JAMES DINICOLANTONIO – Ketogenic keys to unlock the secrets of good fats, bad fats and great health
- *Why We Get Fat* – GARY TAUBES – And what to do about it

Also, check out our *Fat & Furious* podcasts conducted with the contributors. I am confident that you will find it time well spent. You can also watch the webcast version at *www.primalliving.com*.

INDEX

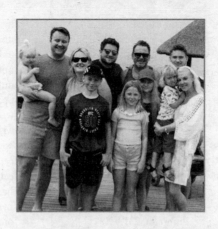

ACKNOWLEDGEMENTS

To my entire family, for always being supportive, especially my wife who has for several years had to put up with my obsessive behaviour in researching and writing about all things primal. To all of the wonderful doctors, authors, nutritionists and medical professionals, for giving up so much of their valuable time.

To my wonderful grandmother and amazing auntie Avis who both sadly died in their fifties from cancer, you will always be remembered. To my incredible dad who two years ago at the age of 77 was diagnosed with type 2 diabetes, and to my loving mother who is suffering with a neurocognitive disorder, this book is dedicated to you. You may never fully appreciate how your illnesses have motivated me to spread the word about how to improve the health of our nation and in some small way I hope that you will find some comfort in how it may help others.

MEET THE AUTHOR

Steve Bennett is a father of seven children and one of the UK's most prominent business leaders, employing more than 1,000 people around the world. Along with his family, in March 2011 he established the charity The Colourful Life Foundation, which to-date has built schools in countries including India, Tanzania and South Africa.

Steve has spent many years in remote countries, and much of the insight in this book has been garnered during his travels. With a keen sense for adventure, Steve and his son-in-law Jake have trekked to the North Pole, and more recently he has walked from the east to the west coast of England with two of his sons, Jack and Tom. He has sailed across the Atlantic with six of his family and ran several marathons.

Steve openly admits to spending most of his adult life overweight, but at the age of 50, he decided that enough was enough. This book details the picture as it unfolded for Steve on his journey to restoring his own health and wellbeing.

Sir Richard Branson